NANOTECHNOLOGICAL MANAGEMENT OF VIRAL INFECTIONS

NANOTECHNOLOGICAL MANAGEMENT OF VIRAL INFECTIONS

Radhakrishnan EK, PhD
Shiji Mathew, PhD
Riya Alex, MSc
Editors

APPLE ACADEMIC PRESS

First edition published 2027

Apple Academic Press Inc.
1265 Goldenrod Circle, NE,
Palm Bay, FL 32905 USA

760 Laurentian Drive, Unit 19,
Burlington, ON L7N 0A4, Canada

CRC Press
2385 NW Executive Center Drive,
Suite 320, Boca Raton FL 33431

4 Park Square, Milton Park,
Abingdon, Oxon, OX14 4RN, UK

Library and Archives Canada Cataloguing in Publication

CIP data on file with Canada Library and Archives

Library of Congress Cataloging-in-Publication Data

CIP data on file with US Library of Congress

ISBN: 978-1-77964-088-8 (hbk)
ISBN: 978-1-77964-089-5 (ebk)

DOI: 10.1201/9781779640895

About the Editors

Radhakrishnan EK, PhD
School of Biosciences, Mahatma Gandhi University, Kottayam, Kerala, India

Radhakrishnan EK, PhD, is currently working as an Associate Professor at the School of Biosciences, Mahatma Gandhi University, Kottayam. He is a multifaceted academic with a distinct research career. He also holds several positions simultaneously, including Hon. Director of the Business Innovation and Incubation Centre (BIIC), Hon. Joint Director of the Inter University Centre for Organic Farming and Sustainable Agriculture (IUCOFSA), Mahatma Gandhi University, Kottayam, and Hon. Director of the Dr. N. Radhakrishnan International Centre for Medical Innovation (NRICMI), as well as Director of the Industry–Academy Interface. He completed his doctoral degree at the Rajiv Gandhi Centre for Biotechnology, Thiruvananthapuram, Kerala, India, in 2008 and his postdoctoral studies at The University of Tokyo, Japan, in 2010. During his 13 years of research, he has published 162 research publications, 38 book chapters, and 3 review papers. He has edited 18 books with Springer Nature, Elsevier, Apple Academic Press (AAP), and CRC Press. He has 4,840 citations and an h-index of 39, and he has delivered 55 invited talks at various national and international conferences and seminars. So far, 16 PhDs have been completed under his guidance. He has completed 14 major research projects and one minor project from various funding agencies and currently has six ongoing projects as Principal Investigator. He was awarded the Kairali Gaveshana Puraskaram in 2023 for research in biological sciences, which included a cash prize and research grant from the Government of Kerala. He has been listed among the top 2% of scientists in the world in the list prepared by Stanford University and Elsevier BV, based on career-long data and single-year impact, for both 2022 and 2023.

Shiji Mathew, PhD
Adjunct Assistant Professor, College of Science and Technology, Temple University, Philadelphia, Pennsylvania, United States

Shiji Mathew, PhD, is currently working as an Adjunct Assistant Professor at Temple University, Philadelphia, Pennsylvania, United States. She completed her doctoral degree in Medical Microbiology at the School of Biosciences, Mahatma Gandhi University, India. Her doctoral thesis was titled "Antimicrobial effects of nanoparticle conjugates." Her MPhil (in Biosciences), MSc, and BSc degrees in Medical Microbiology were also from Mahatma Gandhi University. She worked as a microbiology tutor for over two years at Sri Rajiv Gandhi Dental College, Bangalore, Karnataka, India. From her research work, she has earned several publications in peer-reviewed journals, with 120 citations and an h-index of 6. Dr. Mathew has published numerous research articles in various international peer-reviewed journals. She has also contributed more than ten book chapters in international book volumes from eminent publishers. Her area of research is medical microbiology and nanotechnology, with specialization in the development of nanotechnology-based polymer composites, their characterization, and specialized applications in food packaging and the medical sector.

Riya Alex, MSc
School of Biosciences, Mahatma Gandhi University, Kottayam, Kerala, India

Riya Alex, MSc, is currently a PhD scholar at the School of Biosciences, Mahatma Gandhi University, Kottayam. Prior to this, she held the position of Assistant Professor at St. Berchmans College (Autonomous), Changanassery, Kottayam, Kerala, and worked as a microbiologist at Ananthapuri Hospitals and Research Institute, Thiruvananthapuram, from January 2019 to March 2020. She gained project experience as a trainee at the ICAR–Institute of Spices Research, Kozhikode, in 2018. She is a microbiologist with a diverse background in research and academia. She has published two papers in academic journals and two book chapters. She holds an MSc in General Microbiology and a BSc degree (double main) from Mahatma Gandhi University, Kottayam, Kerala, India.

Contents

Contributors

Jithasha Balan
Post Graduate and Research Department of Microbiology, Sree Sankara College, Kalady, Ernakulam, Kerala, India

Radhakrishnan EK
School of Biosciences, Mahatma Gandhi University, Kottayam, Kerala, India

Sandali Fernando
College of Chemical Sciences, Institute of Chemistry Ceylon, Welikada, Rajagiriya, Sri Lanka

Garima
Chitkara College of Pharmacy, Chitkara University, Punjab, India; M. M. College of Pharmacy, Maharishi Markandeshwar (Deemed to be University), Mullana–Ambala, Haryana, India

Sumi Mary George
Post Graduate and Research Department of Microbiology, Sree Sankara College, Kalady, Ernakulam, Kerala, India

Senuri Hasara
College of Chemical Sciences, Institute of Chemistry Ceylon, Welikada, Rajagiriya, Sri Lanka

U. P. S. Hasara
College of Chemical Sciences, Institute of Chemistry Ceylon, Welikada, Rajagiriya, Sri Lanka

Dona V. Idicula
Post Graduate and Research Department of Microbiology, Sree Sankara College, Kalady, Ernakulam, Kerala, India

Nitin Jain
DSEU Dwarka Campus (formerly Integrated Institute of Technology), New Delhi, India

H. T. D. R. Karunadasa
College of Chemical Sciences, Institute of Chemistry Ceylon, Welikada, Rajagiriya, Sri Lanka

Ravindu Kaveesha
College of Chemical Sciences, Institute of Chemistry Ceylon, Welikada, Rajagiriya, Sri Lanka

Arun Kumar
Chitkara College of Pharmacy, Chitkara University, Punjab, India; Department of Pharmacy, School of Health Sciences, Central University of South Bihar, Gaya, Bihar, India

H. H. Lokuge
College of Chemical Sciences, Institute of Chemistry Ceylon, Welikada, Rajagiriya, Sri Lanka

Jyothis Mathew
School of Biosciences, Mahatma Gandhi University, Kottayam, Kerala, India

Shiji Mathew
Department of Biology, College of Science and Technology, Temple University, Philadelphia, Pennsylvania, United States

Sherin Joy Parappilly
Post Graduate and Research Department of Microbiology, Sree Sankara College, Kalady, Ernakulam, Kerala, India

Ashwini Prabhu
Yenepoya Research Centre, Yenepoya (Deemed to be University), Mangalore, Karnataka, India

Vinitha Rani
Department of Material Science and Engineering, University of Central Florida, Florida, USA

Neethu Sahadevan
School of Biosciences, Mahatma Gandhi University, Kottayam, Kerala, India

Rashmi Sareen
DSEU Dwarka Campus (formerly Integrated Institute of Technology), New Delhi, India

Twinkle Sharma
Chitkara College of Pharmacy, Chitkara University, Punjab, India

Shanali De Silva
College of Chemical Sciences, Institute of Chemistry Ceylon, Welikada, Rajagiriya, Sri Lanka

Binelka Siriwardana
College of Chemical Sciences, Institute of Chemistry Ceylon, Welikada, Rajagiriya, Sri Lanka

Gobika Thiripuranathar
College of Chemical Sciences, Institute of Chemistry Ceylon, Welikada, Rajagiriya, Sri Lanka

N. N. Weeraperuma
College of Chemical Sciences, Institute of Chemistry Ceylon, Welikada, Rajagiriya, Sri Lanka

Foreword

In an era where global health is continuously being challenged by the threat of viral infections, the pursuit of new solutions has never been more crucial. *Nanotechnological Management of Viral Infections* stands at the forefront of this dynamic subject, offering a comprehensive exploration of creative and efficient strategies to combat viral diseases. Within these pages, readers will gain insight into the latest breakthroughs in nano-medicinal approaches, spanning from the utilization of metal nanoparticles to the formulation of natural herbs and spices as potent antiviral agents. Through the lens of nanotechnology, this book illuminates the diverse array of tactics deployed in targeted drug delivery, theragnostics for virus-induced cancer, and the management of notorious viral illnesses such as influenza and coronaviruses. Moreover, it showcases the transformative potential of nano-based analytics for early detection and diagnosis, along-side the promising prospects of nanovaccinology in fortifying our defenses against viral threats. This book gives us encouragement as we navigate the complex web of infectious illnesses by showcasing the inventiveness and tenacity of scientific research in preserving world health.

Abbreviations

ACE2	angiotensin-converting enzyme-2
AFP	alpha-fetoprotein
Ag+	silver particles
AgNPs	silver nanoparticles
AIDS	acquired immunodeficiency syndrome
AlPcSs	aluminum phthalocyanines
AlPcSs	sulfonated aluminum phthalocyanines
APC	antigen presenting cells
ARDS	acute respiratory distress syndrome
ARV	avian reovirus
ASO	antisense oligonucleotides
AuNIs	gold nanoislands
AuNPs	gold nanoparticles
AZT	azidothymidine/zidovudine
BBB	blood-brain barrier
BCS	biopharmaceutics classification system
BL	Burkitt's lymphoma
BRB	berberine
CaP	calcium monophosphate
CAP	cold atmospheric plasma
CAs	contrast agents
CAS-MCs	casein micelles
CCM	cancer cell membranes
CD	Castleman's disease
CDDP	cisplatin
CFR	case fatality rate
CNMs	carbon nanomaterials
CNTs	carbon nanotubes
CNT-STEM	cnt size-tunable enrichment microdevice
CoNS	coagulase-negative *Staphylococci*
CoV	coronavirus
CPT	camptothecin
CQDs	carbon quantum dots

CRB	carboplatin
CS	chitosan
CSCs	cancer stem cells
CSLCs	cancer stem-like cells
CT	computer tomography
CTAB	cetyl trimethyl ammonium bromide
CTAC	cetyltrimethylammonium chloride
CuNPs	copper nanoparticles
CuO	copper oxide
DAF NPs	fullerene-based nanoparticles
DCs	dendritic cells
DIAT	Defense Institute of Advanced Technology
DIP	defective interfering particles
DLS	dynamic light scattering
DMF	dimethylformamide
DOX	doxorubicin
DSN	diosmin
DSPC	distearoylphosphatidylcholine
EBV	Epstein barr virus
EC50	effective concentration
ELISA	enzyme-linked immunosorbent assay
FA	folic acid
Fe3O4	magnetite
FET	field-effect transistor
FGP NPs	gpc3 peptide nanoparticles
FI	fluorescence imaging
FMDV	foot-and-mouth disease virus
FOBT	fecal occult blood test
FRET	fluorescence resonance energy transfer
FRET-C-dots-DDS	fret-based carbon dot drug delivery systems
GAAD	glutamic acid-alginate conjugates
GC	graphene composites
GCDM	gdyo-cddp/dox@dspe-peg-mtx
GDYO	graphdiyne oxide
GLPD	germinotrophic lymphoproliferative disorders
GNPs	gold nanoparticles
GNPs	graphene nanoplatelets
GNRs	graphene nanoribbons

GO	graphene oxide
GOD	glucose oxidase
gp	glycoproteins
GP73	golgi protein-73
GPI	glycosylphosphatidylinositol
GQDs	graphene quantum dots
GQDs	quantum dots from graphene
GRAS	generally recognized as safe
GSJNs	Au-mesoporous silica janus nanoparticles
HA	hemagglutinin
HAdVs	human adenoviruses
HAuCl4	chloroauric acid
HBsAg	hepatitis B surface antigens
HBV	hepatitis B virus
HCC	hepatocellular carcinoma
HCMV	human cytomegalovirus
HCQ	hydroxychloroquine
HCV	hepatitis C virus
HHV-8	herpesvirus-8
HHV-8	human herpes virus
HIFU	high-intensity focused ultrasound
HIV	human immunodeficiency virus
HL	Hodgkin's lymphoma
HLB	hydrophilic-lipophilic balance
HMCSs	hollow mesoporous carbon spheres
HPCPAA	hydroxypropylcellulose-(poly acrylic acid)
HPLC	high-performance liquid chromatography
HPV	human papillomavirus
HSPG	heparin sulphate proteoglycans
HSRV	human respiratory syncytial virus
HSV	herpes simplex virus
HTCC	hydroxy-3-trimethylammonium) propyl] chitosan chloride
HTLV-1	human T-lymphotropic virus type I
IAV	influenza A virus
IBDV	infectious bursal disease virus
IBV	influenza B virus
IC50	inhibition concentration

ICG	indocyanine green
ICV	influenza C virus
IFNα	interferon- α
IIV	inactivated influenza vaccine
IL-2	interleukin 2
INF-α	interferon-alpha
IONPs	iron oxide nanoparticles
ISGs	ifn-stimulating genes
KS	Kaposi sarcoma
KSHV	Kaposi's sarcoma-associated herpesvirus
LA	laser ablation
LA-Au DENPs	lactobionic acid with gold nanoparticles
LAIV	live attenuated influenza vaccine
LPNs	lipid nanoparticles
LSPR	localized surface plasmon resonance
LSTc	liposomal decoys
LUV	large unilamellar vesicles
M1	matrix protein 1
M2	matrix protein 2
MA104	monkey African green kidney
MAPK	mitogen-activated protein kinase
MCC	Merkel cell carcinoma
MCD	multicentric castleman disease
MCNs	mesoporous carbon nanoparticles
MCPyV	Merkel cell polyomavirus
MDCK	Madin-Darby canine kidney cells
MDR	multi-drug-resistant
MERS	middle east respiratory syndrome
MES	mercaptoethanesulfonate
MFe2O4	mixed ferrites
MFH	magnetic fluid hyperthermia
MgO	magnesium oxide
MHA	mesoporous hollow alumina nanoparticles
MHC	major histocompatibility complex
miR-122	microRNA-122
miRNA	microRNA
MNA	methyl-B-neuraminic acid
MNPs	magnetic nanoparticles

MPNs	magneto-plasmonic nanoparticles
MRI	magnetic resonance imaging
MTT	methyl thiazolyl tetrazolium
MTX	methotrexate
MUV	multilamellar vesicles
MVA	modified vaccinia virus ankara
MWCNT	multiwall carbon nanotubes
MX	mitoxantrone
NA	neuraminidase
NaBH4	sodium borohydride
NAI	neuraminidase inhibitors
NCs	nanocomposites
NCS	neocarzinostatin
NDDS	novel drug delivery systems
NDV	newcastle disease virus
NE	nanoemulsions
NG	nanogel
NHL	non-Hodgkin's lymphoma
NIAID	national institute of allergy and infectious diseases
NIR	near-infrared
NK	natural killer
NLCs	nanostructured lipid carriers
NMR	nuclear magnetic resonance
NP	nucleocapsid protein
NPC	nasopharyngeal carcinoma
NPs	nanoparticles
OI	optical imaging
OTPBA–SPION	4-oxo-4-(3-(triethoxysilyl)propylamino) butanoic acid
PA	photoacoustic
PAC	paclitaxel
PAI	photoacoustic imaging
PAMAM	polyamidoamine
PAMPs	pathogen-associated molecular patterns
PAP	phenanthridium
PB	polymerase blockers
PB1-F2	anti-nonstructural proteins
PBAE	poly(beta-amino ester)
PBMCs	peripheral blood mononuclear cells

PC	poly-γ-glutamic acid/chitosan
PDA	polydopamine
PDDA	polydiallyldimethylammonium chloride
PDT	photodynamic therapy
PECL	poly(epsilon-caprolactone)
PEDV	pig epidemic diarrhea virus
PEG 6000	polyethylene glycol 6000
PEG	polyethylene glycol
PEI	polyethylenimine
PEL	primary effusion lymphoma
PERLs	polyunsaturated endoplasmic reticulum liposomes
PET	positron emission tomography
PFP	perfluoropentane
PFU	plaque formation units
PICA	poly(isobutylcyanoacrylate)
PL	polylysine linker
PLA	polylactic acid
PLGA	poly lactic-co-glycolic acid
PMMA	polymethyl methacrylate
PNAs	peptide nucleic acids
PNP	polymeric nanoparticles
PoAuNPs/PoGNPs	porous gold loaded nanoparticles
PPE	personal protective equipment
PR	puerto rico
PRRSV	porcine reproductive and respiratory syndrome virus
PRSs	pattern recognition receptors
PSA	prostate specific antigen
PTLD	post-transplant lymphoproliferative disease
Pt-NA	Pt nanoclusters
PTX	paclitaxel
PVA	polyvinyl alcohol
PVP	polyvinylpyrrolidone
QD	quantum dots
QD-LFIAS	QD-based lateral flow immunoassay system
QDs	quantum dots
qRT-PCR	quantitative reverse transcription polymerase chain reaction
QUT	queensland university of technology

RdRp	RNA-dependent rna polymerase
RFA	radiofrequency ablation
rGO	reduced graphene oxide
RISC	RNA-induced silencing complex
RNA	ribonucleic acid
RNAi	RNA interference
RNase H	ribonuclease H
RNP	ribonucleoprotein
Ro	reproductive number
ROS	reactive oxygen species
RRT-PCR	real-time reverse transcription PCR
RSV	respiratory syncytial virus
RT-PCR	reverse transcriptase-polymerase chain reaction
RVFV	rift valley fever virus
sa-mRNA	self-amplifying mrna
SA-PEG	stearic acid-polyethylene glycol
SARS	severe acute respiratory syndrome
SARS-COV-2	severe acute respiratory syndrome coronavirus 2
Se@OTV NPs	oseltamivir operationalized selenium nanoparticles
SEM	scanning electron microscopy
SeNPs	selenium nanoparticles
SERS	surface-enhanced raman scattering
shRNA	short hairpin RNA
siRNA	short interfering RNA
SLN	sentinel lymph nodes
SLN	solid lipid nanoparticles
SNEDDS	self-nanoemulsifying drug delivery systems
SNFs	silica-based nanoframeworks
SPECT	single-photon emission computed tomography
SpFN	spike protein ferritin nanoparticle
SPIONs	superparamagnetic iron oxide nanoparticles
SPR	surface plasmon resonance
ss-RNA	single-stranded RNA
SUV	unilamellar vesicles
SWCNT	single-wall carbon nanotubes
SwIAV	swine influenza A virus
TC50	toxic concentration
TC-WS-CQDs	trichrome-tryptophan-sorbitol cqds

TDNTs	telodendrimer nanotraps
TEM	transmission electron microscopy
Tf	transferrin
TiO_2	titanium dioxide
TiO_2NPs	titanium dioxide nanoparticles
TSP	tropical spastic paraparesis
UGC	University Grants Commission
US	ultrasound
VEEV	Venezuelan equine encephalitis virus
VLP	virus-like particles
vRNAs	virus RNAs
vRNP	viral ribonucleoprotein complexes
VVV	viral vector vaccines
VZV	varicella-zoster virus
WHO	World Health Organization
ZEN	Zen Graphene Solutions Ltd.
ZnO NPs	zinc oxide nanoparticles
ZnO	zinc oxide
γFe_2O_3	maghemite

Preface

Nanotechnological Management of Viral Infections is a comprehensive exploration of the cutting-edge field where nanotechnology meets virology. In the medical field, the grim evolution of viral pathogens has posed a lasting challenge to human health. Viral infections, in particular, have emerged as a formidable adversary, capable of causing widespread devastation with their swift spread and elusive nature. Throughout history, humanity has grappled with various outbreaks, from the Spanish flu to the more recent COVID-19 pandemic, underscoring the critical need for innovative approaches.

Hence, managing viral infections presents significant challenges due to the rapid emergence of novel viruses, potential pandemics, and limitations of current antiviral therapies. Within these pages, leading experts from around the globe delve into the latest advancements in nano-medicinal approaches for combating viral infections, encompassing a multifaceted array of strategies. These include the utilization of metal-based nanoparticles, nano-formulations derived from oriental herbs and spices, and nanocarriers engineered for targeted drug delivery. Moreover, the promising avenues that nanotechnology offers for theragnostics—particularly in the context of virus-induced cancer—as well as effective treatments for influenza and coronaviruses, have been discussed. Furthermore, innovations in nano-based analytics that enable early detection and diagnosis of viral infections, and nanovaccinology concepts, are a frontier for future approaches in vaccine development against diverse viral threats.

As we stand on the edge of a new era in medicine, marked by unprecedented scientific innovation, it is our hope that this book will serve as a beacon of inspiration for all those dedicated to the pursuit of a world free from the scourge of viral diseases. Together, let us embark on this transformative journey toward a future where nanotechnology stands at the forefront of our defense against infectious agents, safeguarding the well-being of generations to come.

CHAPTER 1

An Overview of Common and Emerging Viral Infections in Humans

NEETHU SAHADEVAN* and JYOTHIS MATHEW

School of Biosciences, Mahatma Gandhi University, Kottayam, Kerala, India

*Corresponding author

ABSTRACT

Human life coexists with all other living organisms, ranging from microorganisms to other animals in the ecosystem. Infectious agents can affect the ecosystem's coherence and remain a significant challenge to human life. Among these, some viruses cause mild infections, while others can have fatal impacts on human life worldwide. Self-acquired genetic variations of viruses pose a significant challenge to efficient control and can trigger severe impacts on human health. The rapid evolution of viruses leads to the emergence of hitherto unknown drug-resistant strains. The current era has witnessed the emergence of several deadly viral infections, such as Corona, Nipah, Ebola, and Zika. Each of these outbreaks underscores the importance of comprehensive research into the improvement of diagnosis, surveillance, treatment, and prevention of the deadliest viral infections. The present chapter outlines viral diseases; Corona, Chikungunya, Ebola, Influenza, and Zika virus infections were selected as representative emerging diseases for detailed discussion.

Nanotechnological Management of Viral Infections.
Radhakrishnan EK, Shiji Mathew, and Riya Alex (Eds.)

DOI: 10.1201/9781779640895-1

1.1 INTRODUCTION

Unicellular microorganisms are classified into prokaryotes and eukaryotes based on their structural complexity. Bacteria, rickettsiae, chlamydiae, and mycoplasmas belong to the prokaryotes, whereas protozoa and fungi belong to the eukaryotes. These microorganisms have cellular organizations, containing both types of nucleic acid, and possess their synthetic machinery for producing macromolecular constituents such as nucleic acid, carbohydrate, protein, and lipid. These unicellular microorganisms multiply by binary fission. On the other hand, viruses do not fall under these categories as they do not possess a cellular organization (Fenner, 1987). They contain only one type of nucleic acid, either RNA or DNA, but never both together. Since viruses have no mitochondria and ribosomes, they completely depend on specialized host cells for their propagation. Viruses are unaffected by antibiotics. Unlike bacteria or other cells, viruses do not reproduce by binary division, but they depend on replication in the living cells of the host that they infect. Viruses encode genetic information for their structural components and possess certain regulatory proteins like transactivators, polymerase, and protease. Furthermore, many viruses can reproduce themselves from their genome, which indicates that their nucleic acid alone is infectious (Lwoff, 1957).

1.2 HISTORY

The history of viruses was just a part of infectious diseases until the end of the 19th century. The concept of a virus as a separate entity originally came to the limelight at the end of the 1800s. The discovery of the Chamber and Pasteur filter in 1884 by Charles Chamberland in Paris paved the way for the recognition of viruses. The Chamber and Pasteur filter consisted of unglazed porcelain candles with a pore size of 0.1–1 micron, which could effectively remove all bacteria and other cells from a suspension. This simple discovery laid the cornerstone for the establishment of virology. Adolf Edward Mayer, in 1886, reported that mosaic disease of tobacco plants could be transmitted to healthy plants by contact with the infected plant extract, though he initially attributed the disease to bacteria. In 1892, Dmitri Ivanovski from Russia filtered infected tobacco plant extract through a Chamber and Pasteur filter and showed that the filtrate remained infectious, thus refuting Adolf Edward Mayer's claim that the causative agent of the mosaic disease was bacteria. Similarly, a Dutch scientist, Martinus

Beijerinck, conducted a similar experiment in 1898 and concluded that the causative agent was a "contagious living fluid," as the bacteria-free fluid he used had a liquid nature. The term "virus," a Latin word meaning slimy fluid, was later coined for this "contagious living fluid." The study of viral morphology became possible after the invention of electron microscopy in 1931. Brenner and Home, in 1959, applied negative staining with potassium phosphotungstate, yielding a more detailed view of the ultrastructure of virus particles (Vigue, 1976).

1.3 VIRUS MORPHOLOGY

Viruses are small, obligate intracellular parasites, with sizes ranging between 20 nm and 300 nm. The infectious virus particle is known as a virion. The virion consists of two basic structural components: a single molecule of nucleic acid and a protein coat, known as the capsid. The nucleic acid-associated protein is called nucleoprotein, and the capsid forms the nucleocapsid. The capsid's function is to protect the enclosed nucleic acid from inactivation by nucleases and other agents. It is composed of a large number of capsomeres connected by noncovalent bonds, either forming rod-shaped or cubic-spherical structures. Rod-shaped capsids exhibit helical symmetry, while spherical capsids exhibit icosahedral symmetry. An icosahedron is a polygon with 12 vertices (corners) and 20 facets, each in the shape of an equilateral triangle.

In nucleocapsids with helical symmetry, the capsomers and nucleic acid molecules are wound together to form a helical or spiral tube structure. In animal viruses, the helical nucleocapsid is enclosed within a lipoprotein envelope, contributing to its stability. However, in plant viruses, the helical nucleocapsids are rod-shaped and non-enveloped (Modrow et al., 2013; Staff, 2008).

The viral genome contains either RNA or DNA and can be single-stranded or double-stranded, circular, linear, or segmented, surrounded by a protective, virus-coded protein coat. The primary function of the virion is to deliver its genome into the host cell, which is subsequently transcribed or translated by the host cell.

Virions can be enveloped or non-enveloped. In some viruses, the nucleocapsid is surrounded by a lipid bilayer derived from the modified host cell membrane, known as an envelope. The envelope's exterior is often studded with virus-coded, glycosylated membrane proteins, sometimes appearing as projecting spikes on the envelope surface called peplomers. Certain viruses, such as the Influenza virus, may possess more than one type of peplomers. The viral envelope confers various chemical, biological, and antigenic properties onto the viruses (Modrow et al., 2013).

1.4 CLASSIFICATION

In the past, viruses were classified based on host, target organ, and vector. Currently, viruses are classified based on the following characteristics:

1. **Type of Nucleic Acid They Possess:** RNA/DNA virus, single-stranded or double-stranded, and their replication strategy;
2. **Capsid Symmetry:** Icosahedral or helical symmetry;
3. **Lipid Envelope:** Presence or absence of lipid envelope;
4. **Virion:** Size and shape of virion (Gelderblom, 1996) (Table 1.1).

TABLE 1.1 The Classification of the Major Group of Medically Important Viruses

Family	Examples of Viruses	Envelope	Genome*	Capsid Morphology
Adenoviridae	Human Adenovirus A-G	No	ds DNA	Icosahedral
Anelloviridae	Torque teno virus	No	ss DNA	Icosahedral
Arenaviridae	Lassa virus, Lymphocytic choriomeningitis virus	Yes	ss RNA	Helical
Astroviridae	Human Astroviruses	No	ss RNA	Icosahedral
Bunyaviridae	California Encephalitis virus, Hantaan virus, Sandfly fever virus, Rift valley fever virus, Crimean-congo hemorrhagic fever	Yes	ss RNA	Helical
Caliciviridae	Norovirus, Sapovirus	No	ds RNA	Icosahedral
Coronaviridae	SARS corona, MERS corona, Human torovirus	Yes	ss RNA	Helical
Filoviridae	Marburg virus, Ebola virus	No	ss RNA	Helical
Flaviviridae	Genus alpha virus: Dengue virus, Yellow fever virus, Japanese encephalitis virus, West Nile virus, Murray Valley encephalitis virus, Zika virus; Genus hepacivirus: Hepatitis C virus	Yes	ds RNA	Icosahedral

TABLE 1.1 *(Continued)*

Family	Examples of Viruses	Envelope	Genome*	Capsid Morphology
Hepadnaviridae	Hepatitis B virus	Yes	ds DNA	Icosahedral
Hepeviridae	Hepatitis E virus	No	ssRNA	Icosahedral
Herpesviridae	Herpes simplex 1, 2, Varicella zoster virus, Cytomegalovirus, Epstein-Barr virus, Human Herpes virus 6,7 and 8	No	ds DNA	Icosahedral
Orthomyxoviridae	Influenza A, B, and C	Yes	ds RNA	Helical
Papillomaviridae	Human papillomaviruses	No	ds DNA	Icosahedral
Paramyxoviridae	Measles, Mumps, Parainfluenza viruses, Nipah virus	Yes	ds RNA	Helical
Parvoviridae	Human Parvovirus B19, Adeno associated viruses	No	ss DNA	Icosahedral
Picobirnaviridae	Human Picobirna virus	No		
Picornaviridae	Genus Enterovirus: Rhinovirus, Enterovirus, Coxsackie virus A, B, Echovirus; Genus Hepatovirus: HAV; Genus Kobu virus: Aichi virus; Genus Cosa virus: Human Cosa viruses	No	ss RNA	Icosahedral
Pneumoviridae	Respiratory Syncytial virus,	Yes	ss RNA	Helical
Polyomaviridae	Human Polyoma virus 6, 7, 9, JC virus, BK virus, KI virus	No	ds DNA	Icosahedral
Poxviridae	Molluscum contagiosum virus, Variola, Monkeypox virus, Vaccinia, Orf virus	Yes	ds DNA	Complex
Reoviridae	Rotavirus	No	ds RNA	Icosahedral
Retroviridae	HIV 1, 2, Human T lymphocyte lymphotropic viruses	Yes	ss RNA	Icosahedral
Rhabdoviridae	Rabies virus, Vesicular stomatitis virus	Yes	ss RNA	Helical
Togaviridae	Rubella virus, Chikungunya virus, Sindbis virus, Semliki virus	Yes	ds RNA	Icosahedral
Delta	Hepatitis delta virus	Yes	ss RNA	Circular

**Abbreviations: ds DNA: Double-stranded DNA; ss DNA: Single stranded DNA; ss RNA: Single stranded RNA; ds RNA: Double-stranded RNA.*

1.5 PATHOGENESIS OF VIRAL INFECTIONS

The key elements of virus-host interactions include:

1. **Size of the Inoculum:** There must be a sufficient amount of virus available to initiate an infection.
2. **Nature of Virus Strain:** Viral strains within a genus may exhibit different cell tropism and replication capacities.
3. **Site of Infection:** Cells at the infection site must be susceptible to the virus and accessible for infection.
4. **Immune Status of the Host:** Initially, local host antiviral defense systems must be absent or ineffective.

The possible outcomes of host-viral interaction are as follows:

- No infection;
- Asymptomatic infection;
- Abortive infection;
- Symptomatic infection;
- Latent infection (Nathanson, 2008).

1.6 VIRUS ENTRY

Viruses enter the body through the respiratory tract, alimentary tract, skin, conjunctiva, and urogenital tracts. Some viruses are also transmitted vertically from mother to child.

1.6.1 RESPIRATORY TRACT

The most common mode of entry of viruses is the respiratory tract. Large numbers of foreign particles and aerosolized droplets are inhaled by the lungs during each breath. A great amount of these particles and droplets contain viruses. However, many of the natural defense mechanisms block the development of infections. The nasal cavity is lined with ciliated cells, goblet cells, and subepithelial mucous-secreting glands. Therefore, any foreign particles that enter through the upper respiratory tract are trapped within the mucus, which either may be coughed out or swallowed. The particles that manage to reach the lower respiratory tract are ingested by macrophages lining the pulmonary alveoli or neutralized by antibody.

1.6.2 ALIMENTARY TRACT

The alimentary tract serves as the most common route of viral entry, although only specific viruses can effectively initiate infection within it. The densely packed microvilli in the intestinal mucosa, along with the surface coat of glycolipids and glycoproteins, act as a barrier to viruses. Despite this protective barrier, certain viruses, including enteroviruses, reoviruses, adenoviruses, and hepatitis viruses, are capable of initiating intestinal infections.

In the case of poliovirus, initial multiplication occurs in the intestinal tract before spreading to other sites and eventually targeting specific organs. Similarly, rotaviruses primarily confine their infection to the gut, leading to local infections. Most enveloped viruses do not typically initiate infection in the intestinal tract due to the susceptibility of their viral envelopes to bile salts. However, enteric coronaviruses represent a notable exception, though the precise mechanisms behind their infection remain unclear (Nathanson, 2008).

1.6.3 UROGENITAL TRACT

The urogenital tract is well protected by physical barriers, such as mucus and the acidic pH of the adult vagina. However, the virus enters the urogenital tract through minute cuts or abrasions in the vaginal epithelium during sexual activities. Some viruses, human papillomavirus, infect the vaginal epithelium and produce local lesions, whereas viruses such as herpes simplex virus and human immunodeficiency virus type 1 infect underlying tissues and cells of immune systems.

1.6.4 SKIN

The intact skin acts as a mechanical barrier around the body and prevents microbial colonization. The microbial invasion takes place only through the skin when its integrity is breached by cuts or abrasions. However, in most cases (vaccinia, papilloma, cowpox, molluscum contagiosum, and orf infections), viral replication will be limited to the site of entry as the epidermis is devoid of blood or lymphatic vessels. In some instances, viruses may enter the circulation through the bite of arthropod vectors such as mosquitos, ticks, mites, and sandflies (arboviruses). Deeper inoculation of viruses into the tissues and muscles takes place through sexual contact (HIV), injections such as skin piercing, tattooing, hypodermic needle punctures (hepatitis B), and animal bites (rabies).

1.6.5 CONJUNCTIVA

Conjunctiva may also act as a mode of entry for certain viruses. The flushing action of tears prevents the entry of any foreign particles into the eyes. Therefore, there is little opportunity for a virus to initiate an infection in the conjunctiva, unless it is abraded or injured. Direct inoculation of viruses through conjunctiva takes place through surgical procedures or improperly sanitized swimming pools (Nathanson, 2008) (Table 1.2).

1.7 EMERGING VIRAL INFECTIONS

In the last two decades, the world has witnessed the rapid spread of emerging and re-emerging viral diseases. Some diseases even led to a dramatic loss of human life and made an unprecedented challenge to the livelihood of the common man. Some of the emerging viral infections are listed in subsections.

1.7.1 INFLUENZA VIRUS

Influenza is an acute, usually self-limiting infectious disease of the respiratory tract. The influenza virus belongs to the family Orthomyxoviridae and is classified into three serotypes: type A, B, and C. These viruses are enveloped and mostly spherical, with a segmented genome consisting of negative-sense single-stranded RNA. The viral genome encodes several proteins, including Hemagglutinin and Neuraminidase (HA and NA), which protrude from the viral envelope and facilitate the virus's attachment to mucoprotein receptors on epithelial cells. HA serves as a primary attachment protein for the influenza virus, mediating the binding between the viral envelope and the endosome to enable viral entry into host cells. NA proteins catalyze the removal of sialic acid residues, facilitating the virus's escape from the host cell and promoting the spread of infection.

TABLE 1.2 Common Portal of Entry of Medically Important Viruses

Route of Infection	Causative Agents	Family	Host	References
Respiratory tract	Adeno-associated virus	Parvoviridae	Vertebrates	Araujo (2022)
	Adenovirus	Adenoviridae	Human	Kajon et al. (2018)
	BK Polyoma virus	Polyomaviridae	Human	Rinaldo et al. (2013)
	Coronavirus	Coronaviridae	Human	Kumar (2020)
	Herpes virus 6	Herpesviridae	Human	Campadelli-Fiume et al. (1999)
	Herpes virus 7	Herpesviridae	Human	Fatkullina et al. (2021)
	Parainfluenza virus	Paramyxoviridae	Human	Branche and Falsey (2016)
	Parvovirus B19	Parvoviridae	Human	Heegaard et al. (2002)
	Respiratory syncytial virus	Pneumoviridae	Human	Eiland (2009)
	Rhinovirus	Picornaviridae	Human	Jacobs et al. (2013)
	Influenza A	Orthomyxoviridae	Humans, pigs, birds	Samji (2009)
	Influenza B	Orthomyxoviridae	Human	Hall et al. (2021)
	Influenza C	Orthomyxoviridae	Human	Hall et al. (2021)
	Measles virus	Paramyxoviridae	Human	Gastanaduy et al. (2018)
	Mumps virus	Paramyxoviridae	Human	Gastanaduy et al. (2018)
	Rubella virus	Togaviridae	Human	Gastanaduy et al. (2018)
	SARS Coronavirus 2	Coronaviridae	Humans, palm civets, bats	Hu et al. (2021)
	WU Polyoma virus	Polyomaviridae	Human	Kleines et al. (2009)
Fecal/oral	Aichi virus	Picornaviridae	Human	Kitajima and Gerba (2015)
	Cosa virus A	Picornaviridae	Human	Smits et al. (2016)
	Coxsackie virus	Picornaviridae	Human	Tahmina (2017)

TABLE 1.2 *(Continued)*

Route of Infection	Causative Agents	Family	Host	References
	Hepatitis A virus	Picornaviridae	Human	Popov et al. (2018)
	Hepatitis E virus	Hepeviridae	Human	Aslan and Balaban (2020)
	Adenovirus	Adenoviridae	Human	Kajon et al. (2018)
	Astrovirus	Astroviridae	Human	Johnson et al. (2017)
	Enterovirus 68, 70	Picornaviridae	Human	Abedi et al. (2018)
	Human Toro virus	Coronaviridae	Human	Jamieson et al. (1998)
	JC Polyoma virus	Polyomaviridae	Human	Diotti et al. (2013)
	KI Polyoma virus	Polyomaviridae	Human	Prezioso et al. (2021)
	Norwalk virus	Caliciviridae	Human	Agency (1972)
	Poliovirus	Picornaviridae	Human, mammals	Estivariz et al. (2021)
	Rota virus A	Reoviridae	Human	Daniel et al. (2019)
	Rota virus B	Reoviridae	Human	Hallowell et al. (2019)
	Rota virus C	Reoviridae	Human	Burke et al. (2018)
	Southampton virus	Caliciviridae	Human	Liu et al. (1996)
Zoonosis/ Arthropod bite	Australian bat Lyssavirus	Rhabdoviridae	Human, bat	Merritt et al. (2018)
	Banna virus	Reoviridae	Humans, pigs, cattle's, mosquitoes	Liu et al. (2010)
	Barmah Forest virus	Togaviridae	Humans, mosquitoes, marsupials	Hills (1996)
	Bunya virus	Bunyaviridae	Humans, mosquitoes, deer's	Briese et al. (2016)
	Chandipura virus	Rhabdoviridae	Humans, sandflies	Menghani et al. (2012)
	Chikungunya virus	Togaviridae	Humans, mosquitoes, monkeys	CDC (2014)
	Cowpox virus	Poxviridae	Humans, mammals	CDC (2014)

TABLE 1.2 *(Continued)*

Route of Infection	Causative Agents	Family	Host	References
	Crimean-Congo Hemorrhagic fever virus	Bunyaviridae	Humans, ticks	Hewson (2019)
	Dengue virus	Flaviviridae	Humans, mosquitoes	Panchangam (2015)
	Dhori virus	Orthomyxoviridae	Humans, ticks	Lledo et al. (2020)
	Dugbe virus	Bunyaviridae	Humans, ticks	Gonzalez et al. (1989)
	Eastern Equine Encephalitis virus	Togaviridae	Humans, mosquitoes, birds	Berlin et al. (2017)
	Ebola virus	Filoviridae	Humans, monkeys, bats	CDC (2018)
	Encephalomyocarditis virus	Picornaviridae	Humans, mouse, pigs, rats	Carocci and Kassimi (2016)
	Hantaan virus	Bunyaviridae	Rodents, humans	Battisti et al. (2011)
	Hepatitis E virus	Hepeviridae	Humans, pigs, monkeys, rodents	Aslan and Balaban (2020)
	Japanese Encephalitis virus	Flaviviridae	Humans, mosquitoes, birds	Thornton et al. (2018)
	Marburg virus	Filoviridae	Humans, monkeys, bats	CDC (1967)
	Lassa virus	Rhabdoviridae	Humans, rats	Thornton et al. (2018)
	Lymphocytic Choriomeningitis virus	Arenaviridae	Humans, rodents	Borrow (2014)
	Monkeypox virus	Poxviridae	Humans, mouse, prairie dogs	Lhamo et al. (2022
	Murray valley virus	Flaviviridae	Humans, mosquitoes	Williams et al. (2016)
	Nipah virus	Paramyxoviridae	Humans, bats	Giangaspero (2015)
	O'nyong-nyong virus	Togaviridae	Humans, mosquitoes	Bessaud et al. (2006)
	Rabies virus	Rhabdoviridae	Humans, mammals	Jackson (2016)
	Rift valley virus	Bunyaviridae	Humans, mammals, mosquitoes, sandflies	Durand et al. (2003)
	Semliki forest virus	Togaviridae	Humans, mosquitoes, birds	Sjo and Ekstro (2014)
	Seoul virus	Bunyaviridae	Humans, rats	Rats (2018)

TABLE 1.2 *(Continued)*

Route of Infection	Causative Agents	Family	Host	References
	Sindbis virus	Togaviridae	Humans, mosquitoes, birds	Arif and Canada (2014)
	Yellow fever virus	Flaviviridae	Humans, mosquitoes, monkeys	Marcelo et al. (2018)
	Zika virus	Flaviviridae	Humans, mosquitoes, monkeys	Shapshak et al. (2015)
Blood/sexual	Hepatitis B	Hepadnaviridae	Humans, chimpanzees	Kodani and Schillie (2016)
	Hepatitis C	Flaviviridae	Human	Morozov and Lagaye (2018)
	Hepatitis D	-	Human	Urban et al (2021)
	Hepatitis G	Flaviviridae	Human	Reshetnyak et al. (2008)
	Human Herpes virus 1	Herpesviridae	Human	Mindel (2014)
	Human Herpes virus 2	Herpesviridae	Human	Mustafa and Elahee (2016)
	Human Herpes virus 8	Herpesviridae	Human	Edelman (2005)
	HIV	Retroviridae	Human	Kapila et al. (2016)
	Papilloma virus 16, 18	Papillomaviridae	Human	Darkuthni et al. (2018)
	Human T-lymphocyte virus	Retroviridae	Human	Leno et al. (1995)
	Torque Teno virus	Anelloviridae	Human	Leno et al. (1995)
Contact	Eastern Chimpanzee Simian foamy virus	Retroviridae	Human	Learn and Easlick (2012)
	Cytomegalovirus	Herpesviridae	Human	Plosa et al. (2014)
	Papilloma virus 2	Papillomaviridae	Human	Russo et al., (2020)
	Molluscum contagiosum virus	Poxviridae	Human	Rao et al. (2013)
	Vaccinia virus	Poxviridae	Human	Bertram et al. (2009)
	Yaba-like disease virus	Poxviridae	Mammals	Yun et al. (2001)

TABLE 1.2 *(Continued)*

Route of Infection	Causative Agents	Family	Host	References
Congenital transmission	Cytomegalovirus	Herpesviridae	Human	Plosa et al. (2014)
	Variola virus	Poxviridae	Human	Babkin and Babkina (2015)
	HSV-1, HSV-2	Herpesviridae	Human	Mustafa and Elahee (2016)
	Measles virus	Paramyxoviridae	Human	Gastanaduy et al. (2018)
	Zika virus	Flaviviridae	Humans, mosquitoes, monkeys	Shapshak et al. (2015)
	Rubella virus	Matonaviridae	Human	Lanzieri et al. (2004)
	Vaccinia virus	Poxviridae	Human	Bertram et al. (2009)
	Herpes simplex virus	Herpesviridae	Human	Mustafa and Elahee (2016)
Central nervous system	Arboviruses (many)	-	Humans, mosquitoes, ticks, sandflies	Tabachnick (2015)
	Coxsackie A virus	Picornaviridae	Human	Tahmina (2017)
	Coxsackie B virus	Picornaviridae	Human	Tahmina (2017)
	Enterovirus	Picornaviridae	Human	Abedi et al. (2018)
	Dengue virus	Flaviviridae	Humans, mosquitoes	Panchangam (2015)
	Lymphocytic Choriomeningitis virus	Arenaviridae	Human	Borrow (2014)
	Herpes viruses	Herpesviridae	Human	Mustafa and Elahee (2016)
	Measles	Paramyxoviridae	Human	Gastanaduy et al. (2018)
	Mumps	Paramyxoviridae	Human	Shuaib et al. (2008)
	Poliovirus	Picornaviridae	Human	Kidd (1996)
	West Nile virus	Flaviviridae	Humans, mosquitoes, birds, ticks	Mcdonald et al. (2019)
Eye	Adenovirus	Adenoviridae	Human	Kajon et al. (2018)
	Cytomegalovirus	Herpesviridae	Human	Plosa et al. (2014)

TABLE 1.2 *(Continued)*

Route of Infection	Causative Agents	Family	Host	References
	Herpes simplex virus	Herpesviridae	Human	Mustafa and Elahee (2016)
	Varicella Zoster virus	Herpesviridae	Human	Pergam and Limaye (2010
	Enterovirus	Picornaviridae	Human	Abedi et al. (2018)
Skin	Varicella zoster virus	Herpesviridae	Human	Pergam and Limaye (2010)
	Coxsackie A virus	Picornaviridae	Human	Tahmina (2017)
	Herpes simplex virus	Herpesviridae	Human	Mustafa and Elahee (2016)

Additionally, the nucleocapsid protein (NP) serves as a ribonucleoprotein that encapsulates the viral genome. The M protein (M), located just beneath the viral envelope, is type-specific and distinct for influenza virus types A, B, and C.

1.7.1.1 CLINICAL MANIFESTATIONS

The onset is abrupt. The incubation period is 1–3 days. The route of entry is the respiratory tract. The disease severity may range from mild coryza to fatal, fulminating pneumonia. Most infections are self-limited. In the typical clinical case, high fever with respiratory symptoms such as cough or nasal discharge, and systemic symptoms such as chills, malaise, or myalgia, are seen. Abdominal pain and vomiting develop in children with type B infections. The most common complication is pneumonia, which can be either viral pneumonia or bacterial superinfection. In the case of viral pneumonia, the virus directly infects the lower respiratory tract, leading to bilateral pneumonia. Viral pneumonia is very fatal and is the major cause of mortality in young adults during flu pandemics. In the case of older patients, most of the mortality is caused by bacterial superinfection with *Streptococcus pneumoniae* or *Staphylococcus aureus*. In such cases, viral infection allows secondary infection with the bacterial pathogens resulting in bacterial pneumonia. Infection with influenza virus type B in young children has been associated with Reye syndrome, which involves acute degenerative changes in the brain and liver dysfunction (Hall et al., 2021; Samji, 2009).

1.7.1.2 BIRD FLU/SWINE FLU

Bird flu, or avian flu, is a disease caused by the Influenza virus type A. Mostly, two different strains of avian-origin influenza A viruses cause bird flu pandemics, with the most mortality cases attributed to the avian influenza virus strain H5N1. The first outbreak was reported in December 2003, and the highest number of infected cases were reported from Indonesia, Egypt, and Vietnam. The most recent case was reported from the United States of America on April 29, 2022, in a poultry farm, where H5N1 was confirmed in the poultry, but no human cases were reported. These viruses naturally spread among wild aquatic birds and eventually spread to farmed poultry and other animals. Human cases of avian influenza H7N9 were reported in China in March 2013. Since then, annual reports of avian influenza H7N9 have resulted in more than 1300 reported cases. The signs and symptoms of avian influenza include fever, headache, cough, malaise, and myalgia. Complications include respiratory failure, fulminant pneumonia, multi-organ failure, septic shock, disseminated intravascular coagulation, and encephalopathy (Ahmed et al., 2017).

1.7.1.3 SWINE FLU

Swine influenza is a respiratory disease of pigs caused by the H1N1 strain of influenza virus type A. The first report came from Mexico in March 2009 and was spread to many countries. The symptoms were similar to those of seasonal influenza, along with gastrointestinal manifestations. The most common findings were fever, sore throat, cough, malaise, vomiting, headache, and diarrhea. Complications include respiratory failure, progressive pneumonia, acute respiratory distress syndrome, and multisystem organ failure (Mujariya and Bodla, 2014).

1.7.2 ZIKA VIRUS

Zika is an acute infection characterized by a generalized maculopapular rash, myalgia, arthralgia, headache, and conjunctivitis. Complications are rare, which include Guillain-Barre syndrome and meningoencephalitis. Zika virus is a single-stranded RNA virus belonging to the family Flaviviridae. The name "Zika" was derived from the Zika forest of Uganda, where the virus was first isolated from the rhesus monkey. The Zika virus was isolated from human cases in 1968. Since then, this virus has caused several outbreaks in different parts of Africa and Asia. In 2015, the Zika virus caused epidemics in Brazil following the 2014 World Cup football. Zika virus is primarily transmitted by the bite of female *Aedes aegypti* mosquitoes; however, *Aedes albopictus* and *Aedes africanus* can also transmit the infection. Musso et al. (2014) reported that the infection can be transmitted through blood and sexual contact. The most alarming aspect of Zika viruses is that they can be transferred from an infected mother to her fetus during pregnancy (Mujariya and Bodla, 2014). Even if Zika virus infections in pregnant women are less severe, the infection may harm the fetus.

There were many reports of microcephaly in infants whose mothers were infected with the Zika virus. Microcephaly may lead to vision or hearing problems, seizures, and developmental disabilities in babies. Zika virus infection in babies may also lead to several brain abnormalities, such as ventriculomegaly, intracranial calcifications, clubfoot, and congenital contractures (Shapshak et al., 2015).

1.7.3 EBOLA VIRUS

Ebola is a deadly disease that mostly occurs in African countries. Ebola virus disease has been seen in humans as well as non-human primates such as monkeys, chimpanzees, and gorillas. Ebola is caused by different members of the genus Ebola virus. The causative agents are the Ebola virus, Sudan virus, Tai Forest virus, Reston virus, Bombali virus, and Bundibugyo virus. Of these, Ebola, Tai Forest, and Bundibugyo viruses cause human cases. Ebola virus is a negative-sense single-stranded RNA virus belonging to the family Filoviridae. Ebola virus infection was first reported in Zaire in 1976. Since then, several epidemics have been reported throughout the African continent. The name "Ebola" was derived from the Ebola River, where it was first reported. Ebola virus disease is animal-borne, with non-human primates and bats being the primary sources. The infection is transmitted through direct contact with the blood or body fluids of the infected person and animals or objects contaminated with them. The virus gets into the body through cuts or abrasions on the skin and mucous membranes. The infection can also be transmitted through sexual contact since the virus can persist in the body fluids after recovery. The symptoms may appear 2–21 days after contact with the virus. The primary symptoms are high fever, aches and pains, sore throat, weakness, fatigue, loss of appetite, rash, gastrointestinal, as well as respiratory symptoms, and bleeding manifestations. Survivors may show antibodies that can be detected in the blood up to 10 years after recovery (Ahmed et al., 2017).

1.7.4 CORONAVIRUS

Coronaviruses are enveloped RNA viruses that cause respiratory and intestinal infections in both humans and animals. The severity of the disease may range from a common cold to fatal pneumonia. The coronavirus family comprises many infectious virus classes that cause severe diseases such as SARS (Severe Acute Respiratory Syndrome) and MERS (Middle East Respiratory Syndrome). A recent report from late December 2019 in Wuhan, Hubei Province of China, revealed new pneumonia-like infections caused by a novel coronavirus (2019-nCoV) (Rothan and Byrareddy, 2020). The infection leads to difficulty in breathing, fever, cough, and invasive lesions in the lungs.

A Public Health Emergency of International Concern declared a lethal outbreak of coronavirus on 30 January 2020. The World Health Organization (WHO) termed the new coronavirus disease acronym as COVID-19 on 11 February 2020, where CO stands for Corona, VI for the virus, D for disease, and 19 for 31/December/2019, when the virus appeared and was first reported (WHO, 2020). The widespread outbreak of the novel coronavirus disease across the globe compelled the WHO to declare the circumstances a pandemic on March 11, 2020 (Livingston et al., 2020). The growth and spread of the novel coronavirus have been exponential ever since its first detection. As of statistics on May 6, 2020, COVID-19 resulted in a total of 628,346,704 infected cases, with 657,968 deaths across 227 countries globally (Livingston et al., 2020).

Coronavirus is commonly found in animals such as cattle and camels. It is believed that the SARS and MERS coronaviruses originated in bats and were directly transmitted to humans through dromedary camels and market civets. COVID-19 transmission was also reported to originate from bats (Zhou et al., 2020). However, the mode of transmission to humans is still unclear. Initial epidemiological investigations in China indicated that pneumonia-like infections originated from a seafood and animal market in Wuhan (Bogoch et al., 2020). The subsequent city shutdown included the termination of all transport links by January 23 in Wuhan, the city of Huanggang, and the city of Ezhou, China, resulting in the quarantine of 18 million people. By January 30, the number of COVID-19 infections had exceeded that of SARS, which had affected 8,096 people worldwide. As time progressed, COVID-19 infections outside China were also reported in the United Kingdom, Russia, Sweden, Canada, and Spain. The first reported instance of human-to-human transmission of COVID-19 was from the USA on January 30. Thank you for watching.

A comprehensive understanding of the lethal pandemic COVID-19 can be achieved by addressing the following questions: How dangerous is the novel coronavirus? What is the case fatality rate of the novel coronavirus? How transmissible is the virus? How does the age of the infected person or the incubation period contribute to the spread and growth of COVID-19? The cumulative impact of all the significant factors that contribute to the spread of COVID-19 can be effectively represented by the basic reproductive number (Ro) and the case fatality rate (CFR). The possibility of asymptomatic transmission is another crucial factor that needs to be taken into account. Ro signifies the average number of people affected by a single infected person (Wang et al., 2020). A Ro value less than one indicates a gradual disappearance of virus transmission, and vice versa. Although the reported absolute Ro values for COVID-19 differ, there is a consensus that the magnitude always remains more than one. For instance, Liu et al. (2020) reported a Ro value of 3.28 with a median of 2.79 for the period of January 1 to February 7, 2020, exceeding the WHO estimates of 1.4–2.5 as of January 23. However, these results unequivocally indicate that COVID-19 has high transmissibility.

According to the World Health Organization's update on January 29, 2020, the novel coronavirus's CFR is approximately 2%. Compared to other similar viral infections, COVID-19 CFR is higher than that of influenza infection (0.1%) but lower than that of SARS disease (9.5%) and Middle East respiratory syndrome (34.4%) (Rajgor et al., 2020). However, the COVID-19 CFR increases to 8.0% for individuals aged 70–79 years and 14.8% for those aged above 80 years (Wang et al., 2020).

In China, approximately 80% of the total deaths were reported for individuals aged above 60, and 70% of those individuals had been suffering from preexisting health problems such as asthma, cardiovascular diseases, or diabetes. The vulnerability of elderly people to COVID-19 is a global trend, particularly for those with preexisting health conditions (Cascella et al., 2020). According to the WHO, as of January 27, the median age of confirmed COVID-19 cases outside China is 45 years, with 71% being males. However, the presence of worse preexisting medical conditions can make younger generations more vulnerable. The incubation period typically ranges between 10 and 14 days but may be as short as 2 days. In rare cases, symptoms may appear after 14 days for one out of every 100 infected individuals.

1.7.4.1 TRANSMISSION OF COVID-19

Evidence indicates three primary modes of virus spread in COVID-19, namely from symptomatic, pre-symptomatic, or asymptomatic infected individuals. Transmission in the symptomatic mode occurs from individuals displaying signs and symptoms of COVID-19 infection (Culp, 2020). The pre-symptomatic phase of affected individuals can also be contagious. An asymptomatic laboratory-confirmed virus case shows COVID-19 infections without any accompanying signs and symptoms. While there have been reports of the asymptomatic presence of the virus, asymptomatic transmission has not been definitively proven (Culp, 2020).

1.7.4.2 SOURCE OF INFECTION

Efforts have been made to locate the reservoir host or an intermediate carrier of COVID-19. Early studies linked infected individuals to the wet animal market of Wuhan city, suggesting the zoonotic origin of the COVID-19 pandemic (Culp, 2020). Additionally, some studies have suggested two species of snakes as possible reservoirs of COVID-19 (Ji et al., 2020; Zhang et al., 2020). A study from the Wuhan Institute of Virology showed a 96.2% similarity between bat coronavirus and SARS-CoV-2 using sequencing technology, indicating that mammals are the most likely link between humans and COVID-19 (Zhou et al., 2020). However, to date, there has been no conclusive evidence for the animal reservoir of COVID-19 other than mammals and birds.

1.7.4.3 MODES OF TRANSMISSION

Infected individuals are more contagious during the initial stage of the disease than later. The COVID-19 virus can spread through respiratory secretions (within three days of the onset of symptoms) of the affected person. Three standard modes of transmission of COVID-19 include direct contact with the infected person, inhalation of respiratory droplets when the infected person coughs, sneezes, or talks, or contact with virus-contaminated surfaces and fomites (WHO, 2020). The most common mode of virus spread occurs through person-to-person contact within a proximity of fewer than six feet. Additionally, researchers have detected the novel coronavirus in stools, saliva, gastrointestinal tract, and urine (Wang et al., 2020). Vertical transmission from mother to infant during the late trimester was ruled out based on a retrospective study conducted on nine pregnant women infected with COVID-19 (Chen et al., 2020).

However, available data on pregnant women with COVID-19 are insufficient to confirm the possibility of vertical transmission of COVID-19.

1.7.4.4 PATHOGENESIS

Clinical studies of COVID-19-infected cases exhibit close similarities to SARS-CoV and MERS-CoV. COVID-19 belongs to the β-coronavirus family and is related to SARS-CoV and MERS-CoV based on genome analysis (Huang et al., 2020). Therefore, the mode of action of SARS-CoV and MERS-CoV can provide insights into the mechanism of COVID-19. Similar to SARS-CoV and MERS-CoV, COVID-19 also uses angiotensin-converting enzyme-2 (ACE2) as the receptor (Huang et al., 2020). The receptor ACE2 is broadly expressed in the respiratory epithelium, vascular endothelium, alveolar monocytes, and macrophages. The envelope glycoprotein of the virus binds to its cellular receptors such as ACE2 (Huang et al., 2020), CD 209 L (C-type lectin) (Williams and Chambers, 2014), and DPP4 (Xu et al., 2020). After binding with the receptors, the entry of COVID-19 into the cells is achieved by the direct fusion of the envelope glycoprotein and the plasma membrane (Simmons et al., 2004). Coronavirus S-protein plays a significant role in the virus's entry into the target cell (Belouzard et al., 2009). After cell fusion, both clathrin-dependent and clathrin-independent endocytosis of COVID-19 occur in the cells (Wang et al., 2008, 2020). Following effective attachment and cell fusion, the virus uncoat's itself to release the viral RNA genome into the host cell's cytoplasm. Viral genome replication ensues, and the viral RNA is translated into two polyproteins and structural proteins (Perlman and Netland, 2009). The assembly of the progeny virions takes place in the endoplasmic reticulum-Golgi intermediate compartment, and the vesicles containing the virus particles fuse with the plasma membrane to release the progeny viruses (De Wit et al., 2016).

The coronavirus in the infected cells is presented to antigen-presenting cells by the major histocompatibility complex (MHC). The antigenic peptides obtained in this manner are recognized by virus-specific cytotoxic T-lymphocytes, which stimulate both humoral and cell-mediated immune responses (Liu et al., 2010). SARS-specific IgM antibodies disappear within 12 weeks, while IgG persists for an extended period (Li et al., 2003). Several reports on cell-mediated immune responses against

COVID-19 outweigh the humoral response. With the progression of the disease, there is a continuous decrease in lymphocyte levels and a significant increase in neutrophils. Subset assays reveal a general decrease in T cells, B cells, and natural killer cells, as well as a decline of both $CD4^+$ and $CD8^+$ lymphocytes in critically ill patients (Xu et al., 2020).

Moreover, several reports indicate that acute respiratory distress syndrome (ARDS) is the leading cause of death in COVID-19 (Huang et al., 2020). Similar immunopathological events have also been observed in SARS-CoV and MERS-CoV infections. An uncontrolled inflammatory response from the immune effector cells during COVID-19 infection can lead to ARDS. This results in a surge of inflammatory markers such as pro-inflammatory cytokines (INF α, INF γ, IL-1β, IL-6, IL-12, IL-18, tumor necrosis factor α, etc.) as well as chemokines (CCL2, CCL3, CCL5, CXCL8, etc.) (Huang et al., 2020). The surge of inflammatory molecules leads to a violent attack of the immune system and eventually results in multiple organ failures or even the death of the patient.

Like SARS-CoV and MERS-CoV, COVID-19 is expected to follow the same strategies for better survival within the host cells. SARS-CoV and MERS-CoV can induce the production of double-layered membrane vesicles, and the replication of the virus takes place within these vesicles. The vesicles lack pathogen-associated molecular patterns (PAMPs), thus evading recognition by pattern recognition receptors (PRSs) of the host cells (Snijder et al., 2006). This allows SARS-CoV and MERS-CoV to evade the host detection of their RNA genome, facilitating their invasion of the host cell's immune defense mechanism. Therefore, understanding the pathogenesis of COVID-19 is imperative for the development of specific treatments.

1.7.4.5 CLINICAL CHARACTERISTICS

COVID-19 causes an acute viral infection in humans. The clinical severity may range from mild symptoms to terminal illness. Severe cases may require mechanical ventilation and support in an intensive care unit. The time from exposure to the onset of clinical signs usually ranges around five days but may extend the range to 2–14 days. The most common symptoms of COVID-19 include fever, cough, dyspnea, loss of appetite, repeated shaking with chills, and a new loss of taste or smell. Some cases in China initially showed only palpitations and chest tightness (Wang et al., 2020).

Approximately 81% of infected individuals showed mild disease with symptoms such as fever, dry cough, sore throat, malaise, headache, and nasal congestion. 14% of infected patients develop severe illness, characterized by dyspnea, respiratory frequency ≥ 30 breaths/min, and hypoxia (SpO_2 < 90% on room air). Critical disease developed in 5% of infected cases and is characterized by pneumonia, respiratory distress syndrome, multiple organ failure, sepsis, and shock. The clinical features of COVID-19 patients with sepsis are serious and involve severe dyspnea, hypoxemia, tachycardia, altered mental status, diarrhea, hyperbilirubinemia, abnormal clotting, renal impairment with reduced urine output, acidosis, thrombocytopenia, and coagulopathy (Chen et al., 2020). In addition to ARDS, severe cases of COVID-19 are also prone to other complications such as acute heart injury, neurological complications, ocular surface infections, arrhythmia, abnormal liver function, and other secondary infections (Cascella et al., 2020) (Figure 1.1).

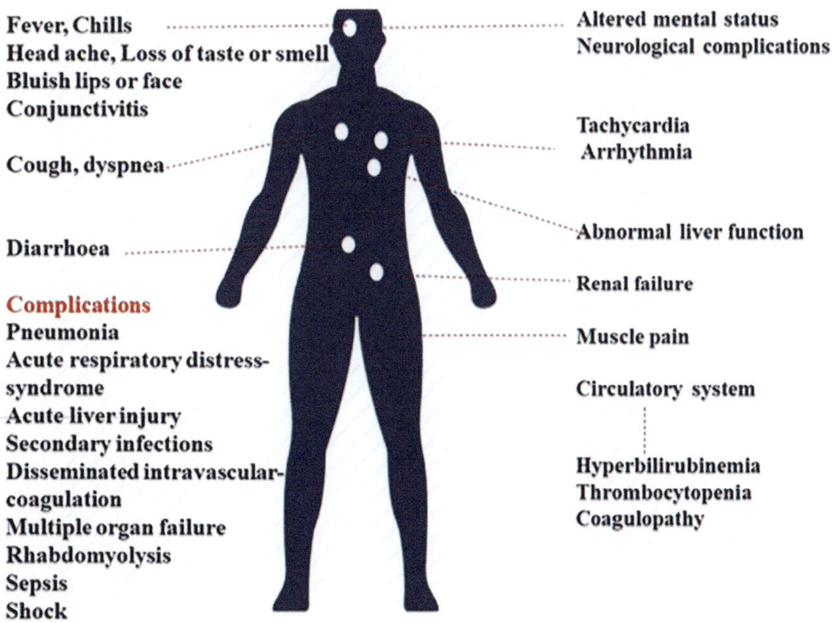

FIGURE 1.1 Clinical symptoms of COVID-19.

1.7.5 CHIKUNGUNYA

Chikungunya virus is primarily transmitted by the bite of infected mosquitoes, mainly *Aedes aegypti* and *Aedes albopictus*. Humans are the primary host for this RNA virus, which belongs to the family Togaviridae and the genus Alphavirus. The virus was first reported along the border of Tanzania and Mozambique in 1952. The term "Chikungunya" originates from a word in the Kimakonde language, meaning "to become contorted," which described the stooped appearance of patients with Chikungunya. The infection is primarily transmitted through the bite of infected female mosquitoes. Cases of transmission through blood have been reported in France. Transmission to the fetus during the second trimester of pregnancy and intrapartum transmission from a viremic mother at the time of delivery have also been documented. Infected individuals typically develop symptoms within 3–7 days after being bitten by the mosquito. Chikungunya manifests as an acute febrile illness with three phases: the acute phase, sub-acute phase, and chronic phase. The acute febrile period is characterized by fever, arthralgia, and rash. The onset of fever is sudden and lasts for 3–5 days, accompanied by joint pain, muscle pain, headache, and rash. The most commonly affected joints are the wrists, hands, and ankles. Complications may include Guillain-Barré syndrome, myocarditis, meningoencephalitis, respiratory failure, and fulminant hepatitis in patients with chronic liver disease. High-risk individuals include infants, older adults, and people with high blood pressure, heart disease, and diabetes (Ganesan et al., 2017).

1.8 CONCLUDING REMARKS

Infectious diseases have posed extreme challenges to life throughout evolution, even risking the existence of living organisms. For humankind, infectious diseases have triggered socio-economic disasters that may reverberate for generations before any meaningful recovery. Viral diseases that frequently emerge pose a major risk to human life and cause significant mortality globally. Some of the deadliest pandemics in human history have been caused by viruses. The current leading infectious agent worldwide, the coronavirus, has caused an estimated 6.5 million deaths since the first cases were reported in 2020. Patterns of disease transmission are continually evolving. Human activities, such as encroaching on and altering wildlife habitats, introducing exotic species, and disrupting environmental homeostasis, play a role in the increased incidence of emerging infections. It is essential to maintain a healthy balance between humans and animals. Therefore, significant attention must be devoted to the prevention and transmission of viral diseases.

KEYWORDS

- **bacteria**
- **contagious**
- **infectious disease**
- **microorganisms**
- **morphology**
- **nucleic acid**
- **viral infections**
- **virion**

REFERENCES

Abedi, G. R., Watson, J. T., Nix, W. A., Oberste, M. S., & Gerber, S. I. (2018). Morbidity and Mortality Weekly Report enterovirus and parechovirus surveillance—United States, 2014–2016. *MMWR. Morbidity and Mortality Weekly Report, 67*(18), 515–518.

Africa, West, United States, Other Orthopoxviruses, Central African, West African, The West African, Is Monkeypox, et al. (2022). *Monkeypox Virus Fact Sheet* (pp. 7–8).

Agency, Human Services. (1972). *State of California—Health and Human Services Agency Department of Health Services Division of Communicable Disease Control* (No. June, pp. 1, 2).

Ahmed, J. U., Rahim, M. A., & Uddin, K. N. (2017). *Emerging Viral Diseases* (No. August). https://doi.org/10.3329/birdem.v7i3.33785 (accessed on 4th July 2025).

Araujo, N. M. (2022). *Adeno-Associated Virus Infection and Its Impact in Human Health: An Overview* (No. November). https://doi.org/10.1186/s12985-022-01900-4 (accessed on 4th July 2025).

Arif, B., & Natural Resources Canada. (2014). *Genome of Sindbis Virus* (No. May). https://doi.org/10.1128/JVI.9.1.102-109.1972 (accessed on 4th July 2025).

Aslan, A. T., & Balaban, H. Y. (2020). Hepatitis E virus: Epidemiology, diagnosis, clinical manifestations, and treatment. *World Journal of Gastroenterology, 26*(37), 5543–5560. https://doi.org/10.3748/wjg.v26.i37.5543 (accessed on 4th July 2025).

Babkin, I. V., & Babkina, I. N. (2015). *The Origin of The Variola Virus*, 1100–1112. https://doi.org/10.3390/v7031100 (accessed on 4th July 2025).

Battisti, A. J., Chu, Y. K., Chipman, P. R., Kaufmann, B., Jonsson, C. B., & Rossmann, M. G. (2011). Structural studies of Hantaan virus. *Journal of Virology, 85*(2), 835–841. https://doi.org/10.1128/jvi.01847-10 (accessed on 4th July 2025).

Belouzard, S., Chu, V. C., & Whittaker, G. R. (2009). Activation of the SARS coronavirus spike protein via sequential proteolytic cleavage at two distinct sites. *Proceedings of the National Academy of Sciences of the United States of America, 106*(14), 5871–5876. https://doi.org/10.1073/pnas.0809524106 (accessed on 4th July 2025).

Berlin, D., Gilani, A. I., Grewal, A. K., & Fowkes, M. (2017). Eastern equine encephalitis. *Practical Neurology, 17*(5), 387–391. https://doi.org/10.1136/practneurol-2017-001659 (accessed on 4th July 2025).

Bessaud, M., Peyrefitte, C. N., Pastorino, B. A. M., Gravier, P., Tock, F., Boete, F., Tolou, H. J., & Grandadam, M. (2006). O'nyong-nyong virus, Chad. *Emerging Infectious Diseases, 12*(8), 1248–1250. https://doi.org/10.3201/eid1208.060199 (accessed on 4th July 2025).

Bogoch, I. I., Watts, A., Thomas-Bachli, A., Huber, C., Kraemer, M. U. G., & Khan, K. (2020). Pneumonia of unknown etiology in Wuhan, China: Potential for international spread via commercial air travel. *Journal of Travel Medicine, 27*(2), 1–3. https://doi.org/10.1093/jtm/taaa008 (accessed on 4th July 2025).

Borrow, P. (2014). Lymphocytic choriomeningitis virus (LCMV). In *Encyclopedia of the Neurological Sciences* (No. Lcm, pp. 942–943). https://doi.org/10.1016/B978-0-12-385157-4.00382-1 (accessed on 4th July 2025).

Branche, A. R., & Falsey, A. R. (2016). Parainfluenza virus infection. *Seminars in Respiratory and Critical Care Medicine, 37*(4), 538–554. https://doi.org/10.1055/s-0036-1584798 (accessed on 4th July 2025).

Briese, T., Williams, D. T., Kapoor, V., Diviney, S. M., Certoma, A., Wang, J., Johansen, C. A., Chowdhary, R., Mackenzie, J. S., & Lipkin, W. I. (2016). Analysis of arbovirus isolates from Australia identifies novel bunyaviruses including a Mapputta group virus from Western Australia that links Gan Gan and Maprik viruses. *PLoS ONE, 11*(10), 1–15. https://doi.org/10.1371/journal.pone.0164868 (accessed on 4th July 2025).

Burke, R. M., Tate, J. E., Barin, N., Bock, C., Bowen, M. D., Chang, D., Gautam, R., et al. (2018). Three rotavirus outbreaks in the postvaccine era—California, 2017. *MMWR. Morbidity and Mortality Weekly Report, 67*(16), 470–472. https://doi.org/10.15585/mmwr.mm6716a3 (accessed on 4th July 2025).

Campadelli-Fiume, G., Mirandola, P., & Menotti, L. (1999). Human herpesvirus 6: An emerging pathogen. *Emerging Infectious Diseases, 5*(3), 353–366. https://doi.org/10.3201/eid0503.990306 (accessed on 4th July 2025).

Carocci, M., & Kassimi, L. B. (2016). Encephalomyocarditis virus. In *Molecular Detection of Human Viral Pathogens* (pp. 13–22). https://doi.org/10.1016/b978-0-12-524180-9.50045-5 (accessed on 4th July 2025).

Cascella, M., Rajnik, M., Cuomo, A., Dulebohn, S. C., & Di Napoli, R. (2020). Features, evaluation and treatment coronavirus (COVID-19). *StatPearls*. http://www.ncbi.nlm.nih.gov/pubmed/32150360 (accessed on 4th July 2025).

CDC National Center for Emerging and Zoonotic Infectious Diseases. (2018). *CDC Fact Sheet: Ebola Virus Disease*. https://www.cdc.gov/vhf/ebola/ (accessed on 4th July 2025).

CDC, Division of Birth Defects and Developmental Disabilities. (2014). *Information for Healthcare Providers*, 1–5. http://www.cdc.gov/ncbddd/heartdefects/hcp.html (accessed on 4th July 2025).

CDC. (1967). *Factsheet—Marburg Hemorrhagic Fever*. https://www.cdc.gov/vhf/marburg/pdf/factsheet.pdf (accessed on 4th July 2025).

Chen, H., Guo, J., Wang, C., Luo, F., Yu, X., Zhang, W., Li, J., et al. (2020). Clinical characteristics and intrauterine vertical transmission potential of COVID-19 infection in nine pregnant women: A retrospective review of medical records. *The Lancet, 395*(10226), 809–815. https://doi.org/10.1016/S0140-6736(20)30360-3 (accessed on 4th July 2025).

Chen, N., Zhou, M., Dong, X., Qu, J., Gong, F., Han, Y., Qiu, Y., et al. (2020). Epidemiological and clinical characteristics of 99 cases of 2019 novel coronavirus pneumonia in Wuhan, China: A descriptive study. *The Lancet, 395*(10223), 507–513. https://doi.org/10.1016/S0140-6736(20)30211-7 (accessed on 4th July 2025).

Culp, W. C. (2020). Coronavirus disease 2019. *A & A Practice, 14*(6), e01218. https://doi.org/10.1213/xaa.0000000000001218 (accessed on 4th July 2025).

Darkuthni, M., Tahir, M., & Tumedia, J. L. (2018). Human papilloma virus 16 and 18 infection and the cervical cytology changes in combined hormonal contraceptive users. 188–192.

Diotti, R. A., Nakanishi, A., Clementi, N., Mancini, N., Criscuolo, E., Solforosi, L., & Clementi, M. (2013). JC polyomavirus (JCV) and monoclonal antibodies: Friends or potential foes? *Clinical and Developmental Immunology, 2013*, Article ID 967581. https://doi.org/10.1155/2013/967581 (accessed on 4th July 2025).

Durand, J. P., Bouloy, M., Richecoeur, L., Peyrefitte, C. N., & Tolou, H. (2003). Rift Valley fever virus infection among French troops in Chad [2]. *Emerging Infectious Diseases, 9*(6), 751–752. https://doi.org/10.3201/eid0906.020647 (accessed on 4th July 2025).

Edelman, D. C. (2005). Human herpesvirus 8–A novel human pathogen. *Virology Journal, 2*, 1–32. https://doi.org/10.1186/1743-422X-2-78 (accessed on 4th July 2025).

Eiland, L. S. (2009). Respiratory syncytial virus: Diagnosis, treatment and prevention. *The Journal of Pediatric Pharmacology and Therapeutics, 14*(2), 75–85. https://doi.org/10.5863/1551-6776-14.2.75 (accessed on 4th July 2025).

Estivariz, C. F., Link-Gelles, R., & Shimabukuro, T. (2021). Pinkbook: Poliomyelitis CDC. *CDC*, 275–288. https://www.cdc.gov/vaccines/pubs/pinkbook/downloads/polio.pdf (accessed on 4th July 2025).

Fatkullina, G. R., Anokhin, V. A., & Musina, A. R. (2021). Human herpes virus 7 infections in children: Clinical and laboratory aspects. *Journal Infectiology, 12*(5), 114–122. https://doi.org/10.22625/2072-6732-2020-12-5-114-122 (accessed on 4th July 2025).

Fenner, F., Bachmann, P. A., Gibbs, E. P. J., Murphy, F. A., Studdert, M. J., & White, D. O. (1987). Structure and composition of viruses. In *Veterinary Virology* (pp. 3–19). https://doi.org/10.1016/B978-0-12-253055-5.50005-0 (accessed on 4th July 2025).

Ganesan, V. K., Duan, B., & Reid, S. P. (2017). Chikungunya virus: Pathophysiology, mechanism, and modeling. *Viruses, 9*(12), 368. https://doi.org/10.3390/v9120368 (accessed on 4th July 2025).

Gastanaduy, P. A., Redd, S. B., & Clemmons, N. S. (2018). VPD surveillance manual. *VPD Surveillance Manual*, 1–22.

Gelderblom, H. R. (1996). Structure and classification of viruses. *Medical Microbiology*. http://www.ncbi.nlm.nih.gov/pubmed/21413309 (accessed on 4th July 2025).

Giangaspero, M. (2015). Tropical Medicine & Surgery: Nipah virus. *Tropical Medicine & Surgery, 1*(April), 1–8. https://doi.org/10.4172/2329-9088 (accessed on 4th July 2025).

Gonzalez, J. P., Cornet, J. P., & Camicas, J. L. (1989). Dogbe virus replication in nymph and adult *Amblyomma variegatum*. *Research in Virology, 140*(C), 333–336. https://doi.org/10.1016/S0923-2516(89)80113-X (accessed on 4th July 2025).

Hall, E., Smith, W., Andrewes, C., & Laidlaw, P. (2021). Influenza. 179–192.

Hallowell, B. D., Parashar, U. D., Curns, A., DeGroote, N. P., & Tate, J. E. (2019). Trends in the laboratory detection of rotavirus before and after implementation of routine rotavirus vaccination–United States, 2000–2018. *MMWR. Morbidity and Mortality Weekly Report, 68*(24), 539–543. https://doi.org/10.15585/mmwr.mm6824a2 (accessed on 4th July 2025).

Heegaard, E. D., & Brown, K. E. (2002). Esportes e classificação funcional paraolímpica. *Clinical Microbiology Reviews, 15*(3), 485–505. https://doi.org/10.1128/CMR.15.3.485 (accessed on 4th July 2025).

Hewson, R. (2019). Crimean-Congo hemorrhagic fever virus. *Microbiology Today, 46*(3), 112–115. https://doi.org/10.2174/156652405774962335 (accessed on 4th July 2025).

Hills, S. (1996). Ross River virus and Barmah Forest virus infection: Commonly asked questions. *Australian Family Physician, 25*(12), 1822–1824.

Hu, B., Guo, H., Zhou, P., & Shi, Z. L. (2021). Characteristics of SARS-CoV-2 and COVID-19. *Nature Reviews Microbiology, 19*(3), 141–154. https://doi.org/10.1038/s41579-020-00459-7 (accessed on 4th July 2025).

Hu, Y., Lee, J., Cart, J. A. M. C., Xu, H. U. I., Moss, B., Alexander, H. R., & Bartlett, D. L. (2001). Yaba-like disease virus: An alternative replicating poxvirus vector for cancer gene therapy. https://doi.org/10.1128/JVI.75.21.10300 (accessed on 4th July 2025).

Huang, C., Wang, Y., Li, X., Ren, L., Zhao, J., Hu, Y., Zhang, L., et al. (2020). Clinical features of patients infected with 2019 novel coronavirus in Wuhan, China. *The Lancet, 395*(10223), 497–506. https://doi.org/10.1016/S0140-6736(20)30183-5 (accessed on 4th July 2025).

Jackson, A. C. (2016). Rabies. https://doi.org/10.1017/S0317167100000998 (accessed on 4th July 2025).

Jacobs, B. L., & Langland, J. O. (2009). NIH public access. *Antiviral Research, 84*(1), 1–13. https://doi.org/10.1016/j.antiviral.2009.06.006.Vaccinia (accessed on 4th July 2025).

Jacobs, S. E., Lamson, D. M., St, K., & Walsh, T. J. (2013). Human rhinoviruses. *Clinical Microbiology Reviews, 26*(1), 135–162. https://doi.org/10.1128/CMR.00077-12 (accessed on 4th July 2025).

Jamieson, F. B., Wang, E. E. L., Bain, C., Good, J., Duckmanton, L., & Petric, M. (1998). Human torovirus: A new nosocomial gastrointestinal pathogen. *Journal of Infectious Diseases, 178*(5 Suppl.), 1263–1269. https://doi.org/10.1086/314434 (accessed on 4th July 2025).

Ji, W., Wang, W., Zhao, X., Zai, J., & Li, X. (2020). Cross-species transmission of the newly identified coronavirus 2019-nCoV. *Journal of Medical Virology, 92*(4), 433–440. https://doi.org/10.1002/jmv.25682 (accessed on 4th July 2025).

Johnson, C., Hargest, V., Cortez, V., Meliopoulos, V. A., & Schultz-Cherry, S. (2017). Astrovirus pathogenesis. *Viruses, 9*(1), 1–10. https://doi.org/10.3390/v9010022 (accessed on 4th July 2025).

Kajon, A. E., Lamson, D. M., Bair, C. R., Lu, X., Landry, M. L., Menegus, M., Erdman, D. D., & St George, K. (2018). Adenovirus type 4 respiratory infections among civilian adults. *Emerging Infectious Diseases, 24*(2), 2011–2015.

Kapila, A., Chaudhary, S., Sharma, R. B., Vashist, H., Sisodia, S. S., & Gupta, A. (2016). A review on: HIV AIDS. *Indian Journal of Pharmaceutical and Biological Research (IJPBR), 4*(3), 69–73.

Kidd, D. (1996). Poliomyelitis. *Postgraduate Medical Journal, 72*(853), 641–647. https://doi.org/10.1136/pgmj.72.853.641 (accessed on 4th July 2025).

Kitajima, M., & Gerba, C. P. (2015). Aichi virus 1: Environmental occurrence and behavior. *Pathogens, 4*(2), 256–268. https://doi.org/10.3390/pathogens4020256 (accessed on 4th July 2025).

Kleines, M., Häusler, M., Krüttgen, A., & Scheithauer, S. (2009). WU polyomavirus (WUPyV): A recently detected virus causing respiratory disease? *Viruses, 1*(3), 678–688. https://doi.org/10.3390/v1030678 (accessed on 4th July 2025).

Kodani, S., & Schillie, M. (2016). Chapter 4: Hepatitis B. In *VPD Surveillance Manual Hepatitis B: Chapter 4.1* (pp. 1–10).

Kumar, D. (2020). Corona virus: A review of COVID-19. *Eurasian Journal of Medicine and Oncology*. https://doi.org/10.14744/ejmo.2020.51418 (accessed on 4th July 2025).

Lanzieri, T., Redd, S., Abernathy, E., & Icenogle, J. (2004). Chapter 14: Rubella (pp. 1–9).

Learn, G., & Easlick, J. (2012). Eastern chimpanzees, but not bonobos, represent a simian immunodeficiency virus reservoir. https://doi.org/10.1128/JVI.01498-12 (accessed on 4th July 2025).

Leno, M., Simpson, R. M., Bowers, F. S., & Kindt, T. J. (1995). Human T lymphocyte virus 1 from a leukemogenic cell line mediates *in vivo* and *in vitro* lymphocyte. *181* (April).

Li, G., Chen, X., & Xu, A. (2003). Profile of specific antibodies to the SARS-associated coronavirus [6]. *New England Journal of Medicine, 349*(5), 508–509. https://doi.org/10.1056/NEJM200307313490520 (accessed on 4th July 2025).

Litvoc, M. N., Novaes, C. T. G., & Lopes, M. I. B. F. (2018). Yellow fever. *64*(2), 106–113.

Liu, B., Clarke, I. N., & Lambden, P. R. (1996). Polyprotein processing in Southampton virus: Identification of 3C-like protease cleavage sites by *in vitro* mutagenesis. *Journal of Virology, 70*(4), 2605–2610. https://doi.org/10.1128/jvi.70.4.2605-2610.1996 (accessed on 4th July 2025).

Liu, H., Li, M. H., Zhai, Y. G., Meng, W. S., Sun, X. H., Cao, Y. X., Fu, S. H., et al. (2010). Banna virus, China, 1987–2007. *Emerging Infectious Diseases, 16*(3), 514–517. https://doi.org/10.3201/eid1603.091160 (accessed on 4th July 2025).

Liu, J., Wu, P., Gao, F., Qi, J., Kawana-Tachikawa, A., Xie, J., Vavricka, C. J., Iwamoto, A., Li, T., & Gao, G. F. (2010). Novel immunodominant peptide presentation strategy: A featured HLA-A*2402-restricted cytotoxic T-lymphocyte epitope stabilized by intrachain hydrogen bonds from severe acute respiratory syndrome coronavirus nucleocapsid protein. *Journal of Virology, 84*(22), 11849–11857. https://doi.org/10.1128/jvi.01464-10 (accessed on 4th July 2025).

Liu, Y., Gayle, A. A., Wilder-Smith, A., & Rocklöv, J. (2020). The reproductive number of COVID-19 is higher compared to SARS coronavirus. *Journal of Travel Medicine, 27*(2), 1–4. https://doi.org/10.1093/jtm/taaa021 (accessed on 4th July 2025).

Livingston, E., Bucher, K., & Rekito, A. (2020). Coronavirus disease 2019 and influenza 2019–2020. *JAMA–Journal of the American Medical Association, 323*(12), 1122. https://doi.org/10.1001/jama.2020.2633 (accessed on 4th July 2025).

Lledó, L., Giménez-Pardo, C., & Gegúndez, M. I. (2020). Epidemiological study of Thogoto and Dhori virus infection in people bitten by ticks, and in sheep, in an area of northern Spain. *International Journal of Environmental Research and Public Health, 17*(7). https://doi.org/10.3390/ijerph17072254 (accessed on 4th July 2025).

Lwoff, A. (1957). The concept of virus. *Journal of General Microbiology, 17*(2), 239–253. https://doi.org/10.1099/00221287-17-2-239 (accessed on 4th July 2025).

McDonald, E., Martin, S. W., Landry, K., Gould, C. V., & Lehman, J. (2019). West Nile virus and other domestic nationally notifiable arboviral diseases–United States, 2018. *MMWR. Morbidity and Mortality Weekly Report, 68*(31).

Menghani, S., Chikhale, R., Raval, A., Wadibhasme, P., & Khedekar, P. (2012). Chandipura virus: An emerging tropical pathogen. *Acta Tropica, 124*(1), 1–14. https://doi.org/10.1016/j.actatropica.2012.06.001 (accessed on 4th July 2025).

Merritt, T., Taylor, K., Cox-Witton, K., Field, H., Wingett, K., Mendez, D., Power, M., & Durrheim, D. (2018). Australian bat lyssavirus. *Australian Journal of General Practice, 47*(3), 93–96. https://doi.org/10.31128/AFP-08-17-4314 (accessed on 4th July 2025).

Mindel, A. (2014). The human herpes viruses. https://doi.org/10.1136/sti.70.1.74-a (accessed on 4th July 2025).

Modrow, S., Falke, D., Truyen, U., & Schätzl, H. (2013). *Molecular Virology* (pp. 1–1016). https://doi.org/10.1007/978-3-642-20718-1 (accessed on 4th July 2025).

Morozov, V. A., & Lagaye, S. (2018). Hepatitis C virus: Morphogenesis, infection and therapy. *World Journal of Hepatology, 10*(2), 186–212. https://doi.org/10.4254/wjh.v10.i2.186 (accessed on 4th July 2025).

Mujariya, R., & Bodla, R. (2014). *Indo-Global Research Library* (No. May). *[Further details not provided].*

Musso, D., Nhan, T., Robin, E., Roche, C., Bierlaire, D., Zisou, K., Yan, A. S., & Broult, J. (2014). Potential for Zika virus transmission through blood transfusion demonstrated during an outbreak in French Polynesia, November 2013 to February 2014. *Eurosurveillance, 19*(14), 20761. https://doi.org/10.2807/1560-7917.ES2014.19.14.20761 (accessed on 4th July 2025).

Mustafa, M., & Elahee, M. I. (2016). Herpes simplex virus infections: Pathophysiology and management. https://doi.org/10.9790/0853-150738591 (accessed on 4th July 2025).

Nathanson, N. (2008). Viral pathogenesis. In *Encyclopedia of Virology* (pp. 314–319). https://doi.org/10.1016/B978-012374410-4.00464-7 (accessed on 4th July 2025).

Panchangam, S. C. (2015). Engineering & science focus, a monthly academic bulletin October issue: 2015 dengue virus. Natural forces within us are true healers of disease and walking is the. https://doi.org/10.13140/RG.2.1.3294.7921 (accessed on 4th July 2025).

Payne, D. C., & Parashar, U. D. (2019). Manual for the surveillance of vaccine-preventable diseases. Chapter 13: Rotavirus. *Manual for the Surveillance of Vaccine-Preventable Diseases, 13*, 1–9. https://stacks.cdc.gov/view/cdc/35646 (accessed on 4th July 2025).

Pergam, S. A., Limaye, A. P., & the AST Infectious Diseases Community of Practice. (2010). NIH public access. *9*(Suppl 4), 1–12. https://doi.org/10.1111/j.1600-6143.2009.02901.x.Varicella (accessed on 4th July 2025).

Perlman, S., & Netland, J. (2009). Coronaviruses post-SARS: Update on replication and pathogenesis. *Nature Reviews Microbiology, 7*(6), 439–450. https://doi.org/10.1038/nrmicro2147 (accessed on 4th July 2025).

Plosa, E. J., Esbenshade, J. C., Fuller, M. P., & Weitkamp, J. H. (2014). Cytomegalovirus infection. https://doi.org/10.1542/pir.33-4-156 (accessed on 4th July 2025).

Popov, G., Baymakova, M., Karcheva, M., Andonova, R., Pishmisheva, M., Pepovich, R., Zaekov, N., Tsachev, I., Pekova, L., & Plochev, K. (2018). Hepatitis A virus infection: General characteristics and prevention. *General Medicine, 20*(2), 68–75.

Prezioso, C., Moens, U., Oliveto, G., Brazzini, G., Piacentini, F., Frasca, F., Viscido, A., et al. (2021). Ki and Wu polyomavirus in respiratory samples of SARS-CoV-2 infected patients. *Microorganisms, 9*(6), 3–10. https://doi.org/10.3390/microorganisms9061259 (accessed on 4th July 2025).

Rajgor, D. D., Lee, M. H., Archuleta, S., Bagdasarian, N., & Quek, S. C. (2020). The many estimates of the COVID-19 case fatality rate. *The Lancet Infectious Diseases, 3099*(20), 30244. https://doi.org/10.1016/S1473-3099(20)30244-9 (accessed on 4th July 2025).

Rats, Pet. (2018). *Preventing Seoul Virus Infection in Pet Rats and People.*

Reshetnyak, V. I., Karlovich, T. I., & Ilchenko, L. U. (2008). Hepatitis G virus. *World Journal of Gastroenterology, 14*(30), 4725–4734. https://doi.org/10.3748/wjg.14.4725 (accessed on 4th July 2025).

Rinaldo, C. H., Tylden, G. D., & Sharma, B. N. (2013). The human polyomavirus BK (BKPyV): Virological background and clinical implications. *APMIS, 121*(8), 728–745. https://doi.org/10.1111/apm.12134 (accessed on 4th July 2025).

Rothan, H. A., & Byrareddy, S. N. (2020). The epidemiology and pathogenesis of coronavirus (COVID-19) outbreak. *Journal of Autoimmunity, 109* (January), 1–4.

Russo, V., Roperto, F., De Biase, D., Cerino, P., Urraro, C., Munday, J. S., & Roperto, S. (2020). Bovine papillomavirus type 2 infection associated with papillomatosis of the amniotic membrane in water buffaloes (*Bubalus bubalis*), 1–15.

Samji, T. (2009). Influenza A: Understanding the viral life cycle. *Yale Journal of Biology and Medicine, 82*(4), 153–159.

Shapshak, P., Somboonwit, C., Foley, B. T., Alrabaa, S. F., Wills, T., & Sinnott, J. T. (2015). Zika virus. https://doi.org/10.1007/978-1-4939-2410-3 (accessed on 4th July 2025).

Shuaib, F., Kimbrough, D., Roofe, M., McGwin, G. Jr., & Jolly, P. (2008). NIH public access. *Bone, 23*(1), 1–7. https://doi.org/10.1002/path.4445.Molecular (accessed on 4th July 2025).

Simmons, G., Reeves, J. D., Rennekamp, A. J., Amberg, S. M., Piefer, A. J., & Bates, P. (2004). Characterization of severe acute respiratory syndrome-associated coronavirus (SARS-CoV) spike glycoprotein-mediated viral entry. *Proceedings of the National Academy of Sciences of the United States of America, 101*(12), 4240–4245. https://doi.org/10.1073/pnas.0306446101 (accessed on 4th July 2025).

Sjö, M., & Ekström, M. (2014). Semliki Forest virus expression system. https://doi.org/10.1038/npg.els.0002661 (accessed on 4th July 2025).

Smits, S. L., Osterhaus, A. D. M. E., & Koopmans, M. P. (2016). Newly identified viruses in human gastroenteritis. *Pediatric Infectious Disease Journal, 35*(1), 104–107. https://doi.org/10.1097/INF.0000000000000950 (accessed on 4th July 2025).

Snijder, E. J., van der Meer, Y., Zevenhoven-Dobbe, J., Onderwater, J. J. M., van der Meulen, J., Koerten, H. K., & Mommaas, A. M. (2006). Ultrastructure and origin of membrane vesicles associated with the severe acute respiratory syndrome coronavirus replication complex. *Journal of Virology, 80*(12), 5927–5940. https://doi.org/10.1128/jvi.02501-05 (accessed on 4th July 2025).

Tabachnick, W. (2015). *Arbovirus Diseases*. https://doi.org/10.1007/978-94-007-1009-2 (accessed on 4th July 2025).

Tahmina, A. (2017). Coxsackie virus: The hand, foot, mouth disease (HFMD). *Juniper Online Journal of Public Health, 1*(4). https://doi.org/10.19080/jojph.2017.01.555566 (accessed on 4th July 2025).

Thornton, K., Chervenak, J., & Neal-Perry, G. (2018). HHS public access. *Physiology & Behavior, 176*(5), 139–148. https://doi.org/10.1016/j.vaccine.2014.11.046.Adverse (accessed on 4th July 2025).

University Health Services, University of California, Berkeley. (2000). *Molluscum Contagiosum*. 94720.

Urban, S., Neumann-, C., & Lampertico, P. (2021). Hepatitis D virus in 2021: Virology, immunology and new treatment approaches for a difficult-to-treat disease, 1782–1794. https://doi.org/10.1136/gutjnl-2020-323888 (accessed on 4th July 2025).

Vigue, C. L. (1976). A short history of the discovery of gene function. *American Biology Teacher, 38*(9), 537–541. https://doi.org/10.2307/4445737 (accessed on 4th July 2025).

Wang, H., Yang, P., Liu, K., Guo, F., Zhang, Y., Zhang, G., & Jiang, C. (2008). SARS coronavirus entry into host cells through a novel clathrin- and caveolae-independent endocytic pathway. *Cell Research, 18*(2), 290–301. https://doi.org/10.1038/cr.2008.15 (accessed on 4th July 2025).

Wang, J., Zhao, S., Liu, M., Zhao, Z., Xu, Y., Wang, P., Lin, M., et al. (2020). ACE2 expression by colonic epithelial cells is associated with viral infection, immunity and energy metabolism. *medRxiv*, 2020.02.05.20020545. https://doi.org/10.1101/2020.02.05.20020545 (accessed on 4th July 2025).

Wang, L., Wang, Y., Ye, D., & Liu, Q. (2020). Review of the 2019 novel coronavirus (SARS-CoV-2) based on current evidence. *International Journal of Antimicrobial Agents, 105948*. https://doi.org/10.1016/j.ijantimicag.2020.105948 (accessed on 4th July 2025).

Williams, A. E., & Chambers, R. C. (2014). The mercurial nature of neutrophils: Still an enigma in ARDS? *American Journal of Physiology–Lung Cellular and Molecular Physiology, 306*(3). https://doi.org/10.1152/ajplung.00311.2013 (accessed on 4th July 2025).

Williams, D. T., Smith, D. W., Harnett, G. B., & Johansen, C. A. (2016). Murray Valley encephalitis virus. In *Molecular Detection of Human Viral Pathogens* (No. November, pp. 219–229). https://doi.org/10.3109/9780203997352.172 (accessed on 4th July 2025).

Wit, E. D., Van Doremalen, N., Falzarano, D., & Munster, V. J. (2016). SARS and MERS: Recent insights into emerging coronaviruses. *Nature Reviews Microbiology, 14*(8), 523–534. https://doi.org/10.1038/nrmicro.2016.81 (accessed on 4th July 2025).

World Health Organization (WHO). (2020). Modes of transmission of virus causing COVID-19: Implications for IPC precaution recommendations. *Scientific Brief*, 1–3.

World Health Organization (WHO). (2020). *Novel Coronavirus–China 11-Fev 2020. WHO Bulletin* (No. February). https://www.who.int/docs/default-source/coronaviruse/situation-reports/20200211-sitrep-22-ncov.pdf?sfvrsn=fb6d49b1_2 (accessed on 4th July 2025).

Xu, Z., Shi, L., Wang, Y., Zhang, J., Huang, L., Zhang, C., Liu, S., et al. (2020). Pathological findings of COVID-19 associated with acute respiratory distress syndrome. *The Lancet Respiratory Medicine, 8*(4), 420–422. https://doi.org/10.1016/S2213-2600(20)30076-X (accessed on 4th July 2025).

Zhang, C., Zheng, W., Huang, X., Bell, E. W., Zhou, X., & Zhang, Y. (2020). Protein structure and sequence reanalysis of 2019-nCoV genome refutes snakes as its intermediate host and the unique similarity between its spike protein insertions and HIV-1. *Journal of Proteome Research, 19*(4), 1351–1360. https://doi.org/10.1021/acs.jproteome.0c00129 (accessed on 4th July 2025).

Zhou, P., Yang, X. L., Wang, X. G., Hu, B., Zhang, L., Zhang, W., Si, H. R., et al. (2020). A pneumonia outbreak associated with a new coronavirus of probable bat origin. *Nature, 579*(7798), 270–273. https://doi.org/10.1038/s41586-020-2012-7 (accessed on 4th July 2025).

CHAPTER 2

Recent Nano-Medicinal Approaches for Antiviral Drugs in the Management of Viral Infections

TWINKLE SHARMA[1] and ARUN KUMAR[1,2,*]

[1]*Chitkara College of Pharmacy, Chitkara University, Punjab, India*

[2]*Department of Pharmacy, School of Health Sciences, Central University of South Bihar, Gaya, Bihar, India*

*Corresponding author

ABSTRACT

Nanotechnology has made significant contributions across all biomedical and paramedical sectors, particularly in the exploration of targeted treatment strategies against various diseases. Viral diseases can potentially transform into life-threatening and chronic conditions. Consequently, easily accessible antiviral medications are used to combat a multitude of viral ailments. However, challenges such as prolonged treatment durations, drug resistance, limited bioavailability, and penetration profiles have rendered the available antiviral formulations less than ideal for administration. To address these complications, the marriage of nanotechnology with the pharmaceutical industry has led to the development of nano-sized formulations for improved treatment outcomes. These formulations, based on organic, inorganic, or biological molecules, exhibit significantly enhanced physicochemical properties, including increased systemic availability, heightened thermodynamic stability, reduced dosing frequency, and improved ability to penetrate biological membranes. These engineered nano-formulations are specifically designed to overcome the

Nanotechnological Management of Viral Infections.
Radhakrishnan EK, Shiji Mathew, and Riya Alex (Eds.)

DOI: 10.1201/9781779640895-2

associated challenges, with the potential to exert a substantial therapeutic effect by reducing the viral load in the host. It is pertinent to acknowledge that, in comparison to conventional antiviral drugs, nanotechnology-based formulations offer multifaceted benefits in treating viral diseases and warrant further investigation and exploration for their efficacy in managing illnesses, both after the onset of the disease and as a prophylactic measure.

2.1 INTRODUCTION

Nanotechnology is a scientific discipline that involves designing and innovating processes, including modeling, controlling, and imaging matter at the nanomolecular level, for the development of various types of active nanoparticles. This technology is often referred to as "technology based on the nanoscale" and is characterized by the molecular size in the order of 100 nm or less (R<100 nm) (Nasrollahzadeh Mahmoud et al., 2019). The presence of these specially sized molecules confers various stabilizing properties, such as a high dispersibility index and a large surface area for absorption on specific planes (Roco, 1999). Additionally, nanoparticles have the significant characteristic of being able to cross the blood-brain barrier (BBB) to exert pharmacological action on encephalic receptors (Sanchez Florence et al., 2010; Tang Jinglong et al., 2010). Thus, nanotechnology is a highly diverse branch incorporated in various sectors such as biomedical and drug delivery, cosmeceuticals, the pharmaceutical industry, biotechnology, and so forth (Nasrollahzadeh Mahmoud et al., 2019).

In recent times, the pharmaceutical industry has been extensively collaborating with nanotechnology, giving rise to the branch known as nanopharmaceuticals. Broadly, nanopharmaceuticals can be classified based on physical structure and complex behavior (Bawa Raj, 2010). They can also be differentiated based on shape, size, and physicochemical characteristics. Nanopharmaceuticals are classified into organic nanocarriers, inorganic nanocarriers, and carbon-based nanoformulations. Organic nanocarriers are primarily derived from natural, semisynthetic, or synthetic origins and are notably characterized as soluble colloids (drug-polymer complexes), biological vesicular structures such as liposomes and phytosomes, or nano-drug condensed entities. These structures are complexed by a phospholipid bilayer, with hydrophobic compounds at the periphery and hydrophilic substances in the core, providing them with amphiphilic, stable, and biocompatible characteristics for administration (Bisso Sofia et al., 2020). Inorganic nanomedicines are systematically prepared from materials containing metallic or non-metallic oxides (Au, Si, Zn, Fe, etc.). The use of these inorganic element oxides in nanoformulations offers clinically enhanced and improved pharmacologically stable responses in various diagnostic processes. They find applications in computed scanning, magnetic imaging, and radiological screening in different types of patients, aiding in the examination of diseases and providing them with intricate and efficacious disease-oriented treatment (Gil Pilar Rivera et al., 2010). Lastly, carbon-based nanostructural formulations are utilized due to their unique properties, such as a conductivity profile, minimal neoplastic effects, high adsorption indices, and certain other promising therapeutic activities against diseases (Polizu Stefania et al., 2006). Nano-pharmaceuticals imply the utilization of numerous nanotechnological approaches to achieve the desired pharmacological targets for patients in the healthcare system. This has led to the enhanced development of nanomedicines with facilitated therapeutic effects, profound safety, toxicological profile, efficacy, and more, making them a novel drug delivery approach. These nanosized delivery systems aim to potentiate the drug-targeted therapeutic effect by circumventing all pharmacokinetic parameters without hindering their biological activity (Owen Andrew et al., 2014).

Likewise, nano-pharmaceutical formulations are being developed with chemotherapeutic potential for the treatment of various ailments, including viral diseases, metabolic syndromes, and genetic-hereditary diseases. Among these, viral infections are particularly concerning, necessitating effective and potent therapeutic strategies for treatment (Bawarski Willie et al., 2008). Therefore, the current prevalent ailment can be addressed by formulating antiviral nanomedicines containing appropriate drugs with particle sizes of 1 billionth meter (10–9) (Bawa Raj, 2010).

Viruses can have a natural or synthetic origin and typically function as obligate parasites, with sizes ranging from 20 nm–300 nm in diameter. Due to their lack of cellular machinery, they are entirely dependent on the host for fulfilling nutritional requirements and completing the life cycle, which includes replication, growth, and development of virus particles (Pradeu Thomas et al., 2016). Therefore, for the relevant treatment and diagnosis of viral diseases, nano-based antiviral preparations specifically target viral enzymes and their life cycle, inhibiting viral growth and replication without causing harm to human cells (Cojocaru Florina-Daniela et al., 2020). Recent approaches involve formulating and aiming to achieve deliberate antiviral outcomes upon administration of nanopharmaceuticals. Overall, the following chapter provides a comprehensive view of various aspects of nanopharmaceuticals, their historical development, scope, and a detailed description of their application in treating various viral manifestations (Mehendale Rujuta et al., 2013).

2.2 HISTORY OF NANOTECHNOLOGY IN MEDICINE

In the early 9th century B.C., the Egyptians and some artisans achieved the production of colored pigments from gold and silver by using finely divided nanomaterials. In 1857, Michael Faraday discovered that the use of metallic-colored pigments had significantly advanced the scientific understanding of the synthesis of nanoparticles through reduction processes (Leon Lorraine et al., 2020). Subsequently, in the early 1900s, Richard Adolf Zsigmondy was the first to conceptualize the idea of nanoparticles. The idea of nanotechnology was initiated in 1959 by the late Nobel Physicist Richard Feynman in his lecture titled "There's Plenty of Room at the Bottom," in which he envisioned the manufacturing of nanoscale machines (Patil Mallanagouda et al., 2008). Later, in 1974, the term "Nanotechnology" was globally introduced by Norio Taniguchi, leading to the establishment of institutions for the advancement of nanotechnology due to the increasing interest in this field. Over the next two to three decades, significant progress was observed in the field of nanotechnology, leading to diverse applications including the development of nanorobots, nano-pharmaceutical formulations, nanosized biomedical equipment, and other electronic devices (Kargozar Saeid et al., 2018). The convergence of pharmaceutical formulations and nanoscience in the 20th century has resulted in productive synergistic approaches for the development of various nanomolecular equipment and products (Hulla et al., 2015). Nanocarriers, with their diverse categories of material and structural components, have the potential to assimilate therapeutically active substances, leading to improved efficacy and systemic distribution profiles. These biologically enhanced parameters have positioned nanosized formulations as a novel delivery approach due to their advanced pharmacological effects and diagnostic characteristics (De Jong et al., 2008).

Research has shown that nanoparticles enhance drug delivery by directly adhering to inflamed sites through perforated vessels, thus exhibiting therapeutic effects. The micromolecular structure of nanoparticles has broadened their applications in the fields of oncology and cardiology (Haley Barbara et al., 2008). Consequently, nanotechnology has emerged as an excellent approach in medical sciences, contributing to advancements in diagnostic imaging techniques such as ultrasound, computed tomography (CT), and magnetic resonance imaging (MRI) (Rosen Joshua et al., 2011). Currently, nanomolecular systems are extensively investigated for imaging, modeling, and manipulating various substances, biomaterials, and other physically compatible substances, leading to advancements in nanoscience and technology. This historical perspective of nanotechnology represents the growing knowledge in various cellular processes, the development of biological agents, significant progress in biotechnology, and various nanoscale-oriented opportunities in the medical and paramedical fields (Caruthers Shelton et al., 2007).

2.2.1 SCOPE OF NANOTECHNOLOGY IN TREATING VIRAL INFECTIONS

The growing optimism and increased interest in nanoscience, combined with its collaboration with pharmaceuticals, have led to unprecedented and significant advancements in the field. Nanotechnology has been integrated into various areas such as biotechnology, biomedicine, and engineering to improve existing biological preparations and develop new products (Caruthers Shelton et al., 2007; Patil Mallanagouda et al., 2008). A wide variety of nanomedications have been formulated against diverse types of viral, bacterial, malignant, and inflammatory diseases (Chakravarty Malobika et al., 2021). Previous outbreaks of various viruses, such as Zika virus, Ebola virus, H1N1 (Hemagglutinin-1 neuraminidase-1) flu, chikungunya virus, and the recent novel coronavirus, have prompted continuous efforts to develop nanoformulations as novel delivery vehicles for effective antiviral agents.

Nanomedicines have garnered attention due to their significant surface area, penetrability, bioavailability, binding, and drug-carrying potential, among other factors (Yang Dongki, 2021). These biopharmaceutical factors make nanosized drug delivery systems compatible with various methods.

The larger surface area of drug particles in nanometers allows a larger number of drug molecules to be carried in the delivery system, leading to enhanced adsorption, improved binding, and increased drug-carrying capacity (Mukherjee Biswajit et al., 2014). Nanomedicines measuring less than the size of body cells can reach and act on inaccessible areas such as tumor cells, necrotic cells, and apoptotic cells due to their intense penetration capacity and efficacy. They can be used for the administration of proteins, genes, and other therapeutic agents. Various types of antiviral nanomedicines include lipid-polymer-based formulations, nanoemulsions, nano injectables, inorganic ion-based formulations, hybrid-based formulations, and nano vaccines, as well as newer methodologies such as nano traps, nanorobotics, and nanofibers (Singh et al., 2017).

Similarly, lipid-polymer-based nanomedicines are lipophilic polymers that are predominantly employed due to their reduced interactions with polypeptides, sustained release capability, long half-life, and limited biodegradability, making them superior delivery systems. Furthermore, multifaceted strategic approaches have been undertaken to produce nanostructured live, recombinant, and attenuated vaccines (Lembo David et al., 2018). These vaccines contain viral particles in live or killed states that are non-pathogenic, replicable, and non-toxic. Nanoscale vaccines provide prolonged bioavailability, long-term stability, and generate effective immune responses and prophylaxis against infections (Singh et al., 2017; Singh Kushagri et al., 2019). These advantageous attributes of nano vaccines aim to elicit a wide spectrum of antiviral activity against diseases and enable the development of a larger number of vectors against various forms of viral ailments (Yezdani Umama et al., 2018). Additionally, nanoemulsions are biphasic homogenized systems in which two immiscible liquid phases remain miscible with the help of suitable emulsifying compounds, with a particle size less than 200 nm. Nanoemulsions are preferred due to their uniformly distributed droplet size and the significant surface tension between the two phases, enabling more efficient drug delivery and use in novel delivery systems (Abolmaali Samira Sadat et al., 2011). They are preferred over other dosage forms due to their kinetic and thermodynamic stability, uniform particle size, and gravitational force, which provide stability and prevent emulsion instabilities such as creaming, phase inversion, and floccule formation (Franklyne Jonathan Sampath et al., 2021).

Consequently, nanotechnology is a revolutionary approach aimed at achieving multifunctional strategies to provide solutions to various health-related issues (Yezdani Umama et al., 2018). The emerging prominence of nanomedicines lies in their ability to provide a broad mode of action without toxicity and complexities in managing viral and other related manifestations. However, other areas of bioscience and technology continue to show interest in nanotechnology and research, exploring more viable, site-specific, and effective treatment methods in the interest of public health (Mukherjee Biswajit et al., 2014).

Based on previous *in vitro* or *ex vivo* cellular analytical investigations, it has been observed that viral infection-coordinated compounds have been identified in infected cells. Some viruses possess multiple enzymes of their own, which may have higher affinities for specific antimetabolites or inhibitors compared to normal cell enzymes. Furthermore, various antiviral drugs are chemosynthesized with specific and diverse pharmacological actions that directly exert proficient antiviral effects during different phases of the viral life cycle, including cell penetration, uncoating, reverse transcriptase, virus assembly or maturation, development, and release from the host cell (Pathak Chandramani et al., 2019).

A critical challenge encountered in acute illness is that symptoms often appear when viral proliferation and growth have reached their peak. To provide effective and meaningful treatment, antiviral agents are classified based on their mechanism of action. These agents need to be administered during the initial ingress of viral particles into the host or during the incubation period, or used as prophylaxis. Some of the accessible targets are illustrated in Figure 2.1. The drugs belonging to their respective categories, incorporated to form nanostructured antiviral formulations, are listed in Table 2.1 (de Souza et al., 2019).

2.3 EXAMPLES OF NANO-ANTIVIRAL AGENTS USED AGAINST EACH FAMILY OF VIRUS

Currently, numerous nano-based antiviral agents are being employed against various types of viral variants, as listed in Table 2.1. These nano-based antiviral drugs are incorporated into specific and suitable types of nano-formulations, taking into account drug compatibility, route of administration, physicochemical attributes, and more (Kerry Rout George et al., 2019). Similarly, the introduction of nanotechnology, along with the presence of nanocarriers in an absolute arrangement for drug delivery, has proven to be an effective therapeutic practice in treating and detecting

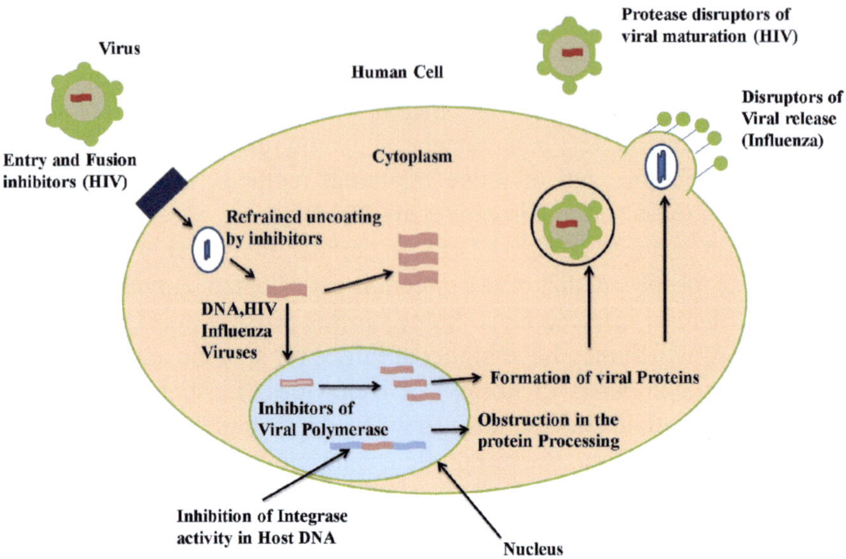

FIGURE 2.1 Different targets of antiviral agents at the different phases of the virus life cycle.

viral infections. Some widely used antiviral nano medications include indinavir nano liposome, acyclovir nano-recombinant molecule, among others (Bamrungsap Suwussa et al., 2012). Several scientists have investigated various nanocarriers such as nanoemulsions, polymeric nanoparticles, nanosuspensions, robust lipid-based nanoparticles, dendrimers, inorganic nanoparticles (such as zinc oxide, gold, and silver), liposomes, chitosan nanoparticles, niosomes, and many others. These drug-based formulations have exhibited activity against various families of viral diseases. However, some therapies have faced challenges due to peculiar or severe adverse drug reactions and the extended duration of drug therapy. Prolonged drug therapy can lead to the development of tolerance, drug resistance, or an increase in the drug toxicity profile (Szunerits Sabine et al., 2015). To maintain drug safety and efficacy parameters, it is crucial to utilize recently advanced and newly formulated nano medications containing aliphatic hydrocarbon chains, as well as organic or inorganic ion-based nanomedicines in the treatment of various types and families of viral illnesses. This ensures accurate, adequate, and targeted treatment, as illustrated in Figure 2.2 (Xu Zhi Ping et al., 2006).

TABLE 2.1 Classification of the Antiviral Therapeutic Agents Utilized as Nanomedicines

Category	Classes of Drugs	Nano- Antiviral Drugs and Their Formulations	Description
Non-retroviral agents	Anti-herpes simplex virus drugs	Acyclovir (ACV), Ganciclovir (GCV) Used as nanospheres and nanoemulsions	Used against herpes and chickenpox; Synthetic analogs of deoxyguanosine
	Anti-influenza virus drugs	Amantadine (AM), Oseltamivir (OTV); OTV-used as nano granules and drug-incorporated silver nanoparticles	Employed to treat German measles and influenza- A and B; OTV – analogs of sialic acid; AM – a tricyclic amine and adamantane derivative
	Anti-hepatitis virus drugs- HBV (Hepatitis B Virus)	Lamivudine (LAM), Tenofovir (TFV); TFV- used as drug-loaded nano spherical globules; LAM- as nanoparticles via IV route administration	LAM – a cytidine analog and RT (Reverse Transcriptase) inhibitor; TFV – prophylaxis against HIV (Human Immunodeficiency Virus) infection
	Anti-hepatitis virus drugs HCV (Hepatitis C Virus)	Interferon alpha (IFN- α), Ribavirin (RBV); RBV – used as biodegradable nano-lipopolymers	IFN α – immunostimulatory cytokine antiviral molecule; RBV – used to treat RSV (Respiratory syncytial virus) infection
	Inhibitor of the release of viral progeny	Oseltamivir (OTV), Zanamivir (ZMV); ZMV- used as nanomolecular inhalation aerosol	Blocks the action of the enzyme neuraminidase. Tend not to disperse and clump the viral particles
Antiretroviral agents	Nucleoside reverse transcriptase inhibitors (NRTIs)	Zidovudine (ZDV), Lamivudine (LAM), Tenofovir (TFV); ZDV- used as encapsulated nanostructured particles	Utilized to prevent and cure HIV-1 and HIV-2 contagions. ZDV and LAM – thymidine analogs
	Non-Nucleoside reverse transcriptase Inhibitors (NNRTIs)	Efavirenz (EFV), Delavirdine (DLV); DLV- is used as a methacrylate or cyanoacrylate nanoparticle; EFV- used as lipo polymer nanoparticles	Portrays the synergistic effect with NRTIs by increasing CD4 cell count and inhibiting the enzyme RT
	Protease inhibitors (PIs)	Saquinavir (SQN), Atazanavir (ATV), Nelfinavir (NFV), Ritonavir (RTV); SQV- used as a methacrylate or cyanoacrylate nanoparticle. RTV- used as polymeric solid nanoparticles. NFV- used as drug-loaded nanoparticles	Impedes the action of protease catalyst that prompts the cleavage of precursor proteins and restricts post-translational processing. Concurrently, used in the treatment of HIV and certain types of hepatic diseases

TABLE 2.1 *(Continued)*

Category	Classes of Drugs	Nano- Antiviral Drugs and Their Formulations	Description
	Fusion, entry, and integrase inhibitors	Enfuvirtide (ENF), Maraviroc (MCV), Raltegravir (RAL); ENF- used as lyophilized and PMA-coated nano entities. MCV- used as a sustained-release nano-injectable; RAL- used as a film-coated tablet and drug-loaded nanoparticles	ENF – obstruct the fusion of virus particle and the cell membrane; MCV – curbs the CCR5 receptor; RAL – hinders the action of integrase and prevents the integration of viral DNA in the host genome
	Multi-drug combinations	Efavirenz + Lopinavir + Ritonavir Zidovudine + Lamivudine + Efavirenz Atazanavir + Ritonavir + Tenofovir Lopinavir + Ritonavir + Tenofovir	Administered as first-line agents in the regimen of HIV infections, hepatitis- B&C and other retroviral diseases

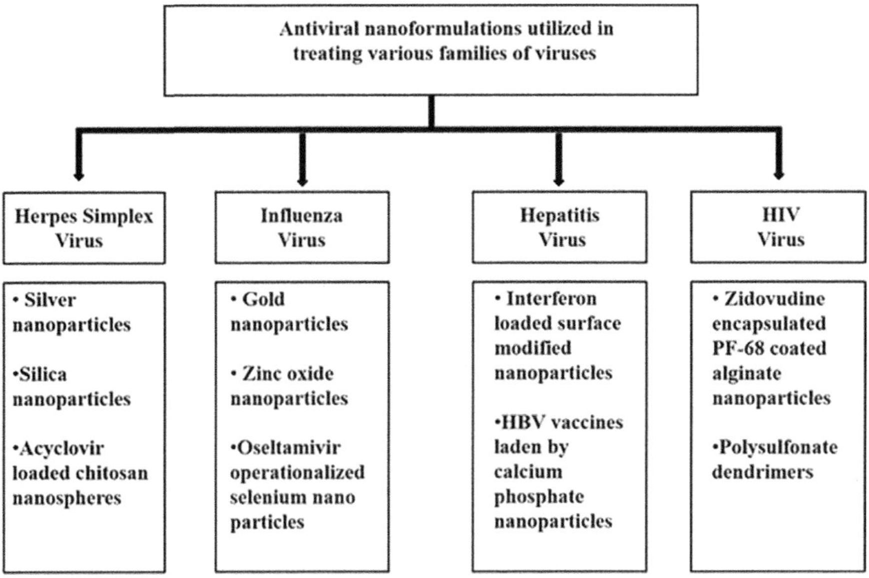

FIGURE 2.2 A flowchart depicting the certain nanoformulation being employed against different types of viruses.

2.3.1 HERPES SIMPLEX VIRUS (HSV)

HSV-1 and 2 are infectious agents that persist as harmful infirmities to human well-being. HSV belongs to the Herpesviridae family. HSV-1 and HSV-2 are widely examined human herpesviruses, where HSV-1 is generally associated with oral or facial disease and encephalitis, though HSV-2 is responsible for genital infection (Whitley Richard et al., 2001). Overall, more than 80% of people are tainted with HSV-1, and generally, 40% have repetitive infections (Fatahzadeh Mahnaz et al., 2007). HSV remains alive by embedding its DNA into the host's body so that, instead of producing cellular proteins, the cell systems produce infectious proteins and prompt its duplication. In the end, the host cell ruptures and delivers all the newly formed viral entities so that they become able to capture the other host cell and can spread further (An anatomical view of HSV is displayed below in Figure 2.3). To cure these life-threatening infections, various inorganic nanoparticles are introduced (Remeijer Lies et al., 2004).

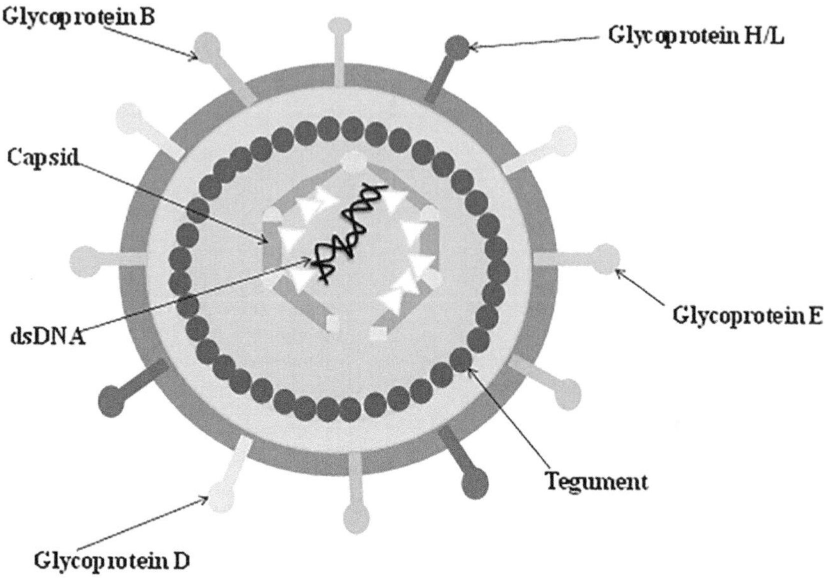

FIGURE 2.3 Herpes simplex virus (HSV).

2.3.1.1 SILVER NANOPARTICLES (AgNPs)

Silver nanoparticles (AgNPs) are widely employed due to their marked antiviral properties. Suriati et al. found that the most common method for the synthesis of silver NPs is a compound reduction by various organic and inorganic reducing agents (Burduşel Alexandra-Cristina et al., 2018). Different reducing agents such as sodium citrate, ascorbate, sodium borohydride ($NaBH_4$), natural hydrogen, polyol measure, Tollen's reagent-dimethylformamide (DMF), and poly (ethylene glycol)-block copolymers are used for the reduction of silver particles (Ag^+) in aqueous or non-aqueous solutions. Researchers observed that by using the bubbling method at various citrate concentrations, AgNPs with a plasmon peak absorbance at 420 nm were produced. By increasing the overall concentration of sodium citrate to silver cation [citrate]/[Ag^+] from 1–10 times, the time for the formation of AgNP was reduced from 40–20 min, respectively, indicating that under equimolar conditions, a portion of the Ag_+ was not reduced (Akbarzadeh Abolfazl et al., 2018).

Hostility in human microbes is a major obstacle in fields like pharmaceuticals and biomedicine. Because of this reason, silver nanoparticles are employed due to their small and uniform particle size (10–9), facilitating their rapid entry into the systemic circulation, and enhancing penetrability into cells for targeted therapeutic effects against diseases. The biocidal activity of AgNPs depends on various morphological and physicochemical attributes (e.g., size, shape, and surface) that contribute to their antiviral properties. Wounds treated with silver nanoparticles display better healing and scarless recovery. Silver nanoparticles inhibit HSV infections by blocking the penetration of the infectious viral agent into cells, thus preventing attachment and inhibiting the virus life cycle (Wei Liuya et al., 2015).

Similarly, the sexually transmitted HSV-2 facilitates the spread of HIV. Presently available antiviral drugs have limitations. The use of silver nanoparticles is gaining attention due to their antiviral and other anti-pathogenic properties. An investigation elucidated the mechanism of action of silver nanoparticles and their inhibitory effects on HSV-2 (Orłowski Piotr et al., 2014). The cytotoxicity of Vero cells induced by various AgNP concentrations was examined using the methyl thiazolyl tetrazolium (MTT) assay. The blocking effect of AgNPs on HSV-2 was also evaluated by performing the plaque assay. The toxicity level was extremely low, reported at 100 μg/ml of AgNPs. The combination of AgNP suspension and HSV-2 before infecting cells significantly inhibited the formation of viral particles. Additionally, AgNPs downregulate the replication of HSV-2 for 24 hours before staining cells with HSV-2. Thus, a 100 μg/mL concentration of AgNPs could prevent the growth and duplication of HSV-2. AgNPs at nontoxic levels were capable of inhibiting HSV-2 spread and growth when administered before viral infection or shortly after the initial exposure to the virus. This analysis explains that the action of AgNPs occurs during the early stages of viral replication (Hu et al., 2014).

2.3.1.2 SILICA NANOPARTICLES USED IN TREATING HERPES VIRUS

Silica nanoparticles have shown promising significance due to their adsorptive capacity, particle size, catalytic functions, dispersive profile, and drug delivery. They have emerged as an efficient nano drug delivery system for various pharmacological agents in the treatment of viral and bacterial ailments. To overcome the unsatisfactory pharmacokinetic characteristics of some antiviral drugs, hollow or mesoporous silica nanoparticles have played a critical role in the treatment of HSV. Various *in vitro* chemosynthetic methods have been reported for the fabrication of silica nanoparticles, such as the modified Stober method, self-assembly, hard and soft templating, and certain aerogel strategies (Mihalcik David et al., 2009).

It is also essential to consider all the necessary attributes of the nanoparticles, such as pore size, area-to-volume ratio, and uniformity of size before the manufacturing process (Fowler et al., 2001). Additionally, the antiviral effect is observed by preventing the entry of viral entities into host cells or by assisting in the detachment of HSV particles from cells during attempted entry. By obstructing the entry of viral particles into host cells, silica nanoparticles can be employed as potent anti-HSV agents for the treatment of the disease. Morphological characteristics and other related attributes of the silica nanoparticles are analyzed by TEM (Transmission Electron Microscopy), X-ray photoelectron spectroscopy, and NMR (Nuclear Magnetic Resonance) techniques. UV Spectrophotometry is also performed at specific wavelengths, and the transmittance is obtained for the qualitative analysis of the gold nanoparticles. All the results obtained satisfy the stability and all restorative and diagnostic parameters of the silica nanoparticles, making them suitable for administration in the treatment of HSV (Lee Edward et al., 2016).

2.3.1.3 ACYCLOVIR-LOADED CHITOSAN NANOSPHERES

Acyclovir alone has limited efficacy as an anti-herpes agent for systemic or topical treatment. Therefore, drug-loaded chitosan nanospheres are prepared to provide efficient topical treatment of HSV infection, as they exhibit highly improved penetration ability, bioavailability, thermodynamic stability, and prolonged contact time of the drug with the body. They are used against both symptomatic and asymptomatic viral infections. The fabrication of chitosan acyclovir-loaded nanospheres followed the nano-emulsion template-based methodology (Prabhu Priyanka et al., 2012).

Manuela Donalisio et al. have explored that the formation of a nano-emulsion is initiated as a template to advance and modify the complete nano-drug delivery system. First, the formation of the template involves the production of a w/o type of emulsion, which is sonicated to uniformly reduce the particle size at the nanomolecular level. Sonication occurs at a specific frequency of 20 MHz. The two immiscible phases are prepared with suitable formulating agents, with the dispersed phase consisting of mineral oil and dodecanol and the dispersing medium containing chitosan acetic acid at a specific concentration (Cavalli Roberta et al., 2014). Furthermore, suitable emulsifying agents or wetting agents are incorporated into the formed solution, followed by the addition of approved excipients that impart stability and long shelf characteristics to the formed nanoemulsion. These two immiscible two-phase systems undergo gradual trituration to form a single biphasic system. This nanoemulsion is then allowed to flow from a syringe through a rotatory roller pump into the sodium citrate solution of the desired molarity. The nanospheres undergo filtration and extraction and then undergo drug (acyclovir) loading procedures. Finally, through various chemical and formulation processes, the acyclovir-loaded chitosan nanospheres are partially obtained in a dried powdered form, ensuring uniform characteristics. The formed nano-based solution is freeze-dried for a specific period, and the chitosan nanospheres with loaded drug are collected in the dried powdered form (Donalisio Manuela et al., 2018).

Lastly, the fabricated nanospheres undergo preliminary screening procedures and various morphological, stability, drug release, qualitative, and quantitative analytical characterization processes. They undergo photon spectroscopy, TEM, HPLC (High-performance Liquid Chromatography) analysis, DLS (Dynamic Light Scattering), and other mandatory *in vitro* drug release, bioassays, and kinetic stability investigations to meet essential standard values. This process allows them to be used in the antiviral regimen against HSV (Cavalli Roberta et al., 2014; Donalisio Manuela et al., 2018). These highly drug-loaded chitosan nanospheres are prepared with improved biocompatibility, polydispersity profiles, particle size, therapeutic activity, dermatological penetrability, cell permeation capacity, and absorptivity index. These biological and physicochemical attributes provide a more effective antiviral effect. Many non-clinical and *in vitro* scientific explorations have illustrated that the incorporation of chitosan, a biodegradable biomaterial, results in high drug loading capacity, reduced toxicity, increased healing tendency, and enhanced permeation, making it highly stable and suitable for dermatological or topical administration. Therefore, it has been reported in numerous *ex vivo*, scientific, and experimental illustrations that these acyclovir-loaded chitosan nanospheres demonstrate potent effectiveness through the topical route of administration against HSV-1 and HSV-2. Hence, these acyclovir-loaded nanospheres have shown improved and marked therapeutic potential for an effective regimen for the prevailing malady (Anton Nicolas et al., 2008; Ferrari Franca et al., 2012).

2.3.2 INFLUENZA VIRUS

Aquatic animals, birds, humans, and pigs serve as the sources of the influenza virus, which has two variants: Influenza A and B. The structure of the Influenza virus is depicted in Figure 2.4 and is classified as a member of the Orthomyxoviridae family. Influenza A has been reported to be more harmful and contagious compared to influenza B and is often recognized as a common cold virus (Ison Michael, 2011). It primarily infects and spreads through the pulmonary tract, nasal cavity, gullet, and lungs. The flu typically manifests with symptoms such as runny noses, chills, and fever. The virus proceeds through the trachea (throat), irritating the ciliated epithelium layer, and subsequently binds to the squamous epithelial lining with the aid of specific molecules (Watanabe Tokiko et al., 2015). This leads to the invasion of viral entities into the host's cells, where they utilize the host's protein factories to release viral-responsive proteins into the body. Consequently, newly formed viral particles are released into the host's body system, allowing the entry of viral molecules into adjacent cells (Englund Janet, 2002).

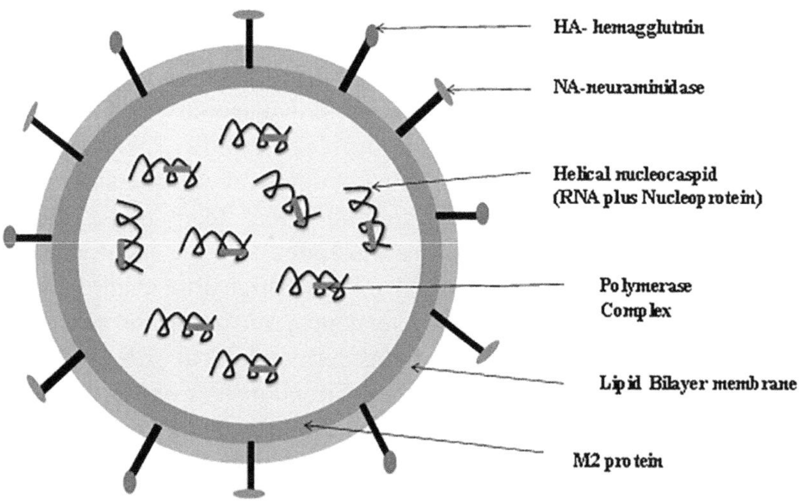

FIGURE 2.4 Influenza virus (Common flu/influenza virus).

2.3.2.1 GOLD NANOPARTICLES (AUNPS)

As stated earlier, influenza is a contagious virus known to cause acute to chronic pulmonary flu infections, which can be fatal in severe cases. To counter this, certain drugs are available for treatment, but their usage is limited due to the increasing hostility and toxic effects associated with these drugs. In the search for a viable and effective treatment, gold nanoparticles were synthesized, garnering substantial attention due to their remarkable characteristics (Sardar Rajesh et al., 2009). Gold nanoparticles are considered for use because they demonstrate enhanced inhibitory activity against the influenza virus and have been reported to reduce the rate of viral multiplication to some extent. Inferences drawn from the scientific literature have justified the diverse applications of gold nanoparticles in fields such as enzyme electrodes, fuel cells, supercapacitors, and Novel Drug Delivery Systems (NDDS) (Ghosh Partha et al., 2008).

2.3.2.1.1 Production and action of gold nanoparticles (AuNPs)

Various methodologies are employed for the synthesis of AuNPs, as indicated in the literature. These methodologies include the use of oligonucleotides in conjunction with AuNPs salt, the aging method, the dealloying of inert metals in a corrosion-promoting environment, and the formation of GNPs through the intervention of specific reducing agents, precursors, and surface-active agents (Brust et al., 1995). Additionally, a variant of gold nanoparticles, known as foraminous or Porous Gold Loaded Nanoparticles (PoAuNPs/PoGNPs), is manufactured using different strategies such as emulsion devoid of a wetting agent, citrated AuNPs, and Tween-capped AuNPs (Nyce Gregory et al., 2007).

Qingfeng Zhang et al. have established that noble gold nanoparticles were synthesized using the conventional seed-mediated process, which involves the use of specific chemical agents such as a precursor, reducing agent, and a surfactant, along with other necessary laboratory equipment and apparatus (Jenkins Julie et al., 2017). Chloroauric acid ($HAuC_{14}$) is utilized as the precursor, while $NaBH_4$ or hydroquinone serves as the reducing agent. The surfactant used is cetyltrimethylammonium chloride (CTAC), or alternatively, a surfactant such as polyvinylpyrrolidone (PVP) may be employed. The generation of the AuNPs takes place in an aqueous medium at the normal laboratory temperature (Zhang Qingfeng et al., 2014).

$HAuCl_4$ is reduced with $NaBH_4$, leading to the formation of colloidal gold seeds. These prepared gold seeds in diluted form are then introduced into a growth medium suitable for the development of AuNPs. This medium comprises chloroauric acid, CTAC, and L-vitamin C, which are responsible for the efficient growth and maturation of the gold nanoparticles. Subsequently, the solution is gently mixed with the incorporation of Au seeds and left undisturbed for a period of 4–6 hours (Sau Tapan et al., 2004). The solution is then centrifuged, causing all the formed nanoparticles to collect on the surface of the supernatant liquid. The obtained Au nanoparticles have exhibited high porosity with improved physicochemical characteristics, such as an enhanced rate of absorption, increased viability, and improved bioavailability (Huang Youju et al., 2013). These AuNPs have also demonstrated an extensive spectrum of activity. This method is commonly employed because it is cost-effective, simple, and less time-consuming (Hakimian Fatemeh et al., 2019).

Furthermore, according to Fatemeh Hakman and Hedayatollah Ghourchian, scientific literature sources suggest that to enhance the functionality and efficacy of these active gold nanoparticles, oligonucleotides (small DNA or RNA molecules with 8–10 nucleotides) play a significant role in the process and are employed in various applications (Hakimian Fatemeh et al., 2019; Huang Youju et al., 2013). Oligonucleotides are coupled with the pre-fabricated AuNPs at susceptible and suitable sites on the nanoparticles. The conjugation of oligonucleotides at the 5' or 3' end occurs using a chemical thiol linker, providing robust proximity to the AuNPs. This entire procedure is followed by the process of salt aging to increase the binding tendency on the surface of GNPs (Qu Xiangmeng et al., 2017). Subsequently, Tween AuNPs are prepared by adding a specific amount of Tween-20 to the previously formed AuNPs, followed by a brief period of swirling for approximately 1–2 minutes. Consequently, Tween AuNPs are successfully synthesized and collected (Zhao Yuyun et al., 2010). The optical absorption was determined using a UV spectrophotometer at specific wavelengths, and the transmittance was obtained for the qualitative analysis of the gold nanoparticles. Scanning Electron Microscopy (SEM) and TEM were performed to determine the morphological characteristics, uniformity in particle size, dispersity, and distribution of particles of narrow size. These investigations hold the potential to be utilized as actuators, catalysts, and efficient restorative agents (Kim Jinyoung et al., 2020).

2.3.2.1.2 Mechanism of action

Fatemeh Hakman and Hedayatollah Ghourchian discovered that gold nanoparticles displayed promising pharmacological activity in combating the zoonotic influenza virus. GNPs linked with thiol-oligonucleotide expressed intense inhibitory action against the disulfide bonds present in the viral molecules. The administration of AuNPs was reported to cleave the disulfide bonds, resulting in the malfunction and distortion of the viral particle. This interaction between gold nanoparticles and the disulfide moiety expedited the restricted activity of the influenza particles, preventing the production of new viral offspring (Kim Jinyoung et al., 2020). Additionally, Jinyoung Kim et al. found that these particles also exhibited inhibitory activity by binding to the RNA of the virus. AuNPs attached to the viral molecule's membrane hindered the unfolding of the viral RNA into the host body cells, inhibiting its replication and obstructing the production of new viral RNA responsible for the infection's spread within the body. This action limited the viral genetic material's quantity in the host cells and blocked the invasion of viral entities into the host body cells (Floyd Daniel et al., 2008; Gubareva Larisa, 2004).

2.3.2.2 ZINC OXIDE NANOPARTICLES (ZNO NPS)

Zinc oxides possess mild to moderate reactive characteristics, but when converted into nanosized particles, they exhibit inertness, easy introduction into the body, and beneficial therapeutic properties. The divalent property and nanostructure of the Zn ion provide high catalytic properties, increased absorption across the biological membrane, and easy transport across cellular junctions, enabling significant pharmacological action (Bedi et al., 2015). Currently, there are mainly two or three approved anti-influenza drugs available to treat the influenza infection, namely amantadine and rimantadine, which act by obstructing the release of the viral nucleic acid into the host's body and prevent the assembly of viral entities. Over time, these drugs have shown side effects such as drug resistance and some observed toxic effects. Hence, to provide a substantial and relevant treatment for this flu virus, ZnO-NPs have demonstrated significant therapeutic effects, including reduced resistance, a less toxic profile, decreased cytotoxic characteristics, and fewer adverse drug reactions (Chen Lu et al., 2020).

Hadi Ghaffari et al. explored that powdered zinc nanoparticles were directly obtained in a pre-manufactured form and incorporated into modified eagle's media to form a uniform biphasic suspension. The suspension was subjected to sonication with a frequency of more than 20 KHz in an automated ultrasonic probe or sonicator to avoid clumping and the accumulation of particles. Subsequently, PEG 6000 (Polyethylene glycol 6000) was used to coat a uniform layer on ZnO-NPs, providing improved efficacy, safety, and reduced toxic effects. The PEGylated zinc oxide nanoparticles were prepared for use and further subjected to qualitative, morphological, and quantitative analysis. These PEGylated ZnO-NPs were then analyzed using plasma spectrometry, gravimetric procedures, TEM, X-ray diffraction tests, and so forth, to determine qualitative and morphological parameters, making them suitable for administration in infected individuals (Ghaffari Hadi et al., 2019; Tavakoli Ahmad et al., 2018).

Through various scientific reports and literary analysis, it has been observed that ZnO-NPs and PEGylated ZnO-NPs are employed at concentrations that are the highest but less than the toxic dose. These ZnO-NPs have shown marked inhibitory effects against the growth and replication of influenza strains. Additionally, these Zn_{2+} ions are released in the body upon the administration of ZnO-NPs, leading to the formation of peroxide radicals, reactive oxygen species (ROS), and inflammatory mediators that degrade fats, proteins, and other cellular contents. Furthermore, they have induced programmed cellular death and the uncontrolled growth of cells, which may increase cytotoxicity (Siddiqi et al., 2018). This is why PEGylated ZnO-NPs are prominently employed, as the presence of the layer of PEG on the nanoparticles prevents the release of free Zn^{+2} ions in the body, thereby avoiding any toxic and unwanted adverse effects. Many *in vitro* studies have claimed that PEGylated ZnO-NPs have shown potent antiviral effects by restraining the growth and assembly of viral entities and inhibiting the exposure of viral molecules to host body cells, preventing the subsequent spread of the flu in the body. Thus, it can be concluded that PEGylated ZnO-NPs possess more potent, enhanced, and effective anti-influenza activity, with very few adverse reactions occurring only after the ingress of viral particles into the body, and have clearly demonstrated inhibitory action against all variants of the influenza virus (Shen Tammy et al., 2015; Soenen Stefaan et al., 2014).

2.3.2.3 OSELTAMIVIR OPERATIONALIZED SELENIUM NANOPARTICLES (SE@OTV NPS)

With the emergence of nanomedicines, the idea of using nanoparticles as therapeutic targets against viral infections has increased manifold. Nanoparticles in the field of nanotechnology have proven to be excellent treatments against various families of viruses. Selenium nanoparticles (SeNPs), due to their lower toxicity, have drawn great interest as significant antiviral, anticancer, and anti-inflammatory agents. SeNPs range in size from 40–100 nm (Nguyen Jack et al., 2012). Yinghua Li et al., 2017, explored in their study that SeNPs were yielded by the following method: the stock solution of Na_2SeO_3 (0.1M) was added gradually to 2 ml of ascorbic acid stock solution. At that instant, a specific amount of OTV was added to the SeNP preparation. An excess of OTV, nutrients, and Na_2SeO_3 was eliminated by dialysis overnight. Se@OTV was sonicated and then filtered through 0.2 μm pores (Li Yinghua et al., 2017). The convergence of SeNPs and OTV was estimated by rationally coupled plasma nuclear outflow spectroscopy. The SeNPs were subjected to various parameters such as TEM, X-ray diffraction, UV optical absorption, calorimeter, and so forth, for identification, characterization, and to obtain the stability profile. These Se@OTV particles were further subjected to energy-dispersive X-ray spectroscopy to determine the uniform metallic elemental organization (Liu Wen et al., 2012).

2.3.2.3.1 Mechanism of action

SeNPs have gained wide attention due to their significant and intricate antiviral potential against the flu virus. They act in the body with the incorporation of OTV, making them less toxic and down-regulating the drug resistance profile. Se@OTV NPs act by restraining the interactivity of influenza viral entities inside the host body, leading to the attenuation of the catalytic action of the H1N1 (hemagglutinin-1 neuraminidase-1) enzyme (Li Yinghua et al., 2017). This results in the shrinkage of the cytoplasm and disruption of cell-to-cell contact in the body. The suppression of the H1N1 enzyme blocks DNA strand segregation, growth, and multiplication, preventing the further spread and duplication of viral molecules in the host cells. Studies have also revealed that Se@

OTV NPs substantially inhibit the generation of some free radicals and ROS, preventing cells from undergoing oxidative stress (Li Yinghua et al., 2017). Additionally, these OTV-functionalized SeNPs have shown a protective action toward pulmonary tissues by inhibiting various molecular and signaling pathways such as Mitogen-Activated Protein Kinase (MAPK) and the proteolytic catalyst caspase-3, thereby reducing the occurrence of apoptosis in host cells and tissues. Therefore, the mode of action of Se@OTV NPs, observed through various pharmacological mechanisms, makes these nanoparticles a promising, potent, and efficacious antiviral agent to treat numerous known strains of H1N1 influenza flu (Li Yinghua et al., 2019).

2.3.3 HEPATITIS VIRUS

Hepatitis viruses are infectious agents that primarily infect the liver, leading to hepatocellular damage and inflammation. These viruses belong to the Hepadnaviridae family. A total of five variants of hepatitis viruses have been discovered, including HBV (Hepatitis B virus), HCV (Hepatitis C virus), HDV, and HEV. Among them, clinical findings have revealed that HBV and HCV are the most common infectious variants, while the remaining three are less frequently encountered (Dehesa-Violante Margarita et al., 2007). Hepatitis B is a severe viral disease that directly targets the liver, causing inflammation and hepatocellular degradation, and may progress to hepatic carcinoma. HBV is a microscopic, enveloped, and the smallest prototype member of the family, completely dependent on the host's liver cells. HBV comprises double-stranded DNA as the genetic material, as shown in Figure 2.5. It is highly communicable and is usually spread through used syringes and needles, infected blood transfusions, sexual contact, from mother to fetus, and through other means of direct contact (Tiollais Pierre et al., 1985). Similarly, HCV is a chronic, blood-borne, and excruciating manifestation, considered the leading cause of liver cancer. It often leads to cirrhosis and, in extreme cases, may cause liver failure (Purcell Robert, 1997). In 2016, WHO statistics revealed that approximately 399,000 people died due to this deadly illness (WHO, 2018). It is a single-stranded RNA (ss-RNA) virus belonging to the Flaviviridae family. HCV spreads similarly to HBV but causes more severe harm, sometimes leading to death.

Currently, there is no explicit and effective treatment available to cure the ailment, prompting continuous clinical studies and investigations to find a pertinent and efficacious regimen against the disease (Op De Beeck Anne et al., 2003).

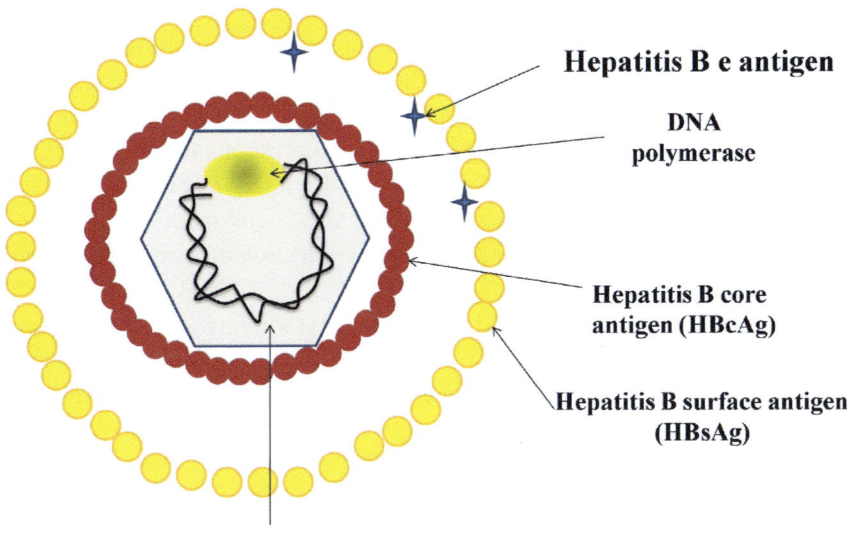

FIGURE 2.5 Structure of hepatitis virus.

2.3.3.1 INTERFERON-LOADED SURFACE-MODIFIED NANOPARTICLES

Interferons are primarily produced in the body and provide protection against viral attacks and malignant cells. The term "interferon" denotes its function in interfering with the growth of carcinogenic cells and the multiplication of viral entities. It also contributes to the prevalence of various hazardous viral illnesses and malignancies in different organs of the gastrointestinal tract (Yang Yuan et al., 2011).

Formulating interferon-loaded surface-modified active nanoparticles significantly enhances the diagnostic process, enabling effective and site-targeted therapeutic action against the HBV. These nanoparticles are developed following the fabrication and manufacturing procedures since interferon- α (IFNα) is the first approved antiviral agent for treating moderate to severe hepatitis B. The process for creating positively charged surface-adsorbed IFNα-loaded nanoparticles is described below (Yang Yuan et al., 2011).

Namita Giri et al. have explored the methodology for producing surface-adsorbed IFNα-loaded nanoparticles, which involves using suitable chemicals and denaturants. Initially, Poly-D, L-lactic-co-glycolic acid (PLGA), octyl glucoside, polyvinyl alcohol (PVA), cetyl trimethyl ammonium bromide (CTAB), IFNα samples, and polypeptide estimating chemicals were collected. The solvent evaporation double emulsification method was employed for forming PLGA nanoparticles (Sanchez Alejandro et al., 2003). These particles were then solubilized in an organic solvent of appropriate solubility and polarity. The organic phase was subjected to sonication with the IFN and sugar solution of specific concentration and molarity, resulting in a biphasic emulsion. This emulsion was mixed well in a solution of PVA and CTAB. Nanoparticles were obtained in pellet form after mechanical stirring and the evaporation of the remaining solvent for four hours. Subsequently, the pellets of nanoparticles were extracted in lyophilized form after multiple washings and dispersion in water (Cun Dongmei et al., 2010; Sanchez Alejandro et al., 2003).

Secondly, Hepatitis B surface antigens (HBsAg) were obtained by depleting most lipids with the help of non-ionic denaturing detergent (octyl glucoside) at neutral pH, followed by high-speed centrifugation with cesium chloride. The positively charged PLGA interferon-loaded nanoparticles were then matured in an incubator in a saline phosphate buffer system. These nanoparticles were subsequently centrifuged, and the collected HBsAg was matured at 25°C, followed by incubation at 4°C for 24 hours (Gavilanes Francisco et al., 1990; Giri Namita et al., 2011). The pellet-form sample was then redispersed in phosphate buffer and lyophilized as described above. Characterization procedures such as biodistribution studies and fluorescence analysis were performed for stability evaluation, including the calculation of zeta potential, light diffraction, particle size, and dispersibility index. Additionally, scanning electron microscopy was conducted to evaluate external surface morphological characteristics (Giri Namita et al., 2011).

These interferon-loaded surface-modified PLGA-coated nanoparticles were primarily developed due to their uniform nanosize and high dispersion profile, facilitating intravenous administration. This targeted administration towards the liver enables the nanoparticles to approach the Kupffer cells and hepatocytes affected by chronic HBV manifestation. They exhibit a profound antiviral effect by inhibiting the conversion of host DNA into viral RNA and proteins, or by reducing the rate of new viral progeny generation. Furthermore, reticuloendothelial cells phagocytose the nanoparticles to inhibit the spread of hepatic viral infection (Cun Dongmei et al., 2010). Consequently, a gradual decline in the viral load was observed, accompanied by the generation of an immune response due to the influence of IFNα, which protects healthy hepatocytes from viral infection and promotes the body's recovery through compensatory molecular and pharmacological mechanisms. In conclusion, numerous clinical or preclinical trials have shown that PLGA-coated cationic IFNα-loaded nanoparticles hold significant potential for liver-specific drug delivery, significantly enhancing the therapeutic index while reducing prominent contraindications and adverse drug reactions (Cun Dongmei et al., 2010; Gavilanes Francisco et al., 1990; Giri Namita et al., 2011).

2.3.3.2 HEPATITIS B VIRUS (HBV) VACCINE LADEN BY CALCIUM PHOSPHATE NANOPARTICLES

Several approved drugs are available for preventing HBV, with some being utilized for treatment and prophylaxis. However, these anti-HBV drugs reportedly have a short biological half-life, low bioavailability, and a narrow therapeutic window (Marohn Mark et al., 2013). This limitation has led to the development of genetically modified nano-dimensional immunizing agents. Immunizing formulations consist of live or killed ineffective viral entities genetically modified for use against hepatic viral infections. The vaccination approach used in generating these vaccines accelerates their action capacity due to the induction of virus-oriented immunogenic responses (Schlickewei Carsten et al., 2019). However, immunized vaccines are prone to catalytic degradation and lack the capacity to withstand the body's metabolic processes. To address this, the need for a stable and inert vehicle arises. Calcium phosphate nanoparticles have shown promising attributes for functioning as a vehicle, providing improved biocompatibility, uniform particle size, resistance to catalytic degradation, efficient loading tendency, and strong binding ability with various biomolecules, among other advantages. HBV vaccines loaded on calcium phosphate nanoparticles have been widely manufactured and utilized to effectively combat contagion (Damm Dominik et al., 2019; Lee Min Sang et al., 2014; Temchura Vladimir et al., 2014).

Kozlova et al. and Rojas-Sanchez et al. found that calcium phosphate nanoparticles were synthesized at room temperature by releasing a calcium lactate solution under pressure into highly pure water, allowing thorough mixing for the required duration (Park In et al., 2009). Subsequently, calcium monophosphate (CaP) was added to the stirred solution, and dispersion was formed by continuous mixing at laboratory temperature conditions for an extended period. Ultrasonication with appropriate chemical agents was used to obtain the prepared calcium phosphate particles (Cui Yan et al., 2011). These calcium phosphate nanoparticles were made functional for use through covalent bonding between silica and calcium particles, a process known as salinization. This process involves providing a uniform coating of alkoxy silane or silica to carry the active ingredient, facilitated by different suitable linker molecules (Kozlova Diana et al., 2012). The bond sharing between silica and calcium provides sufficient stability for use as a vehicle for the nanosized formulation. Salinization enables the loading of pharmacologically active ingredients, such as immunizing agents, nucleic acids, active antigens, and so forth, between the silica coating and the calcium phosphate core. Hepatitis B surface antigens are loaded into the nanoparticles following standard fabrication and loading protocols (Kozlova Diana et al., 2012). After loading the antibodies, the particles are collected in their purest form through filtration, introduced into the designated sections, and finally obtained at the outlets. All these processes were conducted under clean and sterile conditions to avoid any contamination and ensure the preparation's efficiency for consumption. Various morphological, qualitative, and biopharmaceutical procedures, such as spectroscopy, DLS, zeta potential, fluorescence imaging, and so forth, were performed to determine and characterize the formed nanoparticles (Kozlova Diana et al., 2012; Wu Jun et al., 2010).

Encapsulation through salinization makes the nanoparticles resistant to enzymatic degradation and other biological fluids that tend to metabolize the active form, leading to an increased duration of action, biocompatibility, and systemic availability. The administration of hepatitis B surface antigens loaded in calcium phosphate nanoparticles takes place via the intramuscular route (Kozlova Diana et al., 2012). Within 24–48 hours of administering the vaccine, the immunogenic response begins to develop against the HBV virus molecules, activating the antigen-presenting cells

(APCs) of the host body. *Ex vivo* investigations have shown an increase in the expression of fibroblasts, CD80, CD86, B-cells, and T-cells, contributing to the development of the antigen-specific immune response. Subsequently, in the IgG-mediated immune response, B-cells and T-cells contribute to the acquired immune response against the antigen, gradually depleting the viral count and ultimately inhibiting the formation of viral responsive DNA strands in the host body (Knuschke Torben et al., 2013). This phenomenon operates in an extremely sustained manner, depending on the responsiveness of the immunizing nano-entities to the HBV viral molecules in the host body, owing to the prophylactic use of this vaccine. In conclusion, the DNA vaccine fabricated on salinized calcium phosphate nanoparticles has yielded confirmed results, inducing a robust acquired immune response for use with numerous beneficial effects against this hazardous viral disease (Heidegger Simon et al., 2016).

2.3.4 HUMAN IMMUNODEFICIENCY VIRUS (HIV)

Human immunodeficiency virus (HIV) belongs to the family Retroviridae. Failure in detecting and diagnosing HIV in its early stages leads to the chronic autoimmune manifestation known as AIDS (acquired immunodeficiency syndrome), which occurs due to the delayed stage of HIV infection. HIV is a highly infectious agent that can transmit through unprotected sexual contact, infected blood transfusions, and transmission of vaginal fluids from mother to baby (Klimas Nancy et al., 2008). The condition gradually worsens over time, leading to an immune response against the body's own cells, which are responsible for protecting against infection and make the host body highly sensitive to the invasion of other infectious agents. HIV is also known to deplete the count of specific types of blood cells, namely CD^{4+} cells, which play a protective role against infection-causing molecules.

The viral entity is surrounded by a fatty acid covering, within which trimeric structured transmembrane glycoproteins are embedded. Among these proteins are gp 41, to which gp 120 glycoproteins are affixed. HIV possesses a positively sensed diploid viral RNA genome, encoded in the form of two copies of 10 Kb, situated in the core of the viral body (Fanales-Belasio Emanuele et al., 2010).

These two glycoproteins (gp 41 and gp 120) primarily facilitate the attachment of the viral body to the host cell, enabling the easy transfer of the RNA genome into the host machinery, as illustrated in Figure 2.6. This process further leads to the formation of copies of the viral DNA in the host, allowing for replication, growth, and spread within the body. Additionally, three enzymes exist within the virus, namely integrase, protease, and RT, which play significant biological functions in its lifecycle, aiding in growth, multiplication, and development.

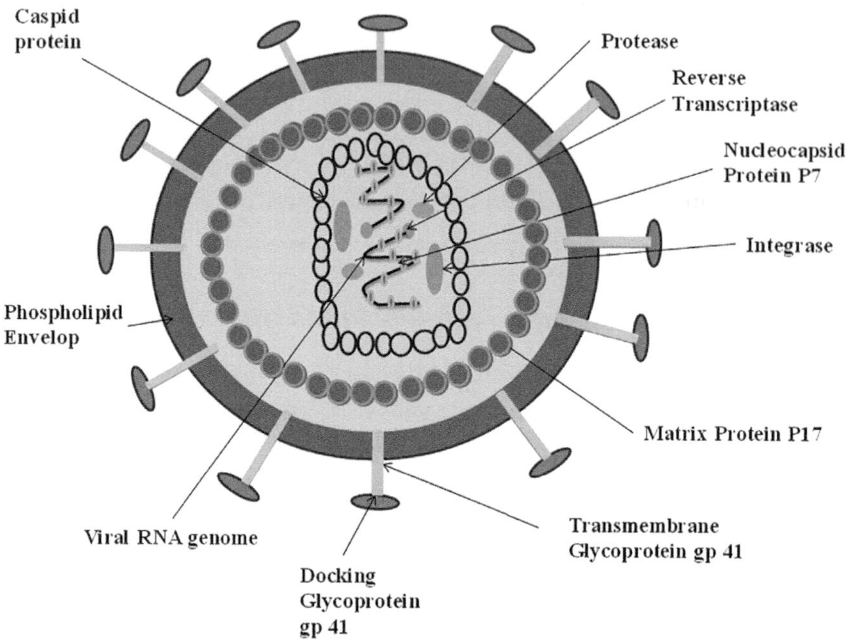

FIGURE 2.6 Human immunodeficiency virus (HIV) (Causative agent of acquired immunodeficiency syndrome (AIDS)).

Due to this specific mechanism of action and replication within the host, this variant of the virus is classified as a retrovirus (Briz Verónica et al., 2006). Retroviruses are characterized by possessing RNA (ribonucleic acid) as their primary genetic material and by their ability to transcribe RNA into viral DNA after invading the host cell, enabling the further spread of infection within the host body. This characteristic is the main reason why no specifically targeted cure is currently available to inhibit the spread of the advancing infection in the body (King Steven, 1994).

In an effort to expedite treatment, nanosized antiretroviral formulations are currently under development to treat the illness to a certain extent.

These formulations aim to decrease the viral load and obstruct the catalytic activity of the enzymes present in the viral molecules (Fanales-Belasio Emanuele et al., 2010).

2.3.4.1 ZIDOVUDINE ENCAPSULATED PF-68 COATED ALGINATE NANOPARTICLES

Antiretroviral therapy continually encounters pharmacokinetic and pharmacodynamic challenges, including reduced systemic availability, drug resistance, high first-pass metabolism, and drug-induced toxic adverse reactions. These drugs must be manufactured in line with specific suitability and targeted pharmaceutical approaches to ensure their safe and effective administration in the form of novel dosage forms, thus utilizing them as a new drug delivery system (George Meera et al., 2006). To overcome these challenges, encapsulated anti-retroviral drug-loaded nanoparticles are synthesized, possessing improved and necessary biopharmaceutical and pharmacokinetic characteristics that enable them to withstand the various challenges associated with the utilization of available anti-HIV agents. These encapsulated nanoparticles have achieved significant therapeutic success due to their efficient stability and biocompatibility, making them extensively employed in HIV therapy (Ruckmani Kandasamy et al., 2010).

Joshy et al. explained that the first step involved the preparation of glutamic acid-alginate conjugates (GAAD) through amidation and the combination of several required chemical compounds in an aqueous solution with a pH ranging from acidic to nearly neutral (Prokop Ales et al., 2008). Precipitates were formed upon complexation of the chemical compounds in the solution, which were then filtered and collected through successive washing with ethyl alcohol. The purified precipitates were lyophilized for further use. Subsequently, the emulsification solvent dissipation strategy was employed to synthesize azidothymidine/zidovudine (AZT) loaded GAAD nanoparticles (Kim Tae Hee et al., 2004). The water-soluble and non-aqueous phases were kept separate. The non-aqueous phase was prepared using a suitable organic solvent at three different concentrations. Meanwhile, GAAD was dissolved in water. The non-aqueous phase was gradually added drop by drop into the aqueous phase. The entire solution underwent sonication and was mixed with the non-organic phase of the wetting agent (PF-68) at a specific concentration, resulting in the formulation of a double emulsion. The mixture was continuously mixed for one hour at 650 rpm, followed by complete dissipation of the undesired solvent (Alex Susan et al., 2011). The AZT-GAAD NPs were then obtained in the biphasic dispersion, and any free AZT was removed using high-speed centrifugation. Finally, they were dissolved in non-ionic water, and the pure impurity-free drug-loaded GAAD nanoparticles were obtained through highly refined filtration and lyophilization for various regimental purposes. To ensure stability and inertness, several morphological, spectroscopic, physicochemical, qualitative, NMR, and biochemical analytical evaluation studies were conducted, yielding valid and justified observations that render them suitable for use (Alex Susan et al., 2011; Joshy et al., 2018).

The study describes that the synthesized nanoparticles have shown exclusive advantageous benefits. The alginate-based encapsulation provides a uniform coating over all the nanoparticles, enabling them to provide long-lasting medication release after entering the gastrointestinal tract. Alginate, known for its inert, non-toxic, and biologically compatible properties, has been used as the encapsulating material (Das Ratul Kumar et al., 2010). This results in reduced dosing frequency, drug clearance rates, and increased bioavailability. Furthermore, this promotes easy penetrability and entry of nanoparticles across the cellular surface, increasing their uptake capacity by host body cells. Simultaneously, the drug is released at a steady rate over an extended duration, inhibiting the activity of the RT catalyst, thereby preventing the production of viral DNA from RNA and ultimately restraining replication, leading to the termination of the DNA strand (Parveen Suphiya et al., 2010). *In vitro* studies have also demonstrated that the sustained presence of AZT in the blood does not lead to toxicity, cytotoxicity, or cellular damage. Instead, it has shown good biostability, minimizing serious drug side effects. Consequently, it can be concluded that AZT-encapsulated PF-68-coated alginate nanoparticles possess profound therapeutic activity, rendering them a potent anti-retroviral pharmacological approach (Joshy et al., 2018; Sahay Gaurav et al., 2008).

2.3.4.2 ANTI-HUMAN IMMUNODEFICIENCY VIRUS (HIV) POLYSULFONATE DENDRIMERS

Dendrimers are extensively branched, rounded, homogeneous, and well-defined mono-dispersed molecules with a radially conforming center and polymeric nanostructure utilized as vehicles to carry lipophilic or hydrophilic active pharmaceutical cargo. They exhibit a range of atomic weights, possessing a three-dimensional bi-layered nano-molecular structure with outer and inner layers and are also termed cascade entities or arborols. Dendrimers are polyvalent macromolecules primarily fabricated through chemosynthetic laboratory methodologies involving alkyne-azide reactions, Diels-Alder reactions, or thiol-yne synthesis. Through continued exploration, these hyperbranched entities have shown remarkable superiority and regimental effectiveness against various retrovirus variants. Polysulfone dendrimers, produced on a large scale, have exhibited a promising anti-HIV effect, providing a potential cure for the syndrome (Kumar Virender et al., 2015; Sepúlveda-Crespo Daniel et al., 2017; Thomas Thea et al., 2007).

Myriam Witvrouw et al. conducted a study wherein dendrimers were produced *in vitro* using two polyanionic compounds, namely, phenyl dicarboxylic acid and naphthyl sulfonic acid, along with a PAMAM (polyamidoamine) solvent, followed by the process of amidation. Naphthyl sulfonic acid and phenyl dicarboxylic acid were obtained as residues separately by dissolving the compounds sodium 3,6-Dimethylthiourea and dicarboxy phenyl isothiocyanate, respectively, in the reaction mixture with the PAMAM solvent. The solutions were heated under nitrogen gas for 2 hours at 53°C. Subsequently, gel filtration was performed on both solutions individually to collect the residues. Gravimetric analysis and NMR spectrometry were conducted to determine the purity, physical, chemical, and biological properties of the resulting dendrimer molecules, validating them for further pharmaceutical and clinical utilization (Witvrouw Myriam et al., 2000; Yoshimura Tomokazu et al., 2004).

Various types of antiviral assays, confocal microscopy, immunological assays, and enzymatic *ex-vivo* reactions were conducted against HIV, revealing that carboxylic and naphthyl sulfonic groups are responsible for exhibiting antiviral activity at certain phases of HIV growth. These microbiological and biological assays have demonstrated the proficient anti-retroviral action of these entities against the virus. Scientific studies have indicated that these dendrimers are primarily formulated to combat NNRTIs or NRTIs resistant strains of HIV. It has been observed that by overcoming developed resistance, these polysulfonate dendrimers are introduced into the viral medium, initiating the formation of an inhibition zone against the virus by disrupting the adsorption of viral molecules, preventing the binding of gp 120 with cells, thereby preventing invasion. Similarly, assays for catalytic activity and replication tendencies have demonstrated the considerable inhibitory action of these polyanionic entities against HIV molecules, leading to the blockade of RT activity, impeding the transcription of RNA into viral DNA and disrupting protein synthesis. This dendrimer action disrupts viral growth, replication, and biological host-dependent viral activity, accountable for the progression of contagion within the host body. Thus, these polyanionic branched loaded particles have demonstrated efficacy against resistant strains, mutated strains, and actively propagating retroviruses by targeting various sites, including proteins, glycoprotein membranes, and adsorption on the host cell membrane. Overall, these nanoparticulated dendrimers, due to the presence of a polysulfone moiety, are considered excellent therapeutic strategies, demonstrating pronounced pharmacological activity against this autoimmune virus with multiple modes of action against viral contagion (Sepúlveda-Crespo Daniel et al., 2017; Thomas Thea et al., 2007; Witvrouw Myriam et al., 2000). Some commonly used and recently developed nanoformulations are depicted below in Figure 2.7.

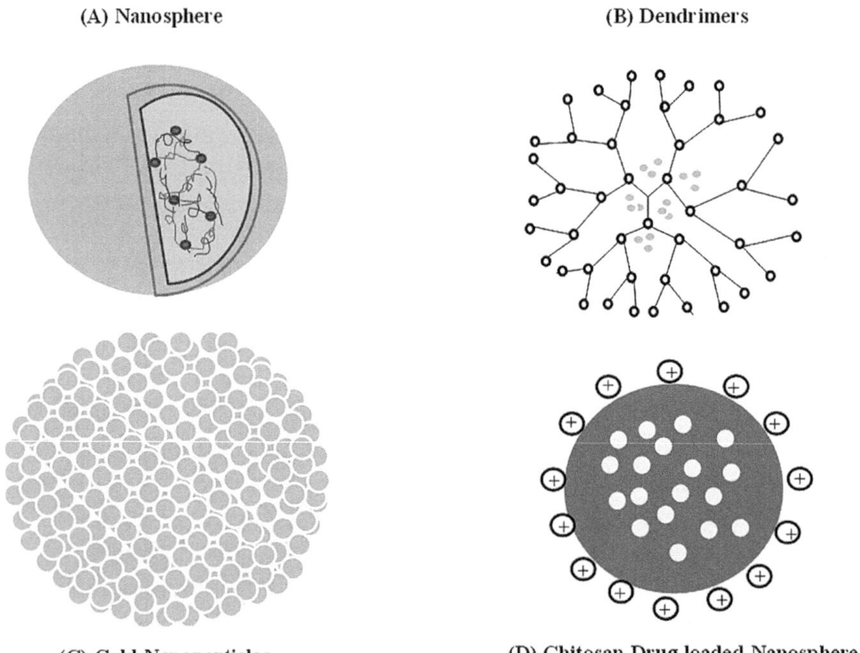

FIGURE 2.7 Diagrammatic representation of various types of antiviral nano formulations or nanovesicles at the molecular level employed against specific types of viral contagions.

2.4 CONCLUSION

Comprehensively, this chapter demonstrates that viral diseases jeopardize large populations. Viral molecules are highly transmissible, easily spreading through shared items, infected materials, and blood transfusions. They invade the host body, causing severe suffering due to the resulting ailment. Nevertheless, nanotechnological formulations offer effective safeguards, surpassing available antiviral therapies. Nanotechnology plays a significant role in various domains such as biotechnology, pharmaceuticals, and paramedical and drug delivery systems. These applications benefit from improved pharmacokinetic and biopharmaceutical characteristics, making them suitable for administration with minimal adverse reactions. A diverse range of organic ions, inorganic ions, active pharmaceutical ingredients, and phyto molecule-based nano-medications have been extensively explored, exhibiting potent and beneficial effects against most excruciating viral contagions. Several formulations, including phospholipid-based, sustained-release, biopolymer-encapsulated, inorganic metal ion-based (Ag NPs, Au NPs, etc.), organic metal ion-based (chitosan nanospheres), and drug-based (Se@OTV NPs), possess justified and stable physicochemical and nanostructural attributes. These attributes include uniform particle size, high systemic availability, uniform dispersity index, improved absorption, and penetrability. Consequently, nanoparticle-based formulations have demonstrated considerable pharmacological potential against various viral and retroviral infections, employing specific pharmacological mechanisms of action. These nanomedicines are increasingly employed as novel drug delivery systems, demanding further exploration in this domain. More sophisticated and efficient nanomedicines are needed to offer more advanced and effective treatment for incurable contagions such as HIV and HBV. Presently, nanotechnology is rapidly advancing and facilitating the development of various nanostructured medications and dosage forms, including nanoapertures, dendrimers, nano-implants, and micelles. These advancements aim to facilitate more advanced and effective therapeutic regimens against current and emerging viral and retroviral manifestations.

KEYWORDS

- **anti-viral**
- **bioavailability**
- **biotechnology**
- **drug resistance**
- **nanocarrier**
- **nanomedicine**
- **nanoparticles**
- **nanotechnology**
- **physicochemical**
- **prophylaxis**

REFERENCES

Abolmaali, S. S., Tamaddon, A. M., Farvadi, F. S., Daneshamuz, S., & Moghimi, H. (2011). Pharmaceutical Nano emulsions and their potential topical and transdermal applications, 139–150. https://www.sid.ir/en/journal/ViewPaper.aspx?id=229489 (accessed on 4th July 2025).

Akbarzadeh, A., Kafshdooz, L., Razban, Z., Dastranj Tbrizi, A., Rasoulpour, S., Khalilov, R., Kavetskyy, T., et al. (2018). An overview application of silver nanoparticles in inhibition of herpes simplex virus. *Artificial Cells, Nanomedicine, and Biotechnology, 46*(2), 263–267. https://doi.org/10.1080/21691401.2017.1307208 (accessed on 4th July 2025).

Alex, S. M., Rekha, M. R., & Sharma, C. P. (2011). Spermine grafted glycosylated chitosan for improved nanoparticle mediated gene delivery. *International Journal of Pharmaceutics, 410*(1, 2), 125–137. https://doi.org/10.1016/j.ijpharm.2011.02.067 (accessed on 4th July 2025).

Anton, N., Benoit, J. P., & Saulnier, P. (2008). Design and production of nanoparticles formulated from nano-emulsion templates—a review. *Journal of Controlled Release, 128*(3), 185–199. https://doi.org/10.1016/j.jconrel.2008.02.007 (accessed on 4th July 2025).

Bamrungsap, S., Zhao, Z., Chen, T., Wang, L., Li, C., Fu, T., & Tan, W. (2012). Nanotechnology in therapeutics: A focus on nanoparticles as a drug delivery system. *Nanomedicine, 7*(8), 1253–1271. https://doi.org/10.2217/nnm.12.87 (accessed on 4th July 2025).

Bawa, R. (2010). Nanopharmaceuticals: Nanopharmaceuticals. *European Journal of Nanomedicine, 3*(1), 34–40. https://doi.org/10.1515/EJNM.2010.3.1.34 (accessed on 4th July 2025).

Bawarski, W. E., Chidlowsky, E., Bharali, D. J., & Mousa, S. A. (2008). Emerging nanopharmaceuticals. *Nanomedicine: Nanotechnology, Biology and Medicine, 4*(4), 273–282. https://doi.org/10.1016/j.nano.2008.06.002 (accessed on 4th July 2025).

Bedi, P., & Kaur, A. (2015). An overview on uses of zinc oxide nanoparticles. *World Journal of Pharmacy and Pharmaceutical Sciences, 4*(12), 1177–1196. https://doi.org/10.2147/IJN.S216204 (accessed on 4th July 2025).

Bisso, S., & Leroux, J. C. (2020). Nanopharmaceuticals: A focus on their clinical translatability. *International Journal of Pharmaceutics, 578*, 119098. https://doi.org/10.1016/j.ijpharm.2020.119098 (accessed on 4th July 2025).

Briz, V., Poveda, E., & Soriano, V. (2006). HIV entry inhibitors: Mechanisms of action and resistance pathways. *Journal of Antimicrobial Chemotherapy, 57*(4), 619–627. https://doi.org/10.1093/jac/dkl027 (accessed on 4th July 2025).

Brust, M., Fink, J., Bethell, D., Schiffrin, D. J., & Kiely, C. (1995). Synthesis and reactions of functionalized gold nanoparticles. *Journal of the Chemical Society, Chemical Communications, 16*, 1655–1656. https://doi.org/10.1039/C39950001655 (accessed on 4th July 2025).

Burduşel, A. C., Gherasim, O., Grumezescu, A. M., Mogoantă, L., Ficai, A., & Andronescu, E. (2018). Biomedical applications of silver nanoparticles: An up-to-date overview. *Nanomaterials, 8*(9), 681. https://doi.org/10.3390/nano8090681 (accessed on 4th July 2025).

Caruthers, S. D., Wickline, S. A., & Lanza, G. M. (2007). Nanotechnological applications in medicine. *Current Opinion in Biotechnology, 18*(1), 26–30. https://doi.org/10.1016/j.copbio.2007.01.006 (accessed on 4th July 2025).

Cavalli, R., Leone, F., Minelli, R., Fantozzi, R., & Dianzani, C. (2014). New chitosan nanospheres for the delivery of 5-fluorouracil: Preparation, characterization and *in vitro* studies. *Current Drug Delivery, 11*(2), 270–278.

Chakravarty, M., & Vora, A. (2021). Nanotechnology-based antiviral therapeutics. *Drug Delivery and Translational Research, 11*(3), 748–787. https://doi.org/10.1007/s13346-020-00818-0 (accessed on 4th July 2025).

Chen, L., & Liang, J. (2020). An overview of functional nanoparticles as novel emerging antiviral therapeutic agents. *Materials Science and Engineering: C, 112*, 110924. https://doi.org/10.1016/j.msec.2020.110924 (accessed on 4th July 2025).

Cojocaru, F. D., Botezat, D., Gardikiotis, I., Uritu, C. M., Dodi, G., Trandafir, L., Rezus, C., Rezus, E., Tamba, B. I., & Mihai, C. T. (2020). Nanomaterials designed for antiviral drug delivery transport across biological barriers. *Pharmaceutics, 12*(2), 171. https://doi.org/10.3390/pharmaceutics12020171 (accessed on 4th July 2025).

Cui, Y., Zheng, X. S., Ren, B., Wang, R., Zhang, J., Xia, N. S., & Tian, Z. Q. (2011). Au@ organosilica multifunctional nanoparticles for the multimodal imaging. *Chemical Science, 2*(8), 1463–1469. https://doi.org/10.1039/C1SC00242B (accessed on 4th July 2025).

Cun, D., Foged, C., Yang, M., Frøkjær, S., & Nielsen, H. M. (2010). Preparation and characterization of poly (DL-lactide-co-glycolide) nanoparticles for siRNA delivery. *International Journal of Pharmaceutics, 390*(1), 70–75. https://doi.org/10.1016/j.ijpharm.2009.10.023 (accessed on 4th July 2025).

Damm, D., Rojas-Sánchez, L., Theobald, H., Sokolova, V., Wyatt, R. T., Überla, K., Epple, M., & Temchura, V. (2019). Calcium phosphate nanoparticle-based vaccines as a platform for improvement of HIV-1 Env antibody responses by infrastructural help. *Nanomaterials, 9*(10), 1389. https://doi.org/10.3390/nano9101389 (accessed on 4th July 2025).

Das, R. K., Kasoju, N., & Bora, U. (2010). Encapsulation of curcumin in alginate-chitosan-pluronic composite nanoparticles for delivery to cancer cells. *Nanomedicine: Nanotechnology, Biology and Medicine, 6*(1), 153–160. https://doi.org/10.1016/j.nano.2009.05.009 (accessed on 4th July 2025).

De Jong, W. H., & Borm, P. J. A. (2008). Drug delivery and nanoparticles: Applications and hazards. *International Journal of Nanomedicine, 3*(2), 133. https://doi.org/10.2147/ijn.s596 (accessed on 4th July 2025).

de Souza, M. E., Verdi, C. M., de Andrade, E. N. C., & Santos, R. C. V. (2019). Antiviral and antimicrobial (antibacterial) potentiality of nano drugs. In *Applications of Targeted Nano Drugs and Delivery Systems* (pp. 327–342). https://doi.org/10.1016/B978-0-12-814029-1.00012-0 (accessed on 4th July 2025).

Dehesa-Violante, M., & Nuñez-Nateras, R. (2007). Epidemiology of hepatitis virus B and C. *Archives of Medical Research, 38*(6), 606–611. https://doi.org/10.1016/j.arcmed.2007.03.001 (accessed on 4th July 2025).

Donalisio, M., Leone, F., Civra, A., Spagnolo, R., Ozer, O., Lembo, D., & Cavalli, R. (2018). Acyclovir-loaded chitosan nanospheres from nano-emulsion templating for the topical treatment of herpesviruses infections. *Pharmaceutics, 10*(2), 46. https://doi.org/10.3390/pharmaceutics10020046 (accessed on 4th July 2025).

Englund, J. A. (2002). Antiviral therapy of influenza. In *Seminars in Pediatric Infectious Diseases, 13*(2), 120–128. https://doi.org/10.1053/spid.2002.122999 (accessed on 4th July 2025).

Fanales-Belasio, E., Raimondo, M., Suligoi, B., & Buttò, S. (2010). HIV virology and pathogenetic mechanisms of infection: A brief overview. *Annali dell'Istituto Superiore di Sanità, 46*, 5–14. https://doi.org/10.4415/ANN_10_01_02 (accessed on 4th July 2025).

Fatahzadeh, M., & Schwartz, R. A. (2007). Human herpes simplex virus infections: Epidemiology, pathogenesis, symptomatology, diagnosis, and management. *Journal of the American Academy of Dermatology, 57*(5), 737–763. https://doi.org/10.1016/j.jaad.2007.06.027 (accessed on 4th July 2025).

Ferrari, F., Bonferoni, M. C., Rossi, S., Sandri, G., & Caramella, C. M. (2012). Manufacture techniques of chitosan-based microparticles and nanoparticles for biopharmaceuticals. In *Chitosan-Based Systems for Biopharmaceuticals: Delivery, Targeting and Polymer Therapeutics* (pp. 137–158). https://doi.org/10.1002/9781119962977.ch9 (accessed on 4th July 2025).

Floyd, D. L., Ragains, J. R., Skehel, J. J., Harrison, S. C., & Van Oijen, A. M. (2008). Single-particle kinetics of influenza virus membrane fusion. *Proceedings of the National Academy of Sciences, 105*(40), 15382–15387. https://doi.org/10.1073/pnas.0807771105 (accessed on 4th July 2025).

Fowler, C. E., Khushalani, D., Lebeau, B., & Mann, S. (2001). Nanoscale materials with mesostructured interiors. *Advanced Materials, 13*(9), 649–652. https://doi.org/10.1002/1521-4095(200105)13:9<649:AID-ADMA649>3.0.CO;2-G (accessed on 4th July 2025).

Franklyne, J. S., Gopinath, P. M., Mukherjee, A., & Chandrasekaran, N. (2021). Nano emulsions: The rising star of antiviral therapeutics and nano delivery systems—Current status and prospects. *Current Opinion in Colloid & Interface Science, 54*, 101458. https://doi.org/10.1016/j.cocis.2021.101458 (accessed on 4th July 2025).

Gavilanes, F., Gomez-Gutierrez, J., Aracil, M., Gonzalez-Ros, J. M., Ferragut, J. A., Guerrero, E., & Peterson, D. L. (1990). Hepatitis B surface antigen. Role of lipids in maintaining the structural and antigenic properties of protein components. *Biochemical Journal, 265*(3), 857–864. https://doi.org/10.1042/bj2650857 (accessed on 4th July 2025).

George, M., & Abraham, T. E. (2006). Polyionic hydrocolloids for the intestinal delivery of protein drugs: Alginate and chitosan—A review. *Journal of Controlled Release, 114*(1), 1–14. https://doi.org/10.1016/j.jconrel.2006.04.017 (accessed on 4th July 2025).

Ghaffari, H., Tavakoli, A., Moradi, A., Tabarraei, A., Bokharaei-Salim, F., Zahmatkeshan, M., Farahmand, M., et al. (2019). Inhibition of H1N1 influenza virus infection by zinc oxide nanoparticles: Another emerging application of nanomedicine. *Journal of Biomedical Science, 26*(1), 1–10. https://doi.org/10.1186/s12929-019-0563-4 (accessed on 4th July 2025).

Ghosh, P., Han, G., De, M., Kim, C. K., & Rotello, V. M. (2008). Gold nanoparticles in delivery applications. *Advanced Drug Delivery Reviews, 60*(11), 1307–1315. https://doi.org/10.1016/j.addr.2008.03.016 (accessed on 4th July 2025).

Gil, P. R., Hühn, D., Loretta, L., Sasse, D., & Parak, W. J. (2010). Nano pharmacy: Inorganic nanoscale devices as vectors and active compounds. *Pharmacological Research, 62*(2), 115–125. https://doi.org/10.1016/j.phrs.2010.01.009 (accessed on 4th July 2025).

Giri, N., Tomar, P., Karwasara, V. S., Pandey, R. S., & Dixit, V. K. (2011). Targeted novel surface-modified nanoparticles for interferon delivery for the treatment of hepatitis B. *Acta Biochemical et Biophysical Sinica, 43*(11), 877–883. https://doi.org/10.1093/abbs/gmr082 (accessed on 4th July 2025).

Gubareva, L. V. (2004). Molecular mechanisms of influenza virus resistance to neuraminidase inhibitors. *Virus Research, 103*(1, 2), 199–203. https://doi.org/10.1016/j.virusres.2004.02.034 (accessed on 4th July 2025).

Hakimian, F., & Ghourchian, H. (2019). Simple and rapid method for synthesis of porous gold nanoparticles and its application in improving DNA loading capacity. *Materials Science and Engineering: C, 103*, 109795. https://doi.org/10.1016/j.msec.2019.109795 (accessed on 4th July 2025).

Haley, B., & Frenkel, E. (2008). Nanoparticles for drug delivery in cancer treatment. In *Urologic Oncology: Seminars and Original Investigations, 26*(1), 57–64. https://doi.org/10.1016/j.urolonc.2007.03.015 (accessed on 4th July 2025).

Heidegger, S., Gößl, D., Schmidt, A., Niedermayer, S., Argyo, C., Endres, S., Bein, T., & Bourquin, C. (2016). Immune response to functionalized mesoporous silica nanoparticles for targeted drug delivery. *Nanoscale, 8*(2), 938–948. https://doi.org/10.1039/C5NR06122A (accessed on 4th July 2025).

Hu, R. L., Li, S. R., Kong, F. J., Hou, R. J., Guan, X. L., & Guo, F. (2014). Inhibition effect of silver nanoparticles on herpes simplex virus 2. *Genetics and Molecular Research, 13*(3), 7022–7028. http://dx.doi.org/10.4238/2014.March.19.2 (accessed on 4th July 2025).

Huang, Y., Wu, L., Chen, X., Bai, P., & Kim, D. H. (2013). Synthesis of anisotropic concave gold nano cuboids with distinctive plasmonic properties. *Chemistry of Materials, 25*(12), 2470–2475. https://doi.org/10.1021/cm400765b (accessed on 4th July 2025).

Hulla, J. E., Sahu, S. C., & Hayes, A. W. (2015). Nanotechnology: History and future. *Human & Experimental Toxicology, 34*(12), 1318–1321. https://doi.org/10.1177/0960327115603588 (accessed on 4th July 2025).

Ison, M. G. (2011). Antivirals and resistance: Influenza virus. *Current Opinion in Virology, 1*(6), 563–573. https://doi.org/10.1016/j.coviro.2011.09.002 (accessed on 4th July 2025).

Jenkins, J. A., Wax, T. J., & Zhao, J. (2017). Seed-mediated synthesis of gold nanoparticles of controlled sizes to demonstrate the impact of size on optical properties. *Journal of Chemical Education, 94*(8), 1090–1093. https://doi.org/10.1021/acs.jchemed.6b00941 (accessed on 4th July 2025).

Joshy, K. S., Alex Susan, M., Snigdha, S., Nandakumar, K., Laly, A. P., & Sabu, T. (2018). Encapsulation of zidovudine in PF-68 coated alginate conjugate nanoparticles for anti-HIV drug delivery. *International Journal of Biological Macromolecules, 107*, 929–937. https://doi.org/10.1016/j.ijbiomac.2017.09.078 (accessed on 4th July 2025).

Kargozar, S., & Mozafari, M. (2018). Nanotechnology and nanomedicine: Start small, think big. *Materials Today: Proceedings, 5*(7), 15492–15500. https://doi.org/10.1016/j.matpr.2018.04.15 (accessed on 4th July 2025).

Kerry, R. G., Malik, S., Redda, Y. T., Sahoo, S., Patra, J. K., & Majhi, S. (2019). Nano-based approach to combat emerging viral (NIPAH virus) infection. *Nanomedicine: Nanotechnology, Biology and Medicine, 18*, 196–220. https://doi.org/10.3390/pharmaceutics12020171 (accessed on 4th July 2025).

Kim, J., Yeom, M., Lee, T., Kim, H. O., Na, W., Kang, A., Lim, J. W., et al. (2020). Porous gold nanoparticles for attenuating infectivity of influenza A virus. *Journal of Nanobiotechnology, 18*(1), 1–11. https://doi.org/10.21203/rs.2.20864/v1 (accessed on 4th July 2025).

Kim, T. H., Park, I. K., Nah, J. W., Choi, Y. J., & Cho, C. S. (2004). Glycosylated chitosan/DNA nanoparticles prepared using water-soluble chitosan as a gene carrier. *Biomaterials, 25*(17), 3783–3792. https://doi.org/10.1016/j.biomaterials.2003.10.063 (accessed on 4th July 2025).

King, S. R. (1994). HIV: Virology and mechanisms of disease. *Annals of Emergency Medicine, 24*(3), 443–449. https://doi.org/10.1016/S0196-0644(94)70181-4 (accessed on 4th July 2025).

Klimas, N., O'Brien Koneru, A., & Fletcher, M. A. (2008). Overview of HIV. *Psychosomatic Medicine, 70*(5), 523–530. https://doi.org/10.1097/PSY.0b013e31817ae69f (accessed on 4th July 2025).

Knuschke, T., Sokolova, V., Rotan, O., Wadwa, M., Tenbusch, M., Hansen, W., Staeheli, P., Epple, M., Buer, J., & Westendorf, A. M. (2013). Immunization with biodegradable nanoparticles efficiently induces cellular immunity and protects against influenza virus infection. *The Journal of Immunology, 190*(12), 6221–6229. https://doi.org/10.4049/jimmunol.1202654 (accessed on 4th July 2025).

Kozlova, D., Chernousova, S., Knuschke, T., Buer, J., Westendorf, A. M., & Epple, M. (2012). Cell targeting by antibody-functionalized calcium phosphate nanoparticles. *Journal of Materials Chemistry, 22*(2), 396–404. https://doi.org/10.1039/C1JM14683A (accessed on 4th July 2025).

Kumar, V., & Mahato, R. I. (2015). Delivery and targeting of miRNAs for treating liver fibrosis. *Pharmaceutical Research, 32*(2), 341–361. https://doi.org/10.1007/s11095-014-1497-x (accessed on 4th July 2025).

Lee, E. C., Davis-Poynter, N., Nguyen, C. T. H., Peters, A. A., Monteith, G. R., Strounina, E., Popat, A., & Ross, B. P. (2016). GAG mimetic functionalized solid and mesoporous silica nanoparticles as viral entry inhibitors of herpes simplex type 1 and type 2 viruses. *Nanoscale, 8*(36), 16192–16196. https://doi.org/10.1039/C6NR03878F (accessed on 4th July 2025).

Lee, M. S., Lee, J. E., Byun, E., Kim, N. W., Lee, K., Lee, H., Sim, S. J., Lee, D. S., & Jeong, J. H. (2014). Target-specific delivery of siRNA by stabilized calcium phosphate nanoparticles using dopa–hyaluronic acid conjugate. *Journal of Controlled Release, 192*, 122–130. https://doi.org/10.1016/j.jconrel.2014.06.049 (accessed on 4th July 2025).

Lembo, D., Donalisio, M., Civra, A., Argenziano, M., & Cavalli, R. (2018). Nanomedicine formulations for the delivery of antiviral drugs: A promising solution for the treatment of viral infections. *Expert Opinion on Drug Delivery, 15*(1), 93–114. https://doi.org/10.1080/17425247.2017.1360863 (accessed on 4th July 2025).

Leon, L., Chung, E. J., & Rinaldi, C. (2020). A brief history of nanotechnology and introduction to nanoparticles for biomedical applications. In *Nanoparticles for Biomedical Applications* (pp. 1–4). Elsevier. https://doi.org/10.1016/B978-0-12-816662-8.00001-1 (accessed on 4th July 2025).

Li, Y., Lin, Z., Gong, G., Guo, M., Xu, T., Wang, C., Zhao, M., et al. (2019). Inhibition of H1N1 influenza virus-induced apoptosis by selenium nanoparticles functionalized with arbidol through ROS-mediated signaling pathways. *Journal of Materials Chemistry B, 7*(27), 4252–4262. https://doi.org/10.1039/c9tb00531e (accessed on 4th July 2025).

Li, Y., Lin, Z., Guo, M., Xia, Y., Zhao, M., Wang, C., Xu, T., Chen, T., & Zhu, B. (2017). Inhibitory activity of selenium nanoparticles functionalized with oseltamivir on H1N1 influenza virus. *International Journal of Nanomedicine, 12*, 5733. https://doi.org/10.2147/IJN.S140939 (accessed on 4th July 2025).

Li, Y., Lin, Z., Xu, T., Wang, C., Zhao, M., Xiao, M., Wang, H., Deng, N., & Zhu, B. (2017). Delivery of VP1 siRNA to inhibit the EV71 virus using functionalized silver nanoparticles through ROS-mediated signaling pathways. *RSC Advances, 7*(3), 1453–1463. https://doi.org/10.1039/C6RA26472G (accessed on 4th July 2025).

Liu, W., Li, X., Wong, Y. S., Zheng, W., Zhang, Y., Cao, W., & Chen, T. (2012). Selenium nanoparticles as a carrier of 5-fluorouracil to achieve anticancer synergism. *ACS Nano, 6*(8), 6578–6591. https://doi.org/10.1021/nn202452c (accessed on 4th July 2025).

Mann, S., Burkett, S. L., Davis, S. A., Fowler, C. E., Mendelson, N. H., Sims, S. D., Walsh, D., & Whilton, N. T. (1997). Sol–gel synthesis of organized matter. *Chemistry of Materials, 9*(11), 2300–2310. https://doi.org/10.1021/cm970274u (accessed on 4th July 2025).

Marohn, M. E., & Barry, E. M. (2013). Live attenuated tularemia vaccines: Recent developments and future goals. *Vaccine, 31*(35), 3485–3491. https://doi.org/10.1016/j.vaccine.2013.05.096 (accessed on 4th July 2025).

Mehendale, R., Joshi, M., & Patravale, V. B. (2013). Nanomedicines for treatment of viral diseases. *Critical Reviews™ in Therapeutic Drug Carrier Systems, 30*(1). (accessed on 4th July 2025).

Mihalcik, D. J., & Lin, W. (2009). Mesoporous silica nanosphere-supported chiral ruthenium catalysts: Synthesis, characterization, and asymmetric hydrogenation studies. *ChemCatChem, 1*(3), 406–413. https://doi.org/10.1002/cctc.200900188 (accessed on 4th July 2025).

Mukherjee, B., Dey, N. S., Magi, R., Bhowmik, P., Das, P. J., & Paul, P. (2014). Current status and future scope for nanomaterials in drug delivery. In *Application of Nanotechnology in Drug Delivery*. IntechOpen. https://doi.org/10.5772/58450 (accessed on 4th July 2025).

Nasrollahzadeh, M., Sajadi, S. M., Sajjadi, M., & Issaabadi, Z. (2019). Applications of nanotechnology in daily life. *Interface Science and Technology, 28*, 113–143. https://doi.org/10.1016/B978-0-12-813586-0.00004-3 (accessed on 4th July 2025).

Nguyen, J. T., Smee, D. F., Barnard, D. L., Julander, J. G., Gross, M., de Jong, M. D., & Went, G. T. (2012). Efficacy of combined therapy with amantadine, oseltamivir, and ribavirin *in vivo* against susceptible and amantadine-resistant influenza A viruses. *PLoS One, 7*(1), e31006. https://doi.org/10.1371/journal.pone.0031006 (accessed on 4th July 2025).

Nyce, G. W., Hayes, J. R., Hamza, A. V., & Satcher, J. H. (2007). Synthesis and characterization of hierarchical porous gold materials. *Chemistry of Materials, 19*(3), 344–346. https://doi.org/10.1021/cm062569q (accessed on 4th July 2025).

Op De Beeck, A., & Dubuisson, J. (2003). Topology of hepatitis C virus envelope glycoproteins. *Reviews in Medical Virology, 13*(4), 233–241. https://doi.org/10.1002/rmv.391 (accessed on 4th July 2025).

Orlowski, P., Tomaszewska, E., Gniadek, M., Baska, P., Nowakowska, J., Sokolowska, J., Nowak, Z., et al. (2014). Tannic acid modified silver nanoparticles show antiviral activity in herpes simplex virus type 2 infection. *PLoS One, 9*(8), e104113. https://doi.org/10.1371/journal.pone.0104113 (accessed on 4th July 2025).

Owen, A., Dufès, C., Moscatelli, D., Mayes, E., Lovell, J. F., Katti, K. V., Sokolov, K., et al. (2014). The application of nanotechnology in medicine: Treatment and diagnostics. *Nanomedicine, 9*(9), 1291–1294. https://doi.org/10.2217/nnm.14.93 (accessed on 4th July 2025).

Park, I., Ko, S. H., An, Y. S., Choi, K. H., Chun, H., Lee, S., & Kim, G. (2009). Monodisperse polystyrene-silica core–shell particles and silica hollow spheres prepared by the Stöber method. *Journal of Nanoscience and Nanotechnology, 9*(12), 7224–7228. https://doi.org/10.1166/jnn.2009.1636 (accessed on 4th July 2025).

Parveen, S., Mitra, M., Krishnakumar, S., & Sahoo, S. K. (2010). Retraction notices to "Enhanced antiproliferative activity of carboplatin loaded chitosan-alginate nanoparticles in retinoblastoma cell line." *Acta Biomaterialia, 6*, 3120–3131. https://doi.org/10.1016/j.actbio.2010.02.010 (accessed on 4th July 2025).

Pathak, C., Vaidya, F. U., & Pandey, S. M. (2019). Mechanism for development of nano-based drug delivery systems. In *Applications of Targeted Nano Drugs and Delivery Systems* (pp. 35–67). https://doi.org/10.1016/B978-0-12-814029-1.00003-X (accessed on 4th July 2025).

Patil, M., Mehta, D. S., & Guvva, S. (2008). Future impact of nanotechnology on medicine and dentistry. *Journal of Indian Society of Periodontology, 12*(2), 34. https://doi.org/10.4103/0972-124X.44088 (accessed on 4th July 2025).

Polizu, S., Savadogo, O., Poulin, P., & Yahia, L. H. (2006). Applications of carbon nanotubes-based biomaterials in biomedical nanotechnology. *Journal of Nanoscience and Nanotechnology, 6*(7), 1883–1904. https://doi.org/10.1166/jnn.2006.197 (accessed on 4th July 2025).

Prabhu, P., Patravale, V., & Joshi, M. (2012). Nanocarriers for effective topical delivery of anti-infectives. *Current Nanoscience, 8*(4), 491–503. https://doi.org/10.2174/157341312801784221 (accessed on 4th July 2025).

Pradeu, T., Kostyrka, G., & Dupré, J. (2016). Understanding viruses: Philosophical investigations. *Studies in History and Philosophy of Science Part C: Studies in History and Philosophy of Biological and Biomedical Sciences, 59*, 57–63. https://doi.org/10.1016/j.shpsc.2016.02.008 (accessed on 4th July 2025).

Prokop, A., & Davidson, J. M. (2008). Nano vehicular intracellular delivery systems. *Journal of Pharmaceutical Sciences, 97*(9), 3518–3590. https://doi.org/10.1002/jps.21270 (accessed on 4th July 2025).

Purcell, R. (1997). The hepatitis C virus: Overview. *Hepatology, 26*(S3), 11S–14S. https://doi.org/10.1002/hep.510260702 (accessed on 4th July 2025).

Qu, X., Zhu, D., Yao, G., Su, S., Chao, J., Liu, H., Zuo, X., et al. (2017). An exonuclease III-powered, on-particle stochastic DNA walker. *Angewandte Chemise, 129*(7), 1881–1884. https://doi.org/10.1002/ange.201611777 (accessed on 4th July 2025).

Remeijer, L., Osterhaus, A., & Verjans, G. (2004). Human herpes simplex virus keratitis: The pathogenesis revisited. *Ocular Immunology and Inflammation, 12*(4), 255–285. https://doi.org/10.1080/092739490500363 (accessed on 4th July 2025).

Roco, M. C. (1999). Nanoparticles and nanotechnology research. *Journal of Nanoparticle Research, 1*(1), 1. https://doi.org/10.1023/A:1010093308079 (accessed on 4th July 2025).

Rosen, J. E., Yoffe, S., Meerasa, A., Verma, M., & Gu, F. X. (2011). Nanotechnology and diagnostic imaging: New advances in contrast agent technology. *Journal of Nanomedicine & Nanotechnology, 2*(5), 1–12. https://doi.org/10.4172/2157-7439.1000115 (accessed on 4th July 2025).

Ruckmani, K., & Sankar, V. (2010). Formulation and optimization of zidovudine noisome. *AAPS PharmSciTech, 11*(3), 1119–1127. https://doi.org/10.1208/s12249-010-9480-2 (accessed on 4th July 2025).

Sahay, G., Batrakova, E. V., & Kabanov, A. V. (2008). Different internalization pathways of polymeric micelles and universe and their effects on vesicular transport. *Bioconjugate Chemistry, 19*(10), 2023–2029. https://doi.org/10.1021/bc8002315 (accessed on 4th July 2025).

Sanchez, A., Tobío, M., González, L., Fabra, A., & Alonso, M. J. (2003). Biodegradable micro-and nanoparticles as long-term delivery vehicles for interferon-alpha. *European Journal of Pharmaceutical Sciences, 18*(3, 4), 221–229. https://doi.org/10.1016/S0928-0987(03)00019-8 (accessed on 4th July 2025).

Sanchez, F., & Sobolev, K. (2010). Nanotechnology in concrete–a review. *Construction and Building Materials, 24*(11), 2060–2071. https://doi.org/10.1016/j.conbuildmat.2010.03.014 (accessed on 4th July 2025).

Sardar, R., Funston, A. M., Mulvaney, P., & Murray, R. W. (2009). Gold nanoparticles: Past, present, and future. *Langmuir, 25*(24), 13840–13851. https://doi.org/10.1021/la9019475 (accessed on 4th July 2025).

Sau, T. K., & Murphy, C. J. (2004). Room temperature, high-yield synthesis of multiple shapes of gold nanoparticles in aqueous solution. *Journal of the American Chemical Society, 126*(28), 8648–8649. https://doi.org/10.1021/ja047846d (accessed on 4th July 2025).

Schlickewei, C., Klatte, T. O., Wildermuth, Y., Laaff, G., Rueger, J. M., Ruesing, J., Chernousova, S., Lehmann, W., & Epple, M. (2019). A bioactive nano-calcium phosphate pastes for *in-situ* transfection of BMP-7 and VEGF-A in a rabbit critical-size bone defect: Results of an *in vivo* study. *Journal of Materials Science: Materials in Medicine, 30*(2), 1–12. https://doi.org/10.1007/s10856-019-6217-y (accessed on 4th July 2025).

Sepúlveda-Crespo, D., Jiménez, J. L., Gomez, R., De La Mata, F. J., Majano, P. L., Muñoz-Fernández, M. Á., & Gastaminza, P. (2017). Polyanionic carbosilane dendrimers prevent hepatitis C virus infection in cell culture. *Nanomedicine: Nanotechnology, Biology and Medicine, 13*(1), 49–58. https://doi.org/10.1016/j.nano.2016.08.018 (accessed on 4th July 2025).

Shen, T. W., Fromen, C. A., Kai, M. P., Luft, J. C., Rahhal, T. B., Robbins, G. R., & DeSimone, J. M. (2015). Distribution and cellular uptake of PEGylated polymeric particles in the lung towards cell-specific targeted delivery. *Pharmaceutical Research, 32*(10), 3248–3260. https://doi.org/10.1007/s11095-015-1701-7 (accessed on 4th July 2025).

Siddiqi, K. S., Rahman, A., Tajuddin, & Husen, A. (2018). Properties of zinc oxide nanoparticles and their activity against microbes. *Nanoscale Research Letters, 13*, 141. https://doi.org/10.1186/s11671-018-2532-3 (accessed on 4th July 2025).

Singh, K., Mishra, A., Sharma, D., & Singh, K. (2019). Antiviral and antimicrobial potentiality of nano drugs. In *Applications of Targeted Nano Drugs and Delivery Systems* (pp. 343–356). Elsevier. https://doi.org/10.1016/B978-0-12-814029-1.00013-2 (accessed on 4th July 2025).

Singh, L., Kruger, H. G., Maguire, G. E. M., Govender, T., & Parboosing, R. (2017). The role of nanotechnology in the treatment of viral infections. *Therapeutic Advances in Infectious Disease, 4*(4), 105–131. https://doi.org/10.1177/2049936117713593 (accessed on 4th July 2025).

Soenen, S. J., Manshian, B. B., Abdelmonem, A. M., Montenegro, J. M., Tan, S., Balcaen, L., Vanhaecke, F., et al. (2014). The cellular interactions of PEGylated gold nanoparticles: Effect of PEGylation on cellular uptake and cytotoxicity. *Particle & Particle Systems Characterization, 31*(7), 794–800. https://doi.org/10.1002/ppsc.201300357 (accessed on 4th July 2025).

Szunerits, S., Barras, A., Khanal, M., Pagneux, Q., & Boukherroub, R. (2015). Nanostructures for the inhibition of viral infections. *Molecules, 20*(8), 14051–14081. https://doi.org/10.3390/molecules200814051 (accessed on 4th July 2025).

Tang, J., Xiong, L., Zhou, G., Wang, S., Wang, J., Liu, L., Li, J., et al. (2010). Silver nanoparticles crossing through and distribution in the blood-brain barrier *in vitro*. *Journal of Nanoscience and Nanotechnology, 10*(10), 6313–6317. https://doi.org/10.1166/jnn.2010.2625 (accessed on 4th July 2025).

Tavakoli, A., Ataei-Pirkooh, A., Sadeghi, G. M. M., Bokharaei-Salim, F., Sahrapour, P., Kiani, S. J., Moghoofei, M., Farahmand, M., Javanmard, D., & Monavari, S. H. (2018). Polyethylene glycol-coated zinc oxide nanoparticle: An efficient nanoweapon to fight against herpes simplex virus type 1. *Nanomedicine, 13*(21), 2675–2690. https://doi.org/10.2217/nnm-2018-0089 (accessed on 4th July 2025).

Temchura, V. V., Kozlova, D., Sokolova, V., Überla, K., & Epple, M. (2014). Targeting and activation of antigen-specific B-cells by calcium phosphate nanoparticles loaded with protein antigen. *Biomaterials, 35*(23), 6098–6105. https://doi.org/10.1016/j.biomaterials.2014.04.010 (accessed on 4th July 2025).

Thomas, T., & Foster, G. (2007). Nanomedicines in the treatment of chronic hepatitis C–focus on pegylated interferon alpha-2a. *International Journal of Nanomedicine, 2*(1), 19. https://doi.org/10.2147/nano.2007.2.1.19 (accessed on 4th July 2025).

Tiollais, P., Pourcel, C., & Dejean, A. (1985). The hepatitis B virus. *Nature, 317*(6037), 489–495. https://doi.org/10.1038/317489a0 (accessed on 4th July 2025).

Watanabe, T., & Kawaoka, Y. (2015). Influenza virus–host interactomes as a basis for antiviral drug development. *Current Opinion in Virology, 14*, 71–78. https://doi.org/10.1016/j.coviro.2015.08.008 (accessed on 4th July 2025).

Wei, L., Lu, J., Xu, H., Patel, A., Chen, Z. S., & Chen, G. (2015). Silver nanoparticles: Synthesis, properties, and therapeutic applications. *Drug Discovery Today, 20*(5), 595–601. https://doi.org/10.1016/j.drudis.2014.11.014 (accessed on 4th July 2025).

Whitley, R. J., & Roizman, B. (2001). Herpes simplex virus infections. *The Lancet, 357*(9267), 1513–1518. https://doi.org/10.1016/S0140-6736(00)04638-9 (accessed on 4th July 2025).

Witvrouw, M., Fikkert, V., Pluymers, W., Matthews, B., Mardel, K., Schols, D., Raff, J., et al. (2000). Polyanionic (ie, polysulfonate) dendrimers can inhibit the replication of human immunodeficiency virus by interfering with both virus adsorption and later steps (reverse transcriptase/integrase) in the virus replicative cycle. *Molecular Pharmacology, 58*(5), 1100–1108. https://doi.org/10.1124/mol.58.5.1100 (accessed on 4th July 2025).

World Health Organization (WHO). (2018). *Hepatitis*. https://www.who.int/hepatitis/news-events/hep-c-scale-up/en/ (accessed on 4th July 2025).

Wu, J., Meng, Z., Jiang, M., Zhang, E., Trippler, M., Broering, R., Bucchi, A., et al. (2010). Toll-like receptor-induced innate immune responses in non-parenchymal liver cells are cell type-specific. *Immunology, 129*(3), 363–374. https://doi.org/10.1111/j.1365-2567.2009.03179.x (accessed on 4th July 2025).

Xu, Z. P., Zeng, Q. H., Lu, G. Q., & Yu, A. B. (2006). Inorganic nanoparticles as carriers for efficient cellular delivery. *Chemical Engineering Science, 61*(3), 1027–1040. https://doi.org/10.1016/j.ces.2005.06.019 (accessed on 4th July 2025).

Yang, D. (2021). Application of nanotechnology in the COVID-19 pandemic. *International Journal of Nanomedicine, 16*, 623. https://doi.org/10.2147/IJN.S296383 (accessed on 4th July 2025).

Yang, Y., Kuang, Y., Liu, Y., Li, W., Jiang, Z., Xiao, L., & Li, M. (2011). Immunogenicity of multiple-epitope antigen gene of HCV carried by novel biodegradable polymers. *Comparative Immunology, Microbiology and Infectious Diseases, 34*(1), 65–72. https://doi.org/10.1016/j.cimid.2010.02.003 (accessed on 4th July 2025).

Yang, Y., Kuang, Y., Yuan, D., Cao, L. L., Wang, B. N., Li, M. Y., & Zhang, Z. W. (2011). Investigation of HCV multi-epitope gene vaccine loaded by CTS-Fe_3O_4. *Sichuan Da Xue Xue Bao. Yi Xue Ban = Journal of Sichuan University. Medical Science Edition, 42*(6), 757–761. https://doi.org/10.3389/fcimb.2021.643953 (accessed on 4th July 2025).

Yezdani, U., Khan, M. G., Kushwah, N., Verma, A., & Khan, F. (2018). Application of nanotechnology in diagnosis and treatment of various diseases and its future advances in medicine. *World Journal of Pharmacy and Pharmaceutical Sciences, 7*(11), 1611–1633. https://doi.org/10.20959/wjpps201818-12703 (accessed on 4th July 2025).

Yoshimura, T., Abe, S., & Esumi, K. (2004). Characterization of quaternized poly (amidoamine) dendrimers of generation 1 with multiple octyl chains. *Colloids and Surfaces A: Physicochemical and Engineering Aspects, 251*(1–3), 141–144. https://doi.org/10.1016/j.colsurfa.2004.09.031 (accessed on 4th July 2025).

Zhang, Q., Large, N., Nordlander, P., & Wang, H. (2014). Porous Au nanoparticles with tunable plasmon resonances and intense field enhancements for single-particle SERS. *The Journal of Physical Chemistry Letters, 5*(2), 370–374. https://doi.org/10.1021/jz402795x (accessed on 4th July 2025).

Zhao, Y., Wang, Z., Zhang, W., & Jiang, X. (2010). Adsorbed Tween 80 is unique in its ability to improve the stability of gold nanoparticles in solutions of biomolecules. *Nanoscale, 2*(10), 2114–2119. https://doi.org/10.1039/C0NR00151A (accessed on 4th July 2025).

CHAPTER 3

Metal and Metal Oxide Nanoparticles as Antiviral Agents

GARIMA[1,2] and ARUN KUMAR[1,3,*]

[1]Chitkara College of Pharmacy, Chitkara University, Punjab, India

[2]M. M. College of Pharmacy, Maharishi Markandeshwar (Deemed to be University), Mullana-Ambala, Haryana, India

[3]Department of Pharmacy, School of Health Sciences, Central University of South Bihar, Gaya, Bihar, India

*Corresponding author

ABSTRACT

Nanotechnology is increasingly influential in various fields, including virology. The utilization of metal or metal oxide nanoparticles in viral targeting formulations is becoming more prevalent, promising to enhance the diagnostic or therapeutic capabilities of agents and improve the prospects of targeted drug delivery. While various nanoparticles with diverse compositions, sizes, shapes, and surface characteristics have been approved for human use, very few candidates are currently under investigation or approved for clinical detection and treatment of viral infections. The sector continues to face challenges due to a lack of essential understanding about the *in vivo* behavior of nanoparticles during viral infections. This literature review provides a comprehensive overview of the current advancements in the use of metal and metal oxide nanoparticles in the diagnosis, prevention, and treatment of HIV, hepatitis, influenza, and herpes infections. The chapter also examines the various types of nanoparticles widely employed as antiviral agents and their diverse applications.

Nanotechnological Management of Viral Infections.
Radhakrishnan EK, Shiji Mathew, and Riya Alex (Eds.)

DOI: 10.1201/9781779640895-3

3.1 INTRODUCTION

Metal oxide nanoparticles hold significant importance in various fields, including chemistry, physics, and materials science (Stanton et al., 2008; Wang et al., 2007). These nanoparticles can be constructed from a wide range of oxide compounds, facilitating various primary applications in electronic architecture, such as semiconductor representation, metallic characteristics, or coverage persona. They are used in the production of microelectronic circuits, switches, piezoelectric modules, energy units, corrosion passivation coatings, and mechanical catalysts (Rao et al., 2017; Yadavalli et al., 2014). Nanotechnology aims to fabricate nano-objects or nanoarrays with distinct properties beyond mass or single molecule species (Peer et al., 2007). Due to their small size and significant surface characteristics, oxide nanoparticles exhibit unique physical and chemical properties (Eng et al., 2011). In recent years, nanomaterials have garnered substantial interest in selective therapeutics and diagnostics. With nanoparticles typically ranging from 10–500 nm, their interactions with human cells are influenced by practical considerations and the size of the molecule (Singh, 2017). Several nanoparticle drug delivery models have been developed and evaluated for the treatment of cancer, diabetes, and bacterial infections (Anselmo and Mitragotri, 2016; Nikalje, 2015).

Emerging quantum mechanical properties exhibited in various size ranges have positioned nanomaterials as a promising area of exploration in medical science (Maila, 2009). The advent of previously unavailable tools such as quantum nanodots, highly paramagnetic nanoparticles, and nano-polymeric suspensions has further expanded the field. Consequently, new research areas, including nanotechnology in vaccine development and nanobiotechnology, have emerged, increasing the application of nanomaterials in the natural sciences (Schwendener, 2014). The significance of nanotechnology in virology has grown significantly over the past decade. Nanoparticles have been utilized for imaging and as medication-delivery adjuvants to enhance virucidal properties in analytic, preventive, and therapeutic approaches. Virucidal nanoparticles have also been explored for the management of infections such as Human Immunodeficiency Virus (HIV), Hepatitis, and Herpes Simplex Virus (HSV). While research on nanoparticles for virucidal effects is ongoing, no clinical or pre-clinical trials have been approved yet (Cruz et al., 2011; Yu et al., 2009). This chapter assesses the methods of formulating nanoparticulate oxides, their fundamental physicochemical properties, and the utilization of several well-known oxides in this domain, with special attention given to their use as antimicrobial and antiviral agents.

3.2 METAL AND METAL OXIDE NANOPARTICLES SYNTHESIS PROTOCOLS

Nanoparticles are integrated using either top-down or bottom-up synthesis methods. Top-down synthesis employs mechanical techniques to reduce the size of bulk materials into nanosized structures one by one. Bottom-up synthesis at the nanoscale stage involves the assembly of atoms or molecules from molecule to molecule (Narayanan and Sakthivel, 2010). Top-down interventions involve reducing the size of a suitable starting material to generate nanoparticles, accomplished through various physical and chemical treatments. Flaws in the surface design of the product are encountered during top-down interventions, posing a significant constraint as surface structure and other real nanoparticle features primarily depend on this structure (Thakkar et al., 2011). In the bottom-up approach, nanoparticles consist of smaller entities like electrons, molecules, and other tiny structures (Hurst et al., 2006). The building blocks for nanoparticles are initially calculated in this nanostructure and then assembled to produce the final particle (Thakkar et al., 2011).

The bottom-up strategy for producing metal nanoparticles involves both chemical and biological techniques. However, this synthesis type employs hazardous chemicals, often leading to unfavorable environmental consequences, as shown in Figure 3.1. Due to these challenges, this synthesis method is seldom used for manufacturing metal nanoparticles. These are among the most commonly employed techniques for nanoparticle production.

3.2.1 PHYSICAL METHOD

Physical methods for the amalgamation of nanoparticles (NPs) include ultraviolet radiation, microwave light, sonochemistry, thermal decomposition (thermolytic), photochemistry, and radical induction (Khandel et al., 2018). These methods utilize a top-down approach to prevent solvent contamination and yield monodisperse NPs. During physical NP

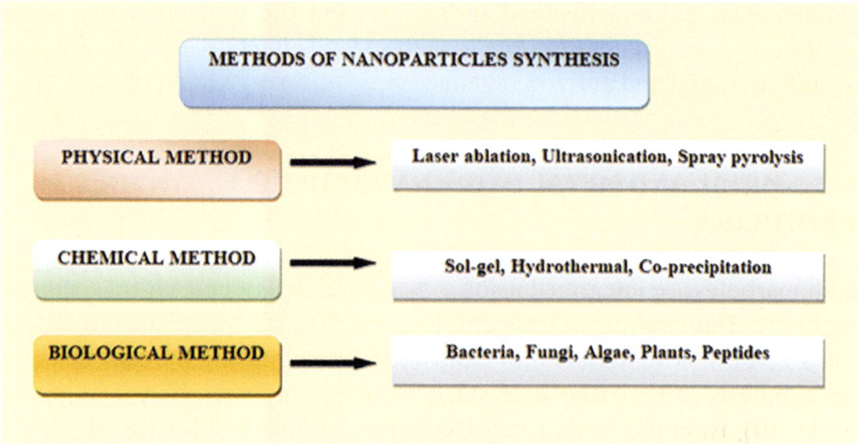

FIGURE 3.1 Various methods of synthesizing metal oxide nanoparticles.

synthesis, metal ions disperse, and the metal atoms reconfigure, forming small clusters of NPs, which are then rapidly condensed under controlled conditions. However, the significant waste generated by physical NP synthesis methods appears to be cost-prohibitive (Online et al., 2015).

3.2.2 CHEMICAL METHOD

The bottom-up approach to metal NP synthesis encompasses various techniques, including hydrothermal blending, the sol-gel technique, chemical vapor synthesis, micro-emulsion, and polyol synthesis (Egorova and Revina, 2000). Chemical synthesis techniques are employed to produce nanoparticles with well-defined size, shape, and structure. This process involves the use of chemical reductants to reduce metal particles or the application of additional energy to decompose metal precursors in the presence of a stabilizer (Patel et al., 2019). Both inorganic and organic solvents serve as reducing agents. Stabilizing agents such as natural/synthetic polymers and organic solvents are utilized to prevent the agglomeration of metal NPs. Surfactants with various functionalities (such as acids, thiols, amines, and alcohols) act as stabilizers, preserving particles from agglomeration, sedimentation, and loss of surface-based properties (Yu et al., 2009). Despite the attractive advantages of chemically synthesized NPs, the use of toxic and non-biodegradable synthetic chemicals presents potential drawbacks (Thevenot et al., 2008).

3.2.3 BIOLOGICAL METHOD

The bottom-up approach to the biological synthesis of metal NPs involves the use of single-cell and multi-cell organic entities, such as microorganisms, actinomycetes, viruses, algae, yeast, and plants (Das et al., 2017; Ingale and Chaudhari, 2013). Biogenic nanoparticles are environmentally friendly, can be produced in large quantities rapidly, are biocompatible, and exhibit distinct size and morphology. Various factors, including pH, temperature, reactant concentration, reaction time, and others, influence the size, morphology, nucleation, and stability of biogenic NPs (Shah et al., 2015). Metal NPs can be generated by microorganisms through two pathways: intracellular and extracellular (Das et al., 2017; Fang et al., 2019). Biological extracts from various plant parts, including leaves, flowers, stems, seeds, and roots, are also considered safe and environmentally friendly. Current metabolites, such as phenolic acids, sugars, proteins, terpenoids, and alkaloids in plants, primarily facilitate the bio-reduction of metal particles and the development of stable NPs. Organic methods are preferred to avoid typical toxicity, cytotoxicity, and disease-causing properties (Majdi et al., 2011).

3.3 METAL AND METAL OXIDE NANOPARTICLES AS ANTIMICROBIAL AGENTS

Metal and metal oxide nanoparticles have gained significant attention from scientists as antibacterial agents due to their distinctive chemical, magnetic, physical, electrical, optical, and biological properties. The primary mechanism of antibacterial action involves the generation of reactive oxygen species (ROS). Various modes of action include photo-killing, genotoxicity, protein toxicity, catalyst poisoning, electrostatic interaction-induced damage to cell membranes, and disturbance of metal/metal particle equilibrium. The attachment of nanoparticles to the bacterial cell wall and their internalization, particularly in Gram-negative bacteria, have been demonstrated. This leads to the inhibition of protein synthesis, inactivation of DNA and enzymes, ultimately resulting in bacterial cell death (Figure 3.2) (Beveridge, 1999). Nanoparticles possess a large surface area, enabling effective interaction with bacteria. Nanotechnology currently offers a robust framework for modifying the physicochemical properties of various materials to produce efficient antimicrobials (Beyth et al., 2015). Silver (Ag), Gold (Au), Zinc Oxide (ZnO), Titanium Dioxide (TiO), Copper Oxide (CuO), and potentially Magnesium Oxide (MgO) are the primary metal NPs utilized as antibacterial agents, as depicted in (Table 3.1) (Zhang, 2015). Metal oxide nanoparticles have exhibited biocidal properties against Gram-positive and Gram-negative bacteria in various studies.

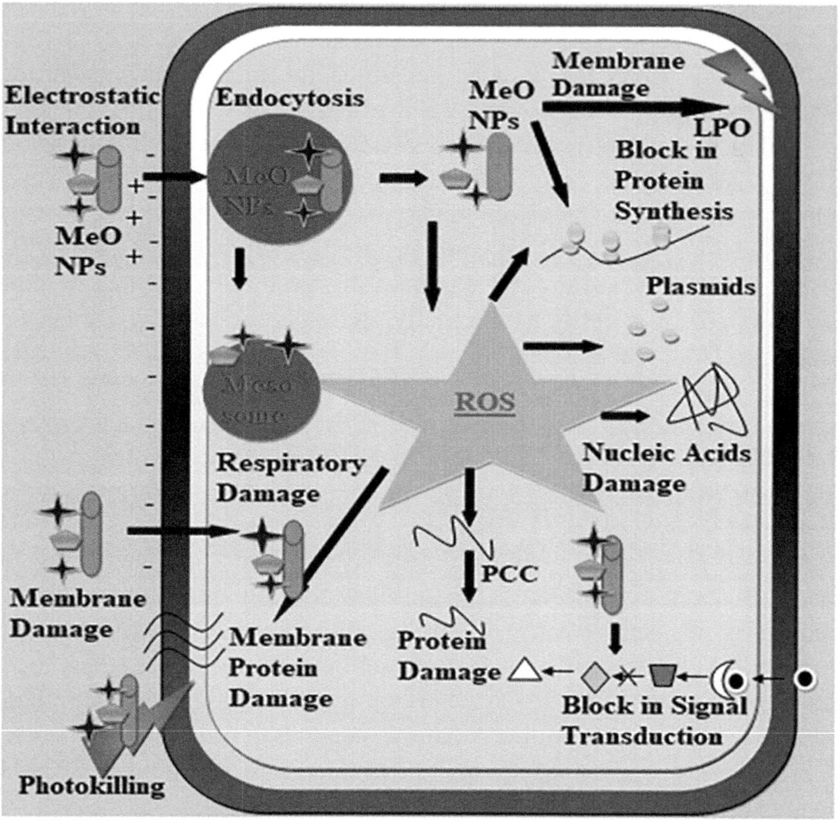

FIGURE 3.2 Outline of antimicrobial systems by metal oxide nanoparticles (MeO-NPs): ROS, reactive oxygen species; LPO, lipid peroxidation.

The surface area in contact with microorganisms is known to influence the antimicrobial action of nanoparticles (Franci et al., 2015; Xiaoming Li et al., 2016). The bactericidal effect of metal nanoparticles is attributed

TABLE 3.1 Metal Oxide Nanoparticles (MeO-NPs) and Their Antimicrobial Potential

MeO-NP	Synthesis	Characterisation	Micro-organisms tested	Outcome	References
Nano silver decorated TiO_2 nanofibers	Electrospinning produces titanium nanofibers. Photochemical process is used to decorate nano silver	SEM (Scanning electron microscopy), XRD	*S. aureus* and *E. coli*	The expansion of nano silver improved the antibacterial activity.	Srisitthiratkul et al. (2011)
Ag-doped and TiO_2 NPs	Modified Sol-gel	UV-Visible, XRD, PL, and TEM	*S. aureus, P. aeruginosa*	It had insignificant imperativeness on *P. aeruginosa* at 40 mg/30 mL, and complete inhibition on *S. aureus* and *E. coli* at 60 mg/30 ml	Gupta et al. (2013)
Silver oxide (AgO) and ZnO NP composite resin	ZnO and AgO	Scanning Electron Microscopy (SEM) with Energy Dispersive X-Ray Analysis (EDX)	*Streptococcus mutans* and Lactobacillus sp	Antibacterial activity against the two microorganisms that were examined in the oral cavity	Kasraei (2014)
ZnO (self-standing agar-based film incorporated with ZnO)	Reflux	SEM and XRD	*E. coli* and *S. aureus*	The nanoparticles were bactericidal in nature towards the tested organisms - *E. coli* and *S. aureus*	Devi and Nagaraj (2014)
Graphene oxide (GO) composites with Cu, Mn, Zn, Ag, AgP, and S	Chemical	AAS, DLS, DPV and SEM	*S. aureus,* MRSA and *E. coli*	Best antibacterial efficiency of all the composites tested against the most common pathogens.	Richtera et al. (2015)
Aluminium oxide (Al_2O_3) NPs	Sigma-Aldrich (purchased)	XRD, HR-TEM and SEM	Clinical isolates of *E. coli*	The growth and multiplication of ESBL-producing *E. coli* were slowed.	Ansari et al. (2013)

TABLE 3.1 *(Continued)*

MeO-NP	Synthesis	Characterisation	Micro-organisms tested	Outcome	References
Bismuth oxide (Bi_2O_3) NPs	Pulsed laser ablation	AAS, AFM and TEM	*E. coli*, *Pseudomonas aeruginosa*, and *Acinetobacter baumannii*	There was no effect on all microorganisms tested at varying concentrations.	Jawad et al. (2022)
Calcium oxide (CaO) NPs	Chemical	XRD, TGA and TEM	*Lactobacillus plantarum*	The bactericidal action of CaO NPs kept in vacuum for 15 hours during planning was more noteworthy.	Artigo (2013)
CaO NPs	Microwave	XRD and HR-TEM	*Candida tropicalis*, *Staphylococcus epidermidis*, and *Pseudomonas aeruginosa*	Stronger antibacterial activity was shown towards Gram-positive strains than Gram-negative ones.	Roy et al. (2013)
CeO_2 NPs	*Aspergillus niger*	UV-Vis, FTIR, XRD, TG/DTA, PL, and TEM	*E. coli*, *Streptococcus pneumoniae*, *B. subtilis*, *Proteus vulgaris*, and *Streptococcus pneumoniae*	Bacterial growth and biofilm biomass were not limited by any of the tested bacterial strains.	Karthika and Gowri (2015)
Cobalt oxide (Co_3O_4) NPs (Co_3O_4-I)	Pyrolytic	TGA, FTIR, SEM, TEM and XRD	*S. aureus* and *E. coli*	Antimicrobial activity was checked against the two microorganisms tested.	Ghosh et al. (2014)

TABLE 3.1 *(Continued)*

MeO-NP	Synthesis	Characterisation	Micro-organisms tested	Outcome	References
CuO NPs	Microwave	SEM, XRD, UV-Vis and FTIR	*Shigella dysenteriae*, *Vibrio cholerae*, *S. pneumoniae*, *S. aureus* and *E. coli*	Antibacterial activity was observed in *S. dysenteriae* and *V. cholerae*	Sutradhar et al. (2014)
CuO NPs	Sigma-Aldrich (Purchased)	-	MRSA, MRSE, VRE, *E. coli*, *K. pneumoniae*, *Pseudomonas* spp., and *Proteus mirabilis*	Uropathogens that produce biofilms were significantly reduced (MRSA and *E. coli*)	Agarwala et al. (2014)
Iron oxide (IO) NPs	Co-precipitation	XRD, SEM and UV-Spectroscopy	*S. aureus*, *Bacillus licheniformis*, *Brevibacillus brevis*, *V. cholerae*, *S. epidermidis*, *B. subtilis* and *E. coli*	Among the 10 microorganisms inspected, it showed moderate antibacterial movement against six Gram-positive and two Gram-negative harmful microbes.	Behera et al. (2012)
α-Fe_2O_3 NPs	Chemical	XRD, BET, XPS and TEM	*P. aeruginosa*	Biofilm development and increased *P. aeruginosa* growth	Jennifer et al. (2015)
NiO NPs	Bio-gel two-step synthesis	XRD, FE-SEM, EDX and TEM	*P. aeruginosa* and *B. subtilis*	Their efficiency against Gram-positive and Gram-negative bacteria indicated a broad spectrum of antibacterial action.	Online et al. (2015)

TABLE 3.1 *(Continued)*

MeO-NP	Synthesis	Characterisation	Micro-organisms tested	Outcome	References
ZnO NPs	-	-	*B. subtilis*, *Bacillus megaterium*, *S. aureus*, *E. coli*, *P. aeruginosa*, and *P. vulgaris*	To the pathogens examined, it had a good bacteriostatic impact but a weak bactericidal impact.	Alekish et al. (2018)
ZnO NPs	Wet chemical precipitation	XRD, TEM and FTIR	*B. subtilis*, *Salmonella paratyphi*, *E. aerogenes*, MRSA, *Candida albicans*, and *Malassezia pachydermatis*	Antimicrobial activity was displayed against normal pathogenic microscopic organisms.	Palanikumar et al. (2014)
ZnO NPs	Standard method	SEM and XRD	*K. pneumonia*	Regardless of medication resistance mechanism, physical and chemical factors inhibited *K. pneumoniae*.	Reddy et al. (2014)
Ag-TiO_2, composite nanostructured samples	Modified sol-gel	EDX, XRD, FTIR, UV-Vis, BET and XPS	*E. coli* cells or *B. subtilis* spores	Increased silver doping had massive antibacterial effects on B. subtilis and E. coli without photoactivation.	Hamal et al. (2010)
Zinc/iron oxide composite NPs	Chemical	ICP, XRD and TEM	*S. aureus* and *E. coli*	With a greater [Zn]/[Fe] weight ratio, *S. aureus* demonstrated the highest antibacterial activity, followed by *E. coli*.	Gordon et al. (2011)

TABLE 3.1 *(Continued)*

MeO-NP	Synthesis	Characterisation	Micro-organisms tested	Outcome	References
ZnO NPs + ultrasound	Alfa Aesar	DLS	*S. aureus* and *P. aeruginosa*	Ultrasound incitement had a higher antibacterial effect than NPs alone on *S. aureus*	Seil and Webster (2012)
Vanadium pentoxide (V_2O_5) nanowires with H_2O_2 and Br	Chemical	TEM and ICP-MS	*E. coli* and *S. aureus*	Strong antibacterial activity against Gram-positive and Gram-negative bacteria, and they could be employed as antifouling agents for marine biota.	Hartog et al. (2012)
Hybrid CH-α-Fe_2O_3 nanocomposite	Self-assembly	XRD, AFM, FTIR, SEMEDX, UV-Vis and UVDRS	*S. aureus* and *E. coli*	Enhanced Antibacterial effectiveness against *S. aureus* and *E. coli*	Halliah et al. (2014)
Zinc-doped CuO nanocomposite	Sonochemical irradiation	XRD, SEM, HRSEM-FEI, DSC and ESR	*S. aureus*, *E. coli* MRSA and MDR *E. coli*	All bacteria tested showed exceptional biocidal activity.	Malka et al. (2013)
Chitosan-based ZnO NPs	Nano spray drying and precipitation	UV-Vis, DLS and SEM	*C. albicans*, *Micrococcus luteus* and *S. aureus*	*M. luteus* and *S. aureus* were found to have antimicrobial and biofilm inhibition properties.	Singh and Surinder (2014)
ZnO NPs are used to embellish a few stacked graphene sheets.	Hydrothermal followed by reduction is the Hummers process (graphene oxide).	XRD, TEM and Raman spectroscopy	*E. coli* and *S. Typhi*	Had substantially stronger antibacterial activity against *S. Typhi* than *E. coli.*	Bykkam et al. (2015)

TABLE 3.1 *(Continued)*

MeO-NP	Synthesis	Characterisation	Micro-organisms tested	Outcome	References
Silver-decorated TiO_2NPs	Chemical	HR-TEM, FEG-SEM, XRD	MRSA and *Candida* spp.	MRSA and *Candida* spp. cells had an antibacterial impact on both planktonic and biofilm-forming cells.	André et al. (2015)
Graphene oxide-modified ZnO NPs	Solution precipitation	FE-SEM, AFM, FTIR and XRD	*E. coli, S. Typhimurium, B. subtilis* and *E. faecalis*	Enhanced antibacterial activity was seen against all microorganisms tested.	Press (2015)

to their small size and high surface-to-volume ratio, allowing them to intimately interact with microbial membranes, rather than just the release of metal particles into the solution (Search et al., 2016). Specific essential metal particles are crucial for the biochemistry of life in all organisms, and their absence can have serious consequences. However, the aggregation of these particles or the presence of other unnecessary particles (like Ag) can lead to protein dysfunction, oxidative stress, or membrane damage, which can be lethal to cells (Lemire et al., 2013). Several metal nanoparticles have demonstrated antimicrobial properties against various pathogenic microorganisms. Moreover, these have found applications in synthetic textiles, water treatment, biomedical and surgical instruments, as well as food processing and packaging (Franci et al., 2015).

3.3.1 SILVER NANOPARTICLES (AgNPs)

Silver nanoparticles (AgNPs) are the most widely used nanomaterials. A wide range of microorganisms, *including Listeria monocytogenes, Escherichia coli, Streptococcus aureus, Enterococcus faecalis, Acinetobacter baumannii, Klebsiella pneumoniae, Salmonella typhi, Micrococcus luteus*, and *Staphylococcus epidermidis*, are susceptible to the antimicrobial effects of silver compounds (Press, 2014; Tamayo et al., 2014; Wang et al., 2014). AgNPs can be incorporated into various matrices such as catheters, bandages, and surgical dressings to control bacterial colonization on different surfaces and prevent infections. Applications of AgNPs include burn treatment, eradication of microorganisms on synthetic fabrics, and water treatment. Although the use of silver in food is prohibited, traces may be present on fruits and vegetables washed with AgNPs suspensions. AgNPs find application in food packaging due to their ability to extend shelf life, yet their use in food packaging is restricted by the EU and the US. Sanitation authorities suggest their cautious use due to the inability to make definitive claims about their toxicity (Antiochia, 2016). Polystyrene with AgNPs has been found to have high temperature stability and low volatility, and AgNPs can be incorporated into various matrices (Kim et al., 2002; Taylor et al., 2013). AgNPs coated on graphene nanosheets have also demonstrated antibacterial and antibiofilm properties. The nanocomposite exhibited antibacterial activity against *Pseudomonas aeruginosa* at a minimum inhibitory concentration and a 100% inhibition rate against bacterial cells adhered to clean surfaces (Alves, 2013). AgNPs can even be incorporated into nanofiber scaffolds, resulting in an intriguing material that could be used as an antimicrobial wound dressing (Dubey et al., 2015).

3.3.2 GOLD NANOPARTICLES (AuNPs)

Gold nanoparticles (AuNPs) have recently been proposed for prophylactic, clinical, sterile, and hygienic applications. Primary uses of AuNPs include diagnostic assays, gene, and drug delivery to various target tissues or specific tumors, as well as radiotherapy enhancers/sensitizers. Specific applications include drug delivery, antigens such as peptides, DNA, identification, and photo-thermolysis of microorganisms as well as cancer cells, biosensors, immunoassays, and clinical science. Broad applications also encompass water purification and the management of various rheumatic diseases (Dykman and Khlebtsov, 2012; Zhang, 2015). AuNPs are generally considered biologically inert but can be modified to have chemical or photothermal properties. The use of functionalized hydrophobic and cationic AuNPs has demonstrated efficacy against 11 clinical multi-drug-resistant (MDR) bacterial strains, with the nanoparticles inhibiting their growth under near-infrared (NIR) light. This highlights the effectiveness of gold-based nanomaterials with characteristic NIR absorption in eradicating cancer cells and diverse bacteria through photothermal heating (Franci et al., 2015; Xiaoning Li et al., 2014). By conjugating antibiotics such as kanamycin and forming kanamycin-coated AuNPs (Kan-AuNPs) against various bacteria such as *S. bovis, S. epidermidis, E. aerogenes, P. aeruginosa*, and *Y. pestis*, it was demonstrated that AuNP conjugation significantly enhanced their effectiveness as antibiotics against both sensitive and resistant bacterial strains (Payne et al., 2016). Highly stable AuNPs prepared against *Bacillus* sp., functionalized with effective antibiotics such as ciprofloxacin, gentamycin, rifampicin, and vancomycin, have shown effectiveness against coagulase-negative staphylococci (CoNS), including *Staphylococcus epidermidis* and *S. haemolyticus* (Roshmi et al., 2015).

3.3.3 COPPER OXIDE NANOPARTICLES

Copper nanoparticles (CuNPs), valuable semiconductors with a variety of functionally potent physical properties, including superconductivity, electron correlation effects, and spin dynamics, have gained increased attention recently, also due to reduced development costs (Ungur and Hrůza, 2017). CuNPs have attracted attention for their catalytic, optical, electrical, and antimicrobial applications (Ingle et al., 2013; Letfullin et al., 2011). Despite their wide range of applications, CuNPs are limited by the inherent reactivity of copper in atmospheric conditions, making them prone to oxidation (Gawande et al., 2016). To address this issue of oxidation, researchers are using inert media such as argon and nitrogen, as well as processes involving reducing, coating, and protecting agents for the reduction of copper salts (Ahmed, 2016). Silver and copper were used for the treatment of microbial infections until the advent of antibiotics and other chemotherapeutics. Copper compounds, unfortunately, are toxic to certain species and can be hazardous to the environment. Copper nanoparticles, on the other hand, can be used as an alternative to mitigate these effects (Ingle et al., 2013). CuNPs have demonstrated their effectiveness against a variety of bacterial pathogens, although they lack the antibacterial efficacy seen in Ag or ZnO. CuNPs have been reported to be effective against bacteria such as *E. coli, S. aureus, B. subtilis, Micrococcus luteus, Klebsiella pneumoniae*, and *Bacillus megaterium* in numerous studies (Ruparelia et al., 2008). *P. aeruginosa* was found to be resistant to CuNPs; however, the antimicrobial activities of CuO nanoparticles are believed to vary significantly depending on the challenged strains of various bacteria (Ramyadevi et al., 2012).

3.3.4 ZINC OXIDE (ZnO) NANOPARTICLES

Zinc oxide (ZNO) nanoparticles are toxic to both Gram-positive and Gram-negative bacteria, as well as heat- and pressure-resistant spores (Ma et al., 2013). ZnO, however, has a negligible effect on human cells, proving to be safe for use as an antimicrobial agent (Judith and Espitia, 2012). Several experiments have shown that ZnO nanoparticles have antimicrobial activity against bacteria such as *E. coli, Pseudomonas fluorescens*, and *S. aureus* (Microbiology and Food, 2009; Zhang et al., 2008). ZnO nanoparticles are effective against biofilm formation, making them suitable for use as coating materials in clinical and other products (Bogutska et al., 2013). Nano zinc compounds have become increasingly important in biomedicine in recent years. For example, nanoparticles of ZnO are typical UV-blocking components due to their excellent reflective properties (in sunscreens, cosmetic creams, and ointments) as well as UV spectrum absorption (Bogutska et al., 2013; Ma et al., 2013). The FDA has approved the use of ZnO in cosmetics (Manuscript, 2014). ZnO nanoparticles can be used as biosensors to detect glucose, H_2O_2, cholesterol, and urea due to their chemical stability and rapid electrochemical response. In the field of biomedicine, it was found that ZnO nanoparticles selectively destroy certain cancer cells, alleviating issues associated with most chemotherapy drugs (Bogutska et al., 2013). Finally, ZnO is one of the five zinc compounds identified by the US Food and Drug Administration as a generally recognized as safe (GRAS) substance and is available as a food additive (Judith and Espitia, 2012).

3.3.5 TITANIUM DIOXIDE NANOPARTICLES (TIO_2NPS)

Titanium dioxide (TiO_2) nanoparticles have gained considerable attention recently due to their unique and enhanced properties compared to their bulk material counterparts. The properties of these substances, both chemically and physically, are significantly influenced by their particle size, demonstrating quantum size effects (Othman et al., 2014). TiO_2NPs have antibacterial activity against multi-antibiotic-resistant strains of *E. coli*, *Pseudomonas aeruginosa*, *Staphylococcus aureus*, and *Pseudomonas putida*, as well as *Bacillus spores* (Bonetta et al., 2013; Yao and Yeung, 2020). Consequently, TiO_2 has been used as an antibacterial agent, as well as self-cleaning and disinfecting materials for surface coatings (ATCC, 2008). TiO_2 also features in wastewater and air purification due to its photocatalytic activity (Weir et al., 2012). In addition to disinfecting equipment in the food industry, TiO_2 can be used in food processing. Recently, researchers developed TiO_2 nanoparticle-coated films, and as the concentration of TiO_2 nanoparticles increased, both fluorescent and UV light enhanced the antibacterial activity of the films. UV light proved more efficient than fluorescent light due to the appropriate band gap, energy spectrum, and increased hydroxyl radical concentration on the surface of the coated films (Othman et al., 2014). TiO_2 nanoparticles have also been shown in some studies to regulate organic molecules such as ethylene, providing yet another compelling reason to use TiO_2 in the food and packaging industries (Li et al., 2018). Silicon dioxide and titanium dioxide are the two nanoparticles often used in food packaging (Pradhan et al., 2015). Biomedical uses of TiO_2 include photodynamic therapy, drug delivery systems, cancer treatments, cell imaging, biosensors in biological testing, and genetic editing (Mahyad, 2020).

3.4 ANTIVIRAL APPLICATIONS OF METAL AND METAL OXIDE NANOPARTICLES

The antiviral activity and efficacy of metal nanoparticles are determined by their shape, size, and various metal ions. Metal-capped NPs have substantially better interaction both with viruses and host cells than bare metal NPs (Galdiero et al., 2011). Their method of action has been found to occur both inside and outside the host cells. Possible methods of action include inactivation of viral particles before cellular entry, interaction with viral DNA, and attachment of viral particles. Furthermore, virally encoded host cellular components essential for viral replication and the formation of progeny virions are highly present in the intracellular compartment of an infected cell. As a result, another antiviral mechanism is the interaction of metal NPs with all these factors of replication. Metal NPs, especially with silver (Ag) and gold (Au), have been shown to exhibit antiviral properties against a variety of infections (Aderibigbe, 2017).

Copper and other metal NPs impede the attachment of the virus, virus-cell interaction, and penetration of the virus into target cells. Copper (Cu) NPs also damage the capsid and kill viral DNA. Zinc (Zn) NPs suppress viral replication by interfering with viral DNA polymerase activity. The capacity of zinc NPs to attach to virions is required to prevent viral entry into target cells. To prevent the virus from connecting with cells, iron (Fe) NPs preferentially bind to it. Selenium NPs, on the other hand, efficiently protect target cells from apoptosis caused by virus infection (Rai et al., 2014). Several publications on the antiviral activity of metal NPs have been released in recent years, and these are described in detail below subsections.

3.4.1 ADENOVIRUSES

Human adenoviruses (HAdVs) are widespread DNA viruses with global pathogenicity. This virus poses a risk to adults, newborns, and immunocompromised individuals, causing respiratory, gastrointestinal, urinary, and ophthalmic disorders (Khanal, 2018). For immunocompromised patients, the clinical treatment of HAdVs contamination focuses on symptom alleviation or the use of antiviral drugs such as ribavirin and cidofovir for severe HAdVs infections (Khanal, 2018). Despite promising treatment results, the therapeutic application of cidofovir is limited due to its low bioavailability and nephrotoxic effects (Nichols et al., 2008). Human adenovirus infections have been studied using silver (Ag), gold (Au), and tungsten (W) carbide NPs as potential treatments (Chen et al., 2013). *In vitro*, silver NPs were found to have dose-dependent inhibitory activity against adenovirus. After 2 hours of incubation, the half-maximal effective concentration (EC50) of the tested silver NPs against virally infected cells was found to be 9.3 g/mL, which was proven to be non-harmful to uninfected cells (Chen et al., 2013). The associated toxicity of gold ions is reduced when gold NPs are escorted by silicon dioxide shells, forming gold-silicon dioxide carrier NPs. Both forms of NPs were found to be effective against adenovirus, with 96% and 100% inhibition. Tungsten carbide NPs were shown to reduce the type 5 Adenovirus infection rate by 50% in 15 minutes. Other viruses that these NPs exhibited antiviral action against included the modified vaccinia virus Ankara (MVA), poliovirus, and norovirus. These NPs could be used as a constructive nanotechnology-based disinfection in this case (Pfaff et al., 2019).

3.4.2 CORONAVIRUS (CoV)

Coronavirus (CoV) is a zoonotic virus with an enclosed positive-sense RNA genome (Singhal, 2020). It comprises a variety of viruses that cause the common cold, as well as severe respiratory problems such as Middle East respiratory syndrome (MERS), severe acute respiratory syndrome (SARS), and COVID-19 in humans (Nikaeen et al., 2020). Nanotechnology has gained significant attention from scientists for use in a coronavirus vaccine (Hasegawa et al., 2019), therapy, diagnostic tool, and protective measure (Nasrollahzadeh et al., 2020; Nikaeen et al., 2020). A novel nanorod-based gold HR1 peptide inhibitor (PIH-Au NRs) for MERS was recently validated in a study. The PIH-Au NRs exhibited a 10-fold greater inhibitory activity than the peptide alone, at a concentration of 1.171 M. Furthermore, the PIH-Au NRs completely prevented cell fusion at the same dose. The researchers also found that the newly produced PIH-Au NRs were biologically compatible, biostable, and an effective anti-MERS agent (Huang et al., 2019). The activity of glutathione-capped silver sulfide nanoclusters of 5.3 nm size against pig epidemic diarrhea virus (PEDV), a coronavirus model, has been confirmed. Plaque formation units (PFU) were reduced from 3.8 (105 per ml) to 2.5 (102 per ml) after 12 hours of treatment using a concentration of 46 g/ml. Treatment with the tested nanoclusters also suppressed PEDV infection by triggering the production of IFN-stimulating genes (ISGs) along with pro-inflammatory cytokines, according to the findings. These nanoclusters also inhibited viral replication and budding. As a result of these findings, further research on additional metal NPs, such as copper and zinc, to prevent coronavirus infections is now possible (Du et al., 2018).

3.4.3 HEPATITIS VIRUS

Virulent hepatitis is one of the leading causes of liver disease, mortality, and disabilities worldwide (Do and Reau, 2020). Liver diseases include cirrhosis, hepatocellular carcinoma, decompensated illness, and extrahepatic symptoms. Hepatitis C is currently curable if detected early and treated with direct-acting antiviral therapies. Oral nucleoside treatments with significant resistance barriers are frequently used to treat hepatitis B. Significant progress has been made in the treatment of hepatitis D infection (Thomas, 2019). Despite suppressive antiviral medication, a viral hepatitis cure remains elusive due to the genetic persistence of the virus within the hepatocyte nucleus. Silver nanoparticles have resurfaced as a promising inhibitor of hepatitis replication. Various sizes of silver NPs ranging from 10–80 nm were tested as antiviral agents against hepatitis B in a study. In this work, AgNPs with a size of around 10 nm caused 38% and 80% virus inhibition at concentrations of 5 M and 50 M, respectively, while silver NPs with a size of 50 nm produced 53% and 92% inhibition at concentrations of 5 M and 50 M, respectively. Copper NPs also prevented hepatitis infection only at the entry and attachment stages, according to the study. These findings suggest that Ag and Cu NPs may have new applications for the treatment of long-persisting/chronic hepatitis patients (Elshamy et al., 2019).

3.4.4 RESPIRATORY SYNCYTIAL VIRUS (RSV)

Infection with the RSV, the ubiquitous RNA-based virus, is the leading causative agent of lower respiratory tract diseases in children and adults (Lanari et al., 2014). Prematurely born babies, elderly adults, infants, adults with chronic respiratory and/or circulatory problems, and immunocompromised patients are all susceptible to severe RSV infections (Meng et al., 2014).

RSV is increasingly recognized as a global health issue and remains a leading cause of mortality. Apart from ribavirin, there are few alternative RSV treatments or licensed vaccines. According to preliminary findings, silver nanoparticles could be used to treat RSV infections (Polak, 2012). Curcumin-modified silver NPs exhibited strong antiviral activity against RSV at concentrations ranging from 0.008–0.12 nM, according to a study. This study found that the curcumin-modified silver NPs directly adhered to the envelope of viral glycoproteins and interfered with the disease pattern of RSV, yielding promising results. As a result, metal NPs, particularly silver, have great potential as antiviral treatments for RSV in the future (Morris et al., 2019).

3.4.5 POLIOVIRUS

Poliovirus has a single-stranded, positively detected RNA genome with 7500 nucleotides, causing poliomyelitis (polio). The wild poliovirus has three serotypes: serotypes two and three were eradicated in 2015 and 2019, respectively, and serotype 1, which is still endemic. Medical manifestations and symptoms range from minor respiratory illness, gastroenteritis, and malaise to severe forms of paralysis (Ghafoor and Sheikh, 2016; Mamun et al., 2020). People of all ages are affected, but it is most common in children under the age of five who have not been vaccinated. Polio is incurable and untreatable (Ghafoor and Sheikh, 2016). The antiviral activity of Ag and W carbide NPs against the poliovirus was studied. Anti-poliovirus action was observed in electrochemically produced 7.1 nm AgNPs with a semi-spherical form and good purity. Within 30 minutes, at a concentration of 3.13 ppm, infectivity of the poliovirus was reduced by 50%. The size of the synthesized NPs was said to be smaller than that of poliovirus particles (20–30 nm) (Huy et al., 2016). Consequently, the NPs could easily engage with viral particles, inhibiting the binding of the virus and its multiplication in host cells. This emphasizes the need for further exploration of the use of metal NPs for poliovirus treatment (Pfaff et al., 2019).

3.5 CONCLUSIONS

The use of metal and metal oxide nanoparticles in clinical research, as well as materials that facilitate both diagnosis and prophylaxis/therapy, has made nanotherapeutics a viable option for the future of drug development.

While a significant number of metals and their oxides can be produced at the nanoscale using nanotechnology, their successful clinical implementation, including modifying their shape, size, and surface, while maintaining them biocompatible and non-toxic, still poses a significant challenge. The growing capabilities of this multidisciplinary field allow for the development of more refined secondary technologies with biomimetic components, as well as improved ligand targeting and multifaceted applications. With optimistic expectations, biomimetic nano-sized metals and metal oxide nanoparticles may one day offer improved diagnostic and antiviral therapies to meet the expanding demand worldwide.

KEYWORDS

- **adenovirus**
- **antimicrobial**
- **antiviral**
- **coronavirus**
- **drug delivery**
- **metal oxide**
- **nanomaterials**
- **nanoparticles**
- **nanotechnology**

REFERENCES

Aderibigbe, B. A. (2017). Metal-based nanoparticles for the treatment of infectious diseases. *Molecules, 22*(8), 1370. https://doi.org/10.3390/molecules22081370 (accessed on 4th July 2025).

Agarwala, M., Choudhury, B., & Yadav, R. N. S. (2014). Comparative study of antibiofilm activity of copper oxide and iron oxide nanoparticles against multidrug resistant biofilm forming uropathogens. *Indian Journal of Microbiology, 54*(3), 365–368. https://doi.org/10.1007/s12088-014-0462-z (accessed on 4th July 2025).

Ahmed, M. Y., & Abdel-Aziz, M. S. (2013). Preparation of polystyrene nanocomposites based on silver nanoparticles using marine bacterium for packaging. *Polymer-Plastics*

Technology and Engineering, 52(6), 607–613. https://doi.org/10.1080/03602559.2012.762658 (accessed on 4th July 2025).

Alekish, M., Ismail, Z. B., Albiss, B., & Nawasrah, S. (2018). *In vitro* antibacterial effects of zinc oxide nanoparticles on multiple drug-resistant strains of *Staphylococcus aureus* and *Escherichia coli*: An alternative approach for antibacterial therapy of mastitis in sheep. *Veterinary World, 11*(10), 1428–1432. https://doi.org/10.14202/vetworld.2018.1428-1432 (accessed on 4th July 2025).

Alves, O. L. (2013). Ac ce p te d us t. *Colloids and Surfaces B: Bio Interfaces*. https://doi.org/10.1016/j.colsurfb.2013.08.006 (accessed on 4th July 2025).

Alzahrani, E. A., & Ahmed, R. A. (2016). Synthesis of copper nanoparticles with various sizes and shapes: Application as a superior non-enzymatic sensor and antibacterial agent. *International Journal of Electrochemical Science, 11*(6), 4712–4713. https://doi.org/10.20964/2016.06.83 (accessed on 4th July 2025).

André, R. S., Zamperini, C. A., Mima, E. G., Longo, V. M., Albuquerque, A. R., Sambrano, J. R., Machado, A. L., et al. (2015). Antimicrobial activity of TiO_2: Ag nanocrystalline heterostructures: Experimental and theoretical insights. *Chemical Physics*. https://doi.org/10.1016/j.chemphys.2015.07.020 (accessed on 4th July 2025).

Ansari, M. A., Khan, H. M., Khan, A. A., Cameotra, S. S., Saquib, Q., & Musarrat, J. (2014). Interaction of Al_2O_3 nanoparticles with *Escherichia coli* and their cell envelope biomolecules. *Journal of Applied Microbiology, 116*(4), 772–783. https://doi.org/10.1111/jam.12423 (accessed on 4th July 2025).

Anselmo, A. C., & Mitragotri, S. (2016). Nanoparticles in the clinic: An update. *Bioengineering and Translational Medicine, 4*(3), e10143. https://doi.org/10.1002/btm2.10003 (accessed on 4th July 2025).

Behera, S. S., Patra, J. K., Pramanik, K., Panda, N., & Thatoi, H. (2012). Characterization and evaluation of antibacterial activities of chemically synthesized iron oxide nanoparticles. *World Journal of Nano Science and Engineering, 2*(4), 196–200.

Beveridge, T. J. (1999). Structures of Gram-negative cell walls and their derived membrane vesicles. *Journal of Bacteriology, 181*(16), 4725–4733. https://doi.org/10.1128/jb.181.16.4725-4733.1999 (accessed on 4th July 2025).

Beyth, N., Houri-Haddad, Y., Domb, A., Khan, W., & Hazan, R. (2015). Alternative antimicrobial approach: Nano-antimicrobial materials. *Evidence-Based Complementary and Alternative Medicine, 2015*, 246012. https://doi.org/10.1155/2015/246012 (accessed on 4th July 2025).

Bogutska, K. I., Sklyarov, Y. P., & Prylutskyy, Y. I. (2013). Zinc and zinc nanoparticles: Biological role and application in biomedicine. *Ukrainica Bioorganica Acta, 1*, 9–16.

Bonetta, S., Bonetta, S., Motta, F., Strini, A., & Carraro, E. (2013). Photocatalytic bacterial inactivation by TiO_2-coated surfaces. *AMB Express, 3*(1), 1. https://doi.org/10.1186/2191-0855-3-59 (accessed on 4th July 2025).

Borcherding, J., Baltrusaitis, J., Chen, H., Stebounova, L., Wu, C. M., Rubasinghege, G., Mudunkotuwa, I. A., et al. (2014). Iron oxide nanoparticles induce *Pseudomonas aeruginosa* growth, induce biofilm formation, and inhibit antimicrobial peptide function. *Environmental Science: Nano, 1*(2), 123–132. https://doi.org/10.1039/C3EN00029J (accessed on 4th July 2025).

Bykkam, S., Narsingam, S., Ahmadipour, M., Dayakar, T., Rao, K. V., Chakra, C. S., & Kalakotla, S. (2015). Few layered graphene sheets decorated by ZnO nanoparticles for anti-bacterial application. *Superlattices and Microstructures, 83*, 776–784. https://doi.org/10.1016/j.spmi.2015.03.063 (accessed on 4th July 2025).

Chen, N., Zheng, Y., Yin, J., Li, X., & Zheng, C. (2013). Inhibitory effects of silver nanoparticles against adenovirus type 3 *in vitro*. *Journal of Virological Methods, 193*(2), 470–477. https://doi.org/10.1016/j.jviromet.2013.07.020 (accessed on 4th July 2025).

Chiriac, V., Stratulat, D. N., Calin, G., Nichitus, S., Burlui, V., Stadoleanu, C., Popa, M., & Popa, I. M. (2016). Antimicrobial property of zinc-based nanoparticles. *IOP Science, 133*(1), 012055. https://doi.org/10.1088/1757-899X/133/1/012055 (accessed on 4th July 2024).

Cruz, L. J., Tacken, P. J., Bonetto, F., Buschow, S. I., Croes, H. J., Wijers, M., De Vries, I. J., & Figdor, C. G. (2011). Multimodal imaging of nano vaccine carriers targeted to human dendritic cells. *Molecular Pharmaceutics, 8*(2), 520–531. https://doi.org/10.1021/mp100356k (accessed on 4th July 2025).

Das, R. K., Laxman, V., & Pachapur, L. (2017). Biological synthesis of metallic nanoparticles: Plants, animals and microbial aspects. *Nanotechnology for Environmental Engineering, 2*(1), 1–21. https://doi.org/10.1007/s41204-017-0029-4 (accessed on 4th July 2025).

Devi, L. G., & Nagaraj, B. (2014). Disinfection of *Escherichia coli* Gram negative bacteria using surface modified TiO_2: Optimization of Ag metallization and depiction of charge transfer mechanism. *Photochemistry and Photobiology, 3*, 1089–1098. https://doi.org/10.1111/php.12308 (accessed on 4th July 2025).

Dhand, C., Dwivedi, N., Loh, X. J., Jie Ying, A. N., Varma, N. K., Beuerman, R. W., Lakshminarayanan, R., & Ramakrishna, S. (2015). Methods and strategies for the synthesis of diverse nanoparticles and their applications: A comprehensive overview. *RSC Advances, 5*, 105003–105037. https://doi.org/10.1039/C5RA19388E (accessed on 4th July 2025).

Do, A., & Reau, N. S. (2020). Chronic viral hepatitis: Current management and future directions. *Hepatology Communications, 4*(3), 329–341. https://doi.org/10.1002/hep4.1480 (accessed on 4th July 2025).

Du, T., Liang, J., Dong, N., Lu, J., Fu, Y., Fang, L., Xiao, S., & Han, H. (2018). Glutathione-capped Ag_2S nanoclusters inhibit coronavirus proliferation through blockage of viral RNA synthesis and budding. *ACS Applied Materials & Interfaces*. https://doi.org/10.1021/acsami.7b13811 (accessed on 4th July 2025).

Dubey, P., Bhushan, B., Sachdev, A., Matai, I., Kumar, S. U., & Gopinath, P. (2015). Silver-nanoparticle-incorporated composite nanofibers for potential wound-dressing applications. *Journal of Applied Polymer Science, 42473*, 1–12. https://doi.org/10.1002/app.42473 (accessed on 4th July 2025).

Dykman, L., & Khlebtsov, N. (2012). Gold nanoparticles in biomedical applications: Recent advances and perspectives. *Chemical Society Reviews*, 2256–2282. https://doi.org/10.1039/c1cs15166e (accessed on 4th July 2025).

Egorova, E. M., & Revina, A. A. (2000). Synthesis of metallic nanoparticles in reverse micelles in the presence of quercetin. *Colloid Journal, 168*, 87–96.

Elshamy, A. M., Rabeh, M. A., Salem, M., Samir, A., Bin Muhsinah, A., & Alsayari, A. (2019). Antiviral potential of green synthesized silver nanoparticles of *Lampranthus coccineus* and *Malephora lutea*. *Molecules*. (accessed on 4th July 2025).

Fang, X., Wang, Y., Wang, Z., Jiang, Z., & Dong, M. (2019). Microorganism-assisted synthesized nanoparticles for catalytic applications. *Energies, 12*(1), 190. https://doi.org/10.3390/en12010190 (accessed on 4th July 2025).

Food Microbiology. (2009). Antimicrobial efficacy of zinc oxide quantum dots against *Listeria monocytogenes*, *Salmonella enteritidis*, and *Escherichia coli* O157:H7. *74*(1). https://doi.org/10.1111/j.1750-3841.2008.01013.x (accessed on 4th July 2024).

Franci, G., Falanga, A., Galdiero, S., Palomba, L., Rai, M., Morelli, G., & Galdiero, M. (2015). Silver nanoparticles as potential antibacterial agents. *Molecules, 20*(5), 8856–8874. https://doi.org/10.3390/molecules20058856 (accessed on 4th July 2025).

Galdiero, S., Falanga, A., Vitiello, M., Cantisani, M., Marra, V., & Galdiero, M. (2011). Silver nanoparticles as potential antiviral agents. *Molecules, 16*(10), 8894–8918. https://doi.org/10.3390/molecules16108894 (accessed on 4th July 2025).

Gawande, M. B., Goswami, A., Asefa, T., Huang, X., Silva, R., Zou, X., Zboril, R., & Varma, R. S. (2016). Cu and Cu-based nanoparticles: Synthesis and applications in catalysis. *Chemical Reviews*. https://doi.org/10.1021/acs.chemrev.5b00482 (accessed on 4th July 2025).

Ghafoor, S., & Sheikh, N. (2016). Eradication and current status of poliomyelitis in Pakistan. *Virology Research Journal, 2016*(May).

Ghosh, T., Dash, K., Chakraborty, P., & Guha, A. (2014). Preparation of antiferromagnetic Co_3O_4 nanoparticles from two different precursors by pyrolytic method: *In vitro* antimicrobial activity. *RSC Advances*, 15022–15029. https://doi.org/10.1039/c3ra47769j (accessed on 4th July 2025).

Gordon, T., Perlstein, B., Houbara, O., Felner, I., Banin, E., & Margel, S. (2011). Synthesis and characterization of zinc/iron oxide composite nanoparticles and their antibacterial properties. *Colloids and Surfaces A: Physicochemical and Engineering Aspects, 374*(1–3), 1–8. https://doi.org/10.1016/j.colsurfa.2010.10.015 (accessed on 4th July 2025).

Gupta, K., Singh, R. P., Pandey, A., & Pandey, A. (2013). Photocatalytic antibacterial performance of TiO_2 and Ag-doped TiO_2 against *S. aureus*, *P. aeruginosa*, and *E. coli*. *Beilstein Journal of Nanotechnology*, 345–351. https://doi.org/10.3762/bjnano.4.40 (accessed on 4th July 2025).

Halliah, G. P., Alagappan, K., & Sairam, A. B. (2014). *Journal of Industrial Textiles*. https://doi.org/10.1177/1528083713485612 (accessed on 4th July 2025).

Hamal, D. B., Haggstrom, J. A., Marchin, G. L., Ikenberry, M. A., Hohn, K., & Klabunde, K. J. (2010). A multifunctional biocide/sporocide and photocatalyst based on titanium dioxide (TiO_2) codoped with silver, carbon, and sulfur. *Langmuir, 26*(25), 2805–2810. https://doi.org/10.1021/la902844r (accessed on 4th July 2025).

Hartog, A. F., Stoll, B., Jochum, K. P., Wever, R., Natalio, F., Andre, R., & Tremel, W. (2012). Vanadium pentoxide nanoparticles mimic vanadium halo peroxidases and thwart biofilm formation. *Nature Nanotechnology, 7*(August), 3–8. https://doi.org/10.1038/nnano.2012.91 (accessed on 4th July 2025).

Huang, X., Li, M., Xu, Y., Zhang, J., Meng, X., An, X., Sun, L., Guo, L., Shan, X., Ge, J., Chen, J., Luo, Y., Wu, H., Zhang, Y., Jiang, Q., & Ning, X. (2019). Novel gold nanorod-based HR1 peptide inhibitor for Middle East respiratory syndrome coronavirus. *ACS Applied Materials & Interfaces, 11*(22), 19799–19807. https://doi.org/10.1021/acsami.9b04240 (accessed on 4th July 2025).

Hurst, S. J., Lytton-Jean, A. K. R., & Mirkin, C. A. (2006). Maximizing DNA loading on a range of gold nanoparticle sizes. *Analytical Chemistry, 78*(24), 8313–8318.

Huy, T. Q., Nguyen, T. H. T., Thuy, N. T., Chung, P. V., Hung, P. N., Le, A. T., & Hanh, N. T. H. (2016). Cytotoxicity and antiviral activity of electrochemical-synthesized silver nanoparticles against poliovirus. *Journal of Virological Methods*. https://doi.org/10.1016/j.jviromet.2016.12.015 (accessed on 4th July 2025).

Ingale, A. G., & Chaudhari, A. N. (2013). Biogenic synthesis of nanoparticles and potential applications: An eco-friendly approach. *Journal of Nanomedicine & Nanotechnology, 4*(2). https://doi.org/10.4172/2157-7439.1000165 (accessed on 4th July 2025).

Ingle, A. P., Duran, N., & Rai, M. (2013). Bioactivity, mechanism of action, and cytotoxicity of copper-based nanoparticles: A review. *Applied Microbiology and Biotechnology*. https://doi.org/10.1007/s00253-013-5422-8 (accessed on 4th July 2025).

Jawad, K. H., Marzoog, T. R., Hasoon, B. A., Sulaiman, G. M., Jabir, M. S., Ahmed, E. M., & Khalil, K. A. A. (2022). Antibacterial activity of bismuth oxide nanoparticles compared to amikacin against *Acinetobacter baumannii* and *Staphylococcus aureus. 2022.*

Judith, P., & Perez Espitia. (2012). Zinc oxide nanoparticles: Synthesis, antimicrobial activity and food packaging applications, 1447–1464. https://doi.org/10.1007/s11947-012-0797-6 (accessed on 4th July 2024).

Karthika, K., Gopinath, V., Sundaravadivelan, C., & Gowri, S. (2015). Myogenesis of cerium oxide nanoparticles using *Aspergillus niger* culture filtrate and their applications for antibacterial and larvicidal activities. *Journal of Nanostructure in Chemistry*. https://doi.org/10.1007/s40097-015-0161-2 (accessed on 4th July 2024).

Kasraei, S. (2014). Antibacterial properties of composite resins incorporating silver and zinc oxide nanoparticles on *Streptococcus mutans* and *Lactobacillus*, *7658*, 109–114.

Khanal, S. (2018). The repertoire of adenovirus in human disease: The innocuous to the deadly. https://doi.org/10.3390/biomedicines6010030 (accessed on 4th July 2024).

Khandel, P., Kumar, R., Deepak, Y., Soni, K., Kanwar, L., Kumar, S., & Silver, A. G. (2018). Biogenesis of metal nanoparticles and their pharmacological applications: Present status and application prospects. *Journal of Nanostructure in Chemistry*, *8*. Springer Berlin Heidelberg. https://doi.org/10.1007/s40097-018-0267-4 (accessed on 4th July 2024).

Kim, Y. B., Kim, H. K., Yoo, J. K., & Hong, J. W. (2002). UV-curable polyurethane dispersion for cationic electrodeposition coating. *Surface and Coatings Technology*, *157*(1), 40–46. https://doi.org/10.1016/S0257-8972(02)00133-0 (accessed on 4th July 2024).

Lanari, M., Vandini, S., Capretti, M. G., Lazzarotto, T., & Faldella, G. (2014). Respiratory syncytial virus infections in infants affected by primary immunodeficiency. *2014*. https://doi.org/10.1155/2014/850831 (accessed on 4th July 2024).

Lemire, J. A., Harrison, J. J., & Turner, R. J. (2013). Antimicrobial activity of metals: Mechanisms, molecular targets and applications. *Nature Reviews Microbiology*, *11*, 371–384. https://doi.org/10.1038/nrmicro3028 (accessed on 4th July 2024).

Letfullin, R. R., Iversen, C. B., & George, T. F. (2011). Modeling nano photothermal therapy: Kinetics of thermal ablation of healthy and cancerous cell organelles and gold nanoparticles. *Nanomedicine: Nanotechnology, Biology, and Medicine*, *7*(2), 137–145. https://doi.org/10.1016/j.nano.2010.06.011 (accessed on 4th July 2024).

Li, D., Ye, Q., Jiang, L., Luo, Z., & Luo, Z. (2016). Effects of nano-TiO_2-LDPE packaging on postharvest quality and antioxidant capacity of strawberry (*Fragaria ananassa* Duch.) stored at refrigeration temperature. *Journal of the Science of Food and Agriculture, 97*(4), 1116–1123. https://doi.org/10.1002/jsfa.7837 (accessed on 4th July 2024).

Li, X., Robinson, S. M., Gupta, A., Saha, K., Jiang, Z., Moyano, D. F., Sahar, A., Riley, M. A., & Rotello, V. M. (2014). Functional gold nanoparticles as potent antimicrobial agents against multi-drug-resistant bacteria.

Li, X., Wei, J., Aifantis, K. E., Fan, Y., Feng, Q., Cui, F. Z., & Watari, F. (2016). Current investigations into magnetic nanoparticles for biomedical applications. *Journal of Biomedical Materials Research. Part A, 104*(5), 1285–1296. https://doi.org/10.1002/JBM.A.35654 (accessed on 4th July 2024).

Ma, H., Williams, P. L., & Diamond, S. A. (2013). Ecotoxicity of manufactured ZnO nanoparticles–A review. *Environmental Pollution, 172*, 76–85. https://doi.org/10.1016/j.envpol.2012.08.011 (accessed on 4th July 2024).

Mahyad, B. (2020). Biomedical applications of TiO_2 nanostructures: Recent advances.

Maila, V. (2009). Interaction of nanoparticles with cells, 2379–2400.

Majdi, A., Aminifard, S., & Zafari, M. (2011). Nanotoxicology and nanoparticle safety in biomedical designs, 1117–1127. https://doi.org/10.2147/IJN.S16603 (accessed on 4th July 2024).

Malka, E., Perelshtein, I., Lipovsky, A., Shalom, Y., Naparstek, L., Perkas, N., Patick, T., et al. (2013). Eradication of multi-drug-resistant bacteria by a novel Zn-doped CuO nanocomposite, 1–8. https://doi.org/10.1002/smll.201301081 (accessed on 4th July 2024).

Mamun, K. Z., Mahboob, N., Mamun, K. T., & Iqbal, H. (2020). Review article: Moving from oral poliovirus vaccine to inactivated poliovirus vaccine–The rationale and challenges, 22–28.

Meng, J., Stobart, C. C., Hotard, A. L., & Moore, M. L. (2014). An overview of respiratory syncytial virus. *10*(4), 10–12. https://doi.org/10.1371/journal.ppat.1004016 (accessed on 4th July 2024).

Morris, D., Ansar, M., Speshock, J., Ivanciuc, T., Qu, Y., Casola, A., & Garofalo, R. (2019). Antiviral and immunomodulatory activity of silver nanoparticles in experimental RSV infection.

Mundargi, R. C., Babu, V. R., Rangaswamy, V., Patel, P., & Aminabhavi, T. M. (2008). Nano/micro technologies for delivering macromolecular therapeutics using poly (D, L-lactide-co-glycolide) and its derivatives. *125*, 193–209. https://doi.org/10.1016/j.jconrel.2007.09.013 (accessed on 4th July 2024).

Narayanan, K. B., & Sakthivel, N. (2010). Phytosynthesis of gold nanoparticles using leaf extract of *Coleus amboinicus* Lour. *Materials Characterization, 61*(11), 1232–1238. https://doi.org/10.1016/j.matchar.2010.08.003 (accessed on 4th July 2024).

Nasrollahzadeh, M., Sajjadi, M., & Jamalipour Soufi, G. (2020). Nanomaterials and nanotechnology-associated innovations against viral infections with a focus on coronaviruses, 1–31. https://doi.org/10.3390/nano10061072 (accessed on 4th July 2024).

Nichols, W. G., Peck Campbell, A. J., & Boeckh, M. (2008). Respiratory viruses other than influenza virus: Impact and therapeutic advances. *Clinical Microbiology Reviews, 21*(2), 274–290. https://doi.org/10.1128/CMR.00045-07 (accessed on 4th July 2024).

Nikaeen, G., Abbaszadeh, S., & Yousefinejad, S. (2020). Application of nanomaterials in treatment, anti-infection and detection of coronaviruses.

Nikalje, A. P. (2015). Nanotechnology and its applications in medicine, *5*, 81–89. https://doi.org/10.4172/2161-0444.1000247 (accessed on 4th July 2024).

Othman, S. H., Raudhah, N., Abd Salam, Zainal, N., Basha, R. K., & Talib, R. A. (2014). Antimicrobial activity of TiO_2 nanoparticle-coated film for potential food packaging applications. *2014*.

Palanikumar, L., Ramasamy, S. N., & Balachandran, C. (2014). Size-dependent antimicrobial response of zinc oxide nanoparticles, 111–117. https://doi.org/10.1049/iet-nbt.2012.0008 (accessed on 4th July 2024).

Patel, P., Agarwal, P., & Kanawaria, S. (n.d.). Plant-based synthesis of silver nanoparticles and their characterization, 271–288. https://doi.org/10.1007/978-3-319-14502-0 (accessed on 4th July 2024).

Payne, J. N., Waghwani, H. K., Connor, M. G., Hamilton, W., Tockstein, S., Moolani, H., Chavda, F., & Badwaik, V. (2016). Novel synthesis of kanamycin conjugated gold nanoparticles with potent antibacterial activity. *Frontiers in Microbiology*, *7*(May), 1–10. https://doi.org/10.3389/fmicb.2016.00607 (accessed on 4th July 2024).

Peer, D., Karp, J. M., Hong, S., Farokhzad, O. C., Margalit, R., & Langer, R. (2007). Nanocarriers as an emerging platform for cancer therapy, 751–760.

Pfaff, F., Hoyer, T., Sauerbrei, A., Zell, R., Eisenberg, W., & Zell, R. (n.d.). Tungsten carbide nanoparticles show a broad spectrum virucidal activity against enveloped and non-enveloped model viruses using a guideline-standardized *in vitro* test, 0–2. https://doi.org/10.1111/lam.13208 (accessed on 4th July 2024).

Polak, M. J. (2012). Original article cost utility of palivizumab prophylaxis among pre-term infants in the United States: A national policy perspective. *Journal of Medical Economics*, *15*(5), 987–996. https://doi.org/10.3111/13696998.2012.690013 (accessed on 4th July 2024).

Pradhan, N., Singh, S., Ojha, N., Shrivastava, A., Barla, A., Rai, V., & Bose, S. (2015). Facets of nanotechnology as seen in food processing, packaging, and preservation industry. *2015*.

Raffi, M., Hussain, F., Bhatti, T. M., Akhter, J. I., Hameed, A., & Hasan, M. M. (2008). Antibacterial characterization of silver nanoparticles against *E. coli* ATCC-15224. *Journal of Materials Science and Technology, 24*(2), 192–196.

Rai, M., Deshmukh, S. D., Ingle, A. P., Gupta, I. R., Galdiero, M., & Galdiero, S. (2014). Metal nanoparticles: The protective nano shield against virus infection, *7828*, 1–11. https://doi.org/10.3109/1040841X.2013.879849 (accessed on 4th July 2024).

Ramyadevi, J., Jeyasubramanian, K., Marikani, A., Rajakumar, G., & Abdul, A. (2012). Synthesis and antimicrobial activity of copper nanoparticles. *Materials Letters*, *71*, 114–116. https://doi.org/10.1016/j.matlet.2011.12.055 (accessed on 4th July 2024).

Rao, L., Cai, B., Bu, L. L., Liao, Q. Q., Guo, S. S., Zhao, X. Z., Dong, W. F., & Liu, W. (2017). Microfluidic electroporation-facilitated synthesis of erythrocyte membrane-coated magnetic nanoparticles for enhanced imaging-guided cancer therapy. *ACS Nano*, *11*(4), 3496–3505. https://doi.org/10.1021/acsnano.7b00133 (accessed on 4th July 2024).

Reddy, L. S., Nisha, M. M., Joice, M., & Shilpa, P. N. (2014). Antimicrobial activity of zinc oxide (ZnO) nanoparticle against *Klebsiella pneumoniae*, 1–10. https://doi.org/10.3109/13880209.2014.893001 (accessed on 4th July 2024).

Richtera, L., Chudobova, D., Cihalova, K., Kremplova, M., Milosavljevic, V., Kopel, P., Blazkova, I., Hynek, D., Adam, V., & Kizek, R. (2015). The composites of graphene oxide with metal or semimetal nanoparticles and their effect on pathogenic microorganisms, 2994–3011. https://doi.org/10.3390/ma8062994 (accessed on 4th July 2024).

Roshmi, T., Soumya, K. R., Jyothis, M., & Radhakrishnan, E. K. (2015). Effect of bio fabricated gold nanoparticle-based antibiotic conjugates on minimum inhibitory concentration of bacterial isolates of clinical origin, 63–71. https://doi.org/10.1007/s13404-015-0162-4 (accessed on 4th July 2024).

Roy, A., Gauri, S. S., Bhattacharya, M., & Bhattacharya, J. (2013). Antimicrobial activity of CaO nanoparticles. https://doi.org/10.1166/jbn.2013.1681 (accessed on 4th July 2024).

Ruparelia, J. P., Kumar, A., & Duttagupta, S. P. (2008). Strain specificity in antimicrobial activity of silver and copper nanoparticles, *4*, 707–716. https://doi.org/10.1016/j.actbio.2007.11.006 (accessed on 4th July 2024).

Salunke, G. R., Ghosh, S., Kumar, R. J. S., Khade, S., Vashisth, P., Kale, T., Chopade, S., Pruthi, V., Kundu, G., Bellare, J. R., & Chopade, B. A. (2014). Rapid efficient synthesis and characterization of silver, gold, and bimetallic nanoparticles from the medicinal plant *Plumbago zeylanica* and their application in biofilm control. *International Journal of Nanomedicine*, *9*, 2635–2653. https://doi.org/10.2147/IJN.S59834 (accessed on 4th July 2024).

Schwendener, R. A. (2014). Liposomes as vaccine delivery systems: A review of the recent advances. *Therapeutic Advances in Vaccines*, *2*(6), 159–182. https://doi.org/10.1177/2051013614541440 (accessed on 4th July 2024).

Seil, J. T., & Webster, T. J. (2012). Antibacterial effect of zinc oxide nanoparticles combined with ultrasound. *Nanotechnology*, *23*, 495101. https://doi.org/10.1088/0957-4484/23/49/495101 (accessed on 4th July 2024).

Shah, M., Fawcett, D., Sharma, S., & Tripathy, S. K. (2015). Green synthesis of metallic nanoparticles via biological entities. https://doi.org/10.3390/ma8115377 (accessed on 4th July 2024).

Simchi, A., Tamjid, E., Pishbin, F., & Boccaccini, A. R. (2011). Recent progress in inorganic and composite coatings with bactericidal capability for orthopedic applications. *Nanomedicine: Nanotechnology, Biology and Medicine, 7*(1), 22–39. https://doi.org/10.1016/j.nano.2010.10.005 (accessed on 4th July 2025).

Singh, G., & Dhillon, S. (2014). Facile fabrication and characterization of chitosan-based zinc oxide nanoparticles and evaluation of their antimicrobial and antibiofilm activity. *International Nano Letters*, *4*(107). https://doi.org/10.1007/s40089-014-0107-6 (accessed on 4th July 2024).

Singhal, T. (2020). A review of coronavirus disease-2019 (COVID-19). *Indian Journal of Pediatrics*, *87*(4), 281–286.

Srisitthiratkul, C., Pongsorrarith, V., & Intasanta, N. (2011). The potential use of nano silver-decorated titanium dioxide nanofibers for toxin decomposition with antimicrobial and self-cleaning properties. *Applied Surface Science*, *257*(21), 8850–8856. https://doi.org/10.1016/j.apsusc.2011.04.083 (accessed on 4th July 2024).

Stanton, J., Korber, B. T. M., Krebs, K., Bogdan, D., Kunstman, K., Wu, S., Phair, J. P., & Mirkin, C. A. (2008). Detection of HIV-1 p24 Gag in plasma by a nanoparticle-based bio-barcode-amplification method. *Nanomedicine (Lond)*, *23*, 293–303.

Sutradhar, P., Saha, M., & Maiti, D. (2014). Microwave synthesis of copper oxide nanoparticles using tea leaf and coffee powder extracts and its antibacterial activity CuO. *Journal of Nanostructure in Chemistry*, *4*(86). https://doi.org/10.1007/s40097-014-0086-1 (accessed on 4th July 2024).

Tamayo, L. A., Zapata, P. A., Vejar, N. D., Azócar, M. I., Gulppi, M. A., Zhou, X., Thompson, G. E., Rabagliati, F. M., & Páez, M. A. (2014). Release of silver and copper nanoparticles from polyethylene nanocomposites and their penetration into *Listeria monocytogenes*. *Materials Science & Engineering C*, *40*, 24–31. https://doi.org/10.1016/j.msec.2014.03.037 (accessed on 4th July 2024).

Thakkar, H. P., Patel, B. V., & Thakkar, S. P. (2011). Development and characterization of nanosuspensions of olmesartan medoxomil for bioavailability enhancement. *Journal of Pharmacy and Bioallied Sciences*, *3*(3), 426–435. https://doi.org/10.4103/0975-7406.84459 (accessed on 4th July 2024).

Thevenot, P., Hu, W., & Tang, L. (2008). Surface chemistry influence implant biocompatibility. *Current Topics in Medicinal Chemistry*, *8*(4), 270. https://doi.org/10.2174/156802608783790901 (accessed on 4th July 2024).

Thomas, D. L. (2019). Global elimination of chronic hepatitis. *New England Journal of Medicine*, *380*(21), 2041–2050. https://doi.org/10.1056/NEJMra1810477 (accessed on 4th July 2024).

Ungur, G., & Hrůza, J. (2017). Modified polyurethane nanofibers as antibacterial filters for air and water purification. *RSC Advances*, *7*(78), 49177–49187. https://doi.org/10.1039/C7RA06317B (accessed on 4th July 2024).

Wang, C., Huang, X., Deng, W., Chang, C., Hang, R., & Tang, B. (2014). A nano-silver composite based on the ion-exchange response for the intelligent antibacterial applications. *Materials Science & Engineering C*, *41*, 134–141. https://doi.org/10.1016/j.msec.2014.04.044 (accessed on 4th July 2024).

Wang, X., Sun, Y., Jing, S., & Zeng, Y. (2007). Combining gold nanoparticles with real-time immuno-PCR for analysis of HIV p24 antigens. *1st International Conference on Bioinformatics and Biomedical Engineering*, 1198–1201. https://doi.org/10.1109/ICBBE.2007.309 (accessed on 4th July 2024).

Weir, A., Westerhoff, P., Fabricius, L., Hristovski, K., & Von Goetz, N. (2012). Titanium dioxide nanoparticles in food and personal care products. *Environmental Science & Technology*, *46*(4), 2242–2250. https://doi.org/10.1021/es204168d (accessed on 4th July 2024).

Yadavalli, T., Ramasamy, S., Chandrasekaran, G., Michael, I., Annal, H., & Chennakesavulu, R. (2014). Dual responsive PNIPAM–chitosan targeted magnetic nano polymers for targeted drug delivery. *Journal of Magnetism and Magnetic Materials*, 1–6. https://doi.org/10.1016/j.jmmm.2014.09.035 (accessed on 4th July 2024).

Yao, N., & Yeung, K. L. (2011). Investigation of the performance of TiO_2 photocatalytic coatings. *Chemical Engineering Journal*. https://doi.org/10.1016/j.cej.2010.11.061 (accessed on 4th July 2024).

Young, M., Willits, D., Uchida, M., & Douglas, T. (2008). Plant viruses as bio templates for materials and their use in nanotechnology. *Annual Review of Phytopathology*, *46*, 361–384. https://doi.org/10.1146/annurev.phyto.032508.131939 (accessed on 4th July 2024).

Yu, C., Tam, K., & Tsang, E. S. C. (2009). Chemical methods for preparation of nanoparticles in solution. In *Handbook of Metal Physics* (Vol. 5, pp. 113–141). https://doi.org/10.1016/S1570-002X(08)00205-X (accessed on 4th July 2024).
Zhang, L., Ding, Y., Povey, M., & York, D. (2008). ZnO nanofluids–A potential antibacterial agent. *Progress in Natural Science*, *18*(8), 939–944. https://doi.org/10.1016/j.pnsc.2008.01.026 (accessed on 4th July 2024).
Zhang, X. (2015). Gold nanoparticles: Recent advances in the biomedical applications. *Cell Biochemistry and Biophysics*, *72*, 771–775. https://doi.org/10.1007/s12013-015-0529-4 (accessed on 4th July 2024).
Zhang, Y., Dong, Y., Zhou, J., Li, X., & Wang, F. (2018). Application of plant viruses as a biotemplate for nanomaterial fabrication. *Molecules*. https://doi.org/10.3390/molecules23092311 (accessed on 4th July 2025).
Zhong, L., & Yun, K. (2015). Graphene oxide-modified ZnO particles: Synthesis, characterization, and antibacterial properties. *International Journal of Nanomedicine*, *10*(sup1), 79–92. https://doi.org/10.2147/IJN.S88319 (accessed on 4th July 2024).

CHAPTER 4

Nano-Formulations of Natural Herbs and Spices as Antiviral Agents

SHIJI MATHEW

Department of Biology, College of Science and Technology, Temple University, Philadelphia, Pennsylvania, United States

ABSTRACT

The re-emergence of viral infections such as SARS-CoV-2, influenza, dengue, and Zika virus has had a profound and discouraging impact on the global community's financial well-being. Compounded by the unavailability of suitable antivirals against these viral infections, the situation has raised significant concerns. Throughout history, plants and their various formulations have been extensively explored and utilized for their medicinal properties. Plant-derived medicines have also demonstrated the potential to act as immunity boosters against common viral infections. As a result, scientists worldwide have intensified their research on plants and their derivative phytopharmaceuticals to develop effective, eco-friendly, and less-toxic therapeutics. This chapter briefly examines the roles of various plant-derived therapeutic strategies, with a primary focus on the use of herbs and spices as antiviral agents. Additionally, the chapter outlines the principles for the development of potential herbs and spices derived nanoformulations, as well as their antiviral efficacies.

Nanotechnological Management of Viral Infections.
Radhakrishnan EK, Shiji Mathew, and Riya Alex (Eds.)

DOI: 10.1201/9781779640895-4

4.1 INTRODUCTION

Viral infections remain a leading cause of mortality and morbidity globally, with an estimated 3–5 million new cases reported each year. For instance, influenza virus alone is responsible for over 3 million new cases and contributes to 300,000–500,000 deaths annually (Gasparini et al., 2012). Despite the progress made in novel drug development and immunization, it is crucial to recognize the continued lack of effective medication for many common viral infections. Moreover, the antivirals available in the market are often prohibitively expensive and associated with adverse effects. Notably, treatments such as interferons and ribavirin, although effective *in vitro*, often demonstrate reduced efficacy in patients (Ben-Shabat et al., 2020). These challenges contribute to the resurgence of viruses and the emergence of viral escape mutants, leading to a significant increase in life-threatening viral infections each year. The economic and societal implications of viral pandemics further exacerbate these concerns (Ben-Shabat et al., 2020). Consequently, exploring the potential of novel therapeutics with enhanced antiviral effectiveness is of utmost importance.

Nearly 200,000 natural compounds derived from plants, animals, fungi, and marine organisms exhibit essential medicinal properties. Herbs and spices, in particular, have been recognized for their therapeutic effects against various viruses for centuries and are extensively used in several Asian and African countries, including China, India, Japan, Thailand, Sri Lanka, and others (Siow et al., 2005). Developing countries are increasingly emphasizing the use of natural antiviral medicines based on plants and their derivatives. Various plant-derived compounds, either alone or in combination, have been recommended for the treatment of human and animal viral infections in the form of leaf powders, pastes, pills, decoctions, and infusions. These natural products contain diverse bioactive phytochemicals, including lignans, sulfides, polyphenols, coumarins, saponins, flavonoids, terpenoids, and organosulfur compounds, all contributing to their potent therapeutic functionality (Aḥmad et al., 2006; Perera et al., 2021). The antiviral properties of these plant extracts/products may vary depending on the molecular mechanisms involved, including scavenging properties, antioxidant activity, inhibition of DNA/RNA synthesis, and inhibition of viral entry and replication (Tolo et al., 2006).

However, the use of natural products faces limitations such as low bioavailability and pharmacokinetics, poor intestinal absorption, and low hydrophilicity and intrinsic dissolution rate. Leveraging the functionalities of nanotechnology offers a promising approach to overcome these limitations. Nanotechnology can be harnessed to develop effective drug delivery systems and nanocarriers, including lipid-based nanocarriers, polymeric nanoparticles, inorganic structures, and hybrid nanocarriers. This chapter aims to provide an overview of the utilization of various natural herbs and spices in the treatment of viral infections, along with a discussion on the applications of various nanoformulations and nanoproducts derived from herbs and spices.

4.2 COMMON HERBS AND SPICES WITH ANTIVIRAL PROPERTY

Bioactive molecules possessing medicinal properties can be derived from various parts of plants, including fruits/vegetables, flowers, seeds, barks, leaves, and roots. These molecules, known as phytochemicals, play a critical role in combating viral infections. Phytochemicals are broadly classified into two categories: primary and secondary metabolites. The secondary metabolites found in these plant structures, such as alkaloids, tannins, saponins, polysaccharides, flavonoids, steroids, coumarins, and terpenes, contribute to the potential antiviral properties. Figure 4.1 provides a summary of some essential herbs and spices and their specific roles in fighting viral infections. Table 4.1 offers an overview of the major phytochemicals known for their potential antiviral activity.

4.2.1 GINGER

Ginger (*Zingiber officinale*) is a common spice and a well-known herbal medicine widely used due to its antioxidant, anti-inflammatory, antimicrobial, anticancer, antidiabetic, anti-obesity, gastrointestinal, cardiovascular, and anti-nausea properties (Han et al., 2013). It belongs to the family Zingiberaceae and genus Zingiber. Ginger is a rich source of phytochemicals such as phenolic groups, alkaloids, and steroids. The bioactive phenolic compounds responsible for elucidating the health benefits of fresh ginger mainly include [4-], [6-], [8-]gingerol, and [6-], [14-]shogaols. Research has shown that fresh ginger could inhibit plaque formation induced by human respiratory syncytial virus (HRSV) in the

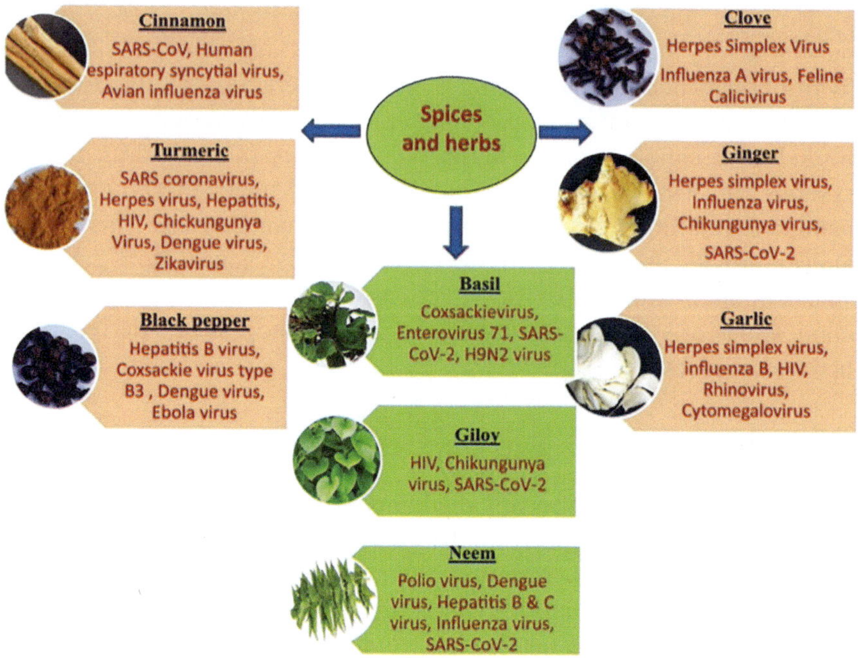

FIGURE 4.1 Antiviral activities of common spices and herbs.

Source: Reprinted and reused with permission from Singh et al. (2021). Copyright © 2021 John Wiley & Sons, Ltd.

respiratory tract cell lineage by blocking the viral penetration and attachment (Chang et al., 2013). Ginger has also exhibited antiviral effects against rhinovirus, SARS-CoV-2, and influenza virus (Imanishi et al., 2006), thereby proving its efficiency in treating respiratory infections. The results of the work done by Hayati et al. (2021) and Kaushik et al. (2020) indicated that [6]-gingerol inhibits the chikungunya virus by inhibiting viral replication. Recently, green-synthesized silver nanoparticles were developed from methanolic extracts of strawberries and ginger. These phytomediated silver nanoparticles were found to be excellent agents exhibiting antiviral activity against SARS-CoV-2 (Al-Sanea et al., 2021).

4.2.2 STAR ANISE (ILLICIUM VERUM)

Star anise is a spice well cultivated in Asian countries. Its dry fruits and seeds are the main condiment in Chinese cuisine. The main

TABLE 4.1 List of Plant Derived Secondary Metabolites with Antiviral Activity Against Major Human Viral Pathogens

Active Compound	Plant	Family	Antiviral Activity Against	References
Polyphenols	*Avicennia marina*	Acanthaceae	Human immunodeficiency virus (HIV) and Herpes simplex virus (HSV)	Namazi et al. (2013)
	Sambucus nigra	Adoxaceae	Dengue virus serotype-2 (DENV-2); Infectious bronchitis virus (IBV) – chicken coronavirus	Castillo-Maldonado et al. (2017); Chen et al. (2014)
	Iresine herbtsii	Amaranthaceae	Newcastle disease virus	Andleeb et al. (2020)
	Anacardium occidentale	Anacardiaceae	Simian (SA-11) virus	Gonçalves et al. (2005)
	Artocarpus integrifolia	Moraceae	SA-11 and human (HCR3) rotavirus	Gonçalves et al. (2005)
	Myristica fragrans	Myristicaceae	Human (HCR3) rotavirus	Gonçalves et al. (2005)
	Psidium guajava	Myrtaceae	Simian (SA-11) virus	Gonçalves et al. (2005)
	Spondias lutea	Anacardiaceae	Simian (SA-11) virus and human (HCR3) rotavirus	Gonçalves et al. (2005)
	Spondias lutea L.	Anacardiaceae	HSV 1 and 2	Gonçalves et al. (2005)
	Rhus aromatica	Anacardiaceae	HSV 1 and 2	Reichling et al. (2009)
	Rhus parviflora	Anacardiaceae	HIV 1	Modi et al. (2013)
	Schinus terebinthifolia	Anacardiaceae	HSV 1	Nocchi et al. (2016)
	Arisaema tortuosum	Araceae	Acyclovir resistant HSV-2 and HSV-1	Rittà et al. (2020)
	Jasonia montana	Asteraceae	Poliomyelitis-1 virus	Soltan and Zaki (2009)
	Baccharis gaudichaudiana DC	Asteraceae	Bovine viral diarrhoea virus (BVDV), HSV-1, Poliovirus type 2 (PV-2) and vesicular stomatitis virus (VSV)	Visintini Jaime et al. (2013)
	Pluchea sagittalis (Lam.) Cabrera	Asteraceae	BVDV, HSV-1, PV-2 VSV	Visintini Jaime et al. (2013)
	Tagetes minuta L	Asteraceae	BVDV, HSV-1, PV-2 VSV	Visintini Jaime et al. (2013)

TABLE 4.1 *(Continued)*

Active Compound	Plant	Family	Antiviral Activity Against	References
	Eupatorium perfoliatum	Asteraceae	Influenza A virus (IAV) H1NI	Derksen et al. (2016)
	Silybum marianum	Asteraceae	Chikungunya virus (CHIKV), Hepatitis C virus (HCV)	Lani et al. (2015)
	Tanacetum parthenium	Asteraceae	HSV-1	Benassi-Zanqueta et al. (2019)
	Taraxacum officinale	Asteraceae	HCV	Rehman et al. (2016)
	Senna augustifolia	Fabaeceae	DENV-2	Rothan et al. (2014)
	Tridax procumbers	Asteraceae	DENV-2	Rothan et al. (2014)
	Vernonia cinerea	Asteraceae	DENV-2	Rothan et al. (2014)
	Epimedium koreanum nakai	Berberidaceae	Porcine epidemic diarrhoea virus (PEDV)	Cho et al. (2012)
	Canarium album (Lour.)	Burseraceae	IAV	Chen et al. (2020)
	Cistus incanus	Cistaceae	HIV-1 and 2, Filoviruses, Ebola and Marbung virus	Rebensburg et al. (2016)
	Combretum adenogonium	Combreteceae	HIV-1	Mushi et al. (2012)
	Cornus canadensis	Cornaceae	HSV-1	Lavoie et al. (2017)
	Taxodium distichum	Cupressaceae	Influenza A and B	Hsieh et al. (2016)
	Cyperus rotundus	Cyperaceae	HSV-1, HBV	Xu et al. (2015)
	Equisetum giganteum	Equisetaceae	HSV-2	Churqui et al. (2018)
	Euphorbia hirta	Euphorbiaceae	HIV-1, 2 and SIV mac 251	Gyuris et al. (2009)
	Euphorbia sikkimensis	Euphorbiaceae	HIV-1	Jiang et al. (2016)
	Acacia arabica	Fabaceae	Influenza A virus H9N2	Ghoke et al. (2018)
	Aspalathus linearis	Fabaceae	Rhesus rotavirus (RRV), Simian rotavirus (SA-11),	
	Vachellia nilotica	Fabaceae	HSV-2	Donalisio et al. (2018)
	Acacia catechu	Fabaceae	HIV-1	Nutan et al. (2013)

TABLE 4.1 *(Continued)*

Active Compound	Plant	Family	Antiviral Activity Against	References
	Geranium thunbergii	Geranicaceae	Influenza, HINI, H3N2, Influenza type B	
	Quercus persica	Fagaceae	HSV-1	Rafieian-kopaei et al. (2013)
	Anthemis hyalina	Asreraceae	SARS-CoV	Ulasli et al. (2014)
	Alnus japonica	Betulaceae	SARS-CoV	
	Cassia tora	Fabaceae	SARS-CoV	
	Psolarea corylifolia	Fabaceae	SARS-CoV	Kim et al. (2014)
	Taxillus chinensis	Loranthaceae	SARS-CoV	
	Citrus sinensis	Rutaceae	SARS-CoV	Ulasli et al. (2014)
	Polygorum multiflorum	Polygonaceae	SARS-CoV	Ho et al. (2007)
	Rheum officinale	Polygonaceae	SARS-CoV	Ho et al. (2007)
	Rheum palmatum	Polygonaceae	SARS-CoV	Luo et al. (2009)
Alkaloids	*Sambucus nigra*	Adoxaceae	DENV-2	Castillo-Maldonado et al. (2017)
	Iresine herbistii	Amaranthaceae	NDV	Andleeb et al. (2020)
	Combretum adegonium	Combretaceae	HIV-1	Mushi et al. (2012)
	Cyperus rodundus	Cyperaceae	HSV-1, HBV	Xu et al. (2015)
	Equisetum giganteum	Equisetaceae	HSV-2	Churqui et al. (2018)
	Cissampelos pareira Linn	Menispermaceae	DENV 1–4	Sood et al. (2015)
	Ficus religiosa	Moraceae	HSV-2	Ghosh et al. (2016)
	Phyllanthus amarus	Phyllanthaceae	HCV	Ravikumar et al. (2011)
	Plumbago indica	Plumbaginaceae	Influenza A (H1N1)	Chavan et al. (2016)

TABLE 4.1 *(Continued)*

Active Compound	Plant	Family	Antiviral Activity Against	References
	Pavetta tomentosa	Rubiaceae	DENV	Pratheeba et al. (2019)
	Tarenna asiatica	Rubiaceae	DENV	Pratheeba et al. (2019)
	Moringa peregrina	Moringaceae	HSV	Shi et al. (2020) and Soltan and Zaki (2009)
	Capparis sinaica	Capparaceae	HSV	Soltan and Zaki (2009)
	Balanites aegyptiaca	Balanitaceae	VSV	Maregesi et al. (2008)
	Lycoris radiata	Amaryllis	SARS-CoV	Kim et al. (2015)
	Acanthopanacis cortex	Araliaceae	SARS-CoV	Li et al. (2005)
Saponins	*Iresine herbstii*	Amaranthaceae	NDV	Andleeb et al. (2020)
	Anacardium occidentale	Anacardaceae	Simian (SA-11) virus	Gonçalves et al. (2005)
	Panax ginseng	Araliaceae	RSV	Lee et al. (2014)
	Panax ginseng	Araliaceae	Murine norovirus (MNV) and feline calcivirus (FCV)	Lee et al. (2011)
	Balanites aegyptiaca	Balanitaceae	VSV	Maregesi et al. (2008)
	Capparis sinaica	Capparaceae	HSV	Soltan and Zaki (2009)
	Combretum adegonium	Combretaceae	HIV-1	Mushi et al. (2012)
	Vachellia nilotica	Fabaceae	HSV-2	Donalisio et al. (2018)
	Lindernia crustaceae	Linderniaceae	Epstein Barr virus (EBV)	Tsai et al. (2020)
	Artocarpus integrifolia	Moraceae	SA-11 and human (HCR3) rotavirus	Gonçalves et al. (2005)
	Ficus religiosa	Moraceae	HSV-2	Ghosh et al. (2016)
	Ficus sycomorus	Moraceae	HSV-1	Maregesi et al. (2008)
	Moringa peregrina	Moringceae	HSV	Soltan and Zaki (2009)

TABLE 4.1 *(Continued)*

Active Compound	Plant	Family	Antiviral Activity Against	References
	Plumbago indica	Plumbaginaceae	Influenza A (H1N1)	Chavan et al. (2016)
	Pavetta tomentosa	Rubiaceae	DENV	Pratheeba et al. (2019)
	Tarenna asiatica	Rubiaceae	DENV	Pratheeba et al. (2019)
Carbohydrates	*Panax ginseng*	Araliaceae	Human rotavirus	
	Panax notoginseng	Araliaceae	Influenza A (H1N1)	Choi et al. (2017)
	Equisetum giganteum	Equisetaceae	HSV-2	
	Prunella vulgaris	Lamiaceae	HSV-1 and 2 viral antigens in verso cells	Chi-Ming Chiu et al. (2004)
	Prunellae spica	Lamiaceae	HSV	Ma et al. (2016)
	Laminaria japonica	Laminaraceae	RSV	Cao et al. (2016)
	Plumbago indica	Plumbaginaceae	Influenza A (H1N1)	Chavan et al. (2016)
	Ardisia chinensis Benth	Primulaceae	Coxsackie B3 virus	Su et al. (2006)
	Capparis sinaica	Capparaceae	HSV	Soltan and Zaki (2009)
	Balanites aegyptiaca	Balanitaceae	RSV	Maregesi et al. (2008)
	Carissa edulis	Apocynaceae	HSV, chicken pox, shingles	Tolo et al. (2006)
Terpenoids	*Andrographis paniculata*	Acanthaceae	DENV-1	Anna Pick Kiong LING et al. (2014)
	Baccharis gaudichaudiana DC	Asteraceae	BVD, HSV-1, poliovirus type 2 (PV-2) and VSV	Visintini Jaime et al. (2013)
	Baccharis spicata (Lam.) Baill	Asteraceae	BVD, HSV-1, poliovirus type 2 (PV-2) and VSV	Visintini Jaime et al. (2013)
	Taxodium distichum	Cupresseceae	Influenza A and B	Hsieh et al. (2016)
	Euphorbia hirta	Euphorbiaceae	HIV-1, HIV-2, SIV mac 251	Gyuris et al. (2009)

TABLE 4.1 *(Continued)*

Active Compound	Plant	Family	Antiviral Activity Against	References
	Jatropha multiphida	Euphorbiaceae	Influenza A (H1N1)	Shoji et al. (2017)
	Torreya nucifera	Taxaceae	SARS-CoV 3CLPro	Ryu et al. (2010)
	Agrimonium pilosa	Rosaceae	Influenza (H1N1 and H3N2)	Shin et al. (2010)
	Tripterigium regelli	Celastraceae	SARS-CoV	Ryu et al. (2010)
	Gentiana scabra	Gentianaceae	SARS-CoV	Wen et al. (2011)

Source: Adapted and modified from Bhuiyan et al. (2020). Open access journal under Creative Commons Attribution License (CC BY).

phytochemical that contributes to the medicinal effect of star anise is shikimic acid. Shikimic acid is the main component of oseltamivir, the antiviral drug for influenza A and B. The essential oil from star anise is composed of sesquiterpenes, prenylated C6-C3 compounds, lignans, and flavonoids, which deliver the medicinal property. A study conducted by Alhajj et al. reported the inhibitory effects of star anise extracts against avian reovirus (ARV), Infectious Bursal Disease virus (IBDV), Newcastle disease virus (NDV), and infectious laryngotracheitis virus (ILTV) (Alhajj et al., 2020).

4.2.3 TURMERIC (CURCUMA LONGA L.)

Turmeric belongs to the Zingiberaceae family and is abundantly cultivated in Southeast Asia and India. One of its major active ingredients is curcumin, a polyphenol, which is the most studied among the dietary natural products. Curcumin is already well-known for its therapeutic effects against inflammation, cancer, depression, and other ailments. Among its varied medicinal uses, its most important one is the antiviral activity. Studies have reported the notable antiviral properties of curcumin against noroviruses (Yang et al., 2016), HIV viruses (Prasad and Tyagi, 2015), zika, and chikungunya viruses (Mounce et al., 2017), herpes virus (Šudomová and Hassan, 2021), hepatitis virus (Wei et al., 2017), influenza viruses (Chen et al., 2010), and even SARS-CoV-2. The mechanism of the antiviral activity of curcumin is mediated by several molecular targets, resulting in the suppression of intercellular signaling cascades, thereby inhibiting the viral replication cycle (Ferreira et al., 2015). The main mode of antiviral activity includes inhibiting viral attachment, penetration, and entry into host cells (Chen et al., 2013). Other mechanisms include the regulation of transcription and replication (Narayan et al., 2011), inhibition of protease enzymes (Sui et al., 1993), and inactivation of the virus structures (Chen et al., 2013). Table 4.2 summarizes the antiviral properties and mechanism of action of curcumin.

The reduced bioavailability of curcumin, however, limits its usage in biopharmaceuticals. Researchers have found that these limitations of curcumin can be overcome by the hydrophobic nature of nanoparticles, which can be designed as curcumin carriers. The application of nanocarriers in the form of nanoemulsions, nanogels, and liposomes has been

TABLE 4.2 Antiviral Activity of *Curcuma longa* Against Common Viral Pathogens

Sl. No.	Type of Virus	Mechanism of Action	References
1	SARS coronavirus	Inhibition of replication and protease activity	Wen et al. (2007)
2	Herpes virus	Inhibition of gene expression	Kutluay et al. (2008)
3	Hep B virus	Inhibition of replication; Inhibition of cccDNA replication	Mouler Rechtman et al. (2010); Wei et al. (2017)
4	Hep C virus	Inhibition of viral entry	Anggakusuma et al. (2014)
5	HIV virus	Protease inhibitor, Integrase inhibitor; Tat protein inhibitor	Ali and Banerjea (2016); Balasubramanyam et al. (2004)
6	Human papilloma virus	Inhibition of gene expression	Maher et al. (2011); Mishra (2015)
7	Chikungunya virus	Inhibition of viral entry	Mounce et al. (2017); von Rhein et al. (2016)
8	Dengue virus	Inhibition of viral entry; Inhibition of particle formation	Chen et al. (2013)
9	Zika virus	Inhibition of viral entry	Mounce et al. (2017)
10	Influenza A	Inhibition of viral entry, replication, and particle formation	Dai et al. (2018)

Source: Reused and reprinted from Singh et al. (2021). Copyright © 2021 John Wiley & Sons, Ltd. Open access journal.

found to be effective in loading and carrying curcumin, thereby increasing its bioavailability and transportation, protecting it from degradation, and improving its solubility (Zeng et al., 2022). During the COVID-19 pandemic, three curcumin-based oral nanotechnology formulations were available in the market, demonstrating benign therapeutic effects. These products were Nanocurc™ (polymer nanoparticles), Lipocurc™ (liposomes), and Sinacurcumin™ (nanoparticles) (Ahmadi et al., 2021; Saber-Moghaddam et al., 2021; Tahmasebi et al., 2021; Valizadeh et al., 2020). Various nano-based formulations of curcumin are also available, exhibiting a significant impact on pharmaceutical industries due to their anticancer, analgesic, antioxidant, anti-inflammatory, and antimicrobial properties. Figure 4.2 demonstrates the different applications of curcumin nano-formulations in pharmaceutical industries.

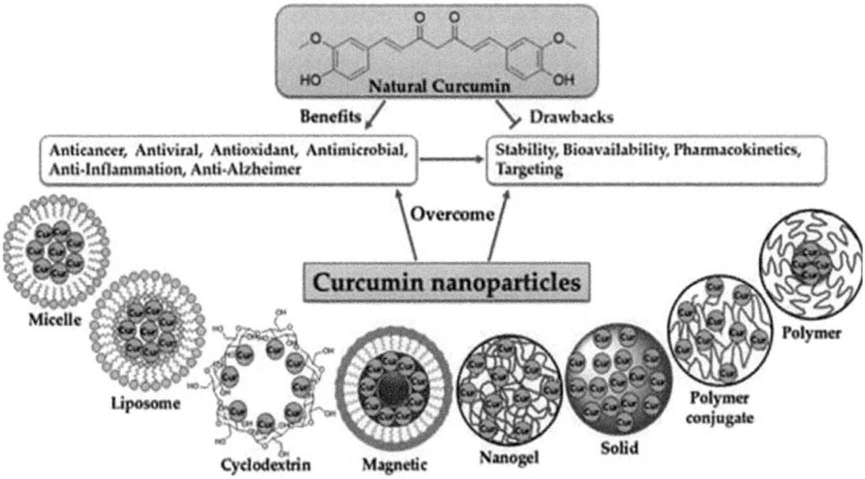

FIGURE 4.2 Applications of nanocurcumin formulations.

Source: Reprinted and reused with permission from Hafez Ghoran et al. 2022; https://creativecommons.org/licenses/by/4.0/.

4.2.4 CINNAMON (CINNAMOMUM CASSIA)

Cinnamon is an aromatic spice belonging to the family *Lauraceae*. It is a common ingredient in traditional Chinese, Indian, Unani, and Persian medicine. Cinnamon is obtained from the bark of young branches and is a common condiment. For many years, cinnamon has been used as a medicine for toothache, diarrhea, flatulence, amenorrhea, fever, the common cold, and headache (Hajimonfarednejad et al., 2019). In a study, silver nanoparticles were synthesized from cinnamon extract and tested against the H7N3 Influenza A virus in Vero cells. The viability of the cells was determined by the tetrazolium dye (MTT assay). The silver nanoparticles synthesized from cinnamon extract were found to have enhanced antiviral activity, ensuring their potential use as an antiviral agent (Fatima et al., 2016). In another recent study, a suspension containing selenium sulfide nanoparticles stabilized by spice extracts (cinnamon, curcumin, and pepper) was found to be highly active (99% reduction) against the influenza virus and B-coronavirus (Długosz et al., 2022).

4.2.5 GARLIC (ALLIUM SATIVUM)

Allium sativum is one of the most common herbal medicines used since ancient times. The major bioactive compound of garlic is allicin. Several organosulfur compounds extracted from *A. sativum* have also been found to be active against common pathogenic viruses (*see* Table 4.3). Fresh garlic extract and garlic oil have shown potential antiviral activity against human cytomegalovirus (HCMV) and influenza A virus. Several preclinical studies have been conducted on different aqueous extracts of *A. sativum*. A plaque reduction study with Vero and HeLa cells demonstrated that the aqueous extract of *A. sativum* in gold nanoparticles exhibited antiviral activity against the measles virus, HSV-1, and HSV-2. The mechanism of antiviral action was found to be the inhibition of viral entry via the disruption of the viral envelope and cell membrane (Weber et al., 1992). In another similar study, the results of a toxicity assay carried out in chicken embryos demonstrated that the aqueous extract of *A. sativum* had a promising antiviral effect against coronavirus (Mohajer Shojai et al., 2016). The oil extracted from garlic is also found to have potential antiviral activities. Recently, a transdermal nanoemulsion film loaded with garlic oil and acyclovir was synthesized and assessed for activity against Herpes simplex virus (HSV) cold sore infection. This study provided strong preclinical evidence of enhanced pharmacokinetic potential of the developed formulation (Almehmady and Ali, 2021).

4.2.6 CHINESE SKULLCAP (SCUTELLARIA BAICALENSIS)

Scutellaria baicalensis has been a part of traditional Chinese medicine for 200 years. The root of this plant is rich in steroids, flavonoids, essential oils, and has anti-inflammatory and anti-cancer properties. Additionally, it has been found effective against many viral infections. The most active component of *Scutellaria baicalensis* is baicalin. Various studies have demonstrated that this plant has the potential to inhibit the replication of SARS-CoV-2 (Liu et al., 2021) and HIV (Li et al., 1993). It has shown both *in vitro* and *in vivo* activity against Dengue (Zandi et al., 2013), RSV (Shi et al., 2016), H1N1 (Ding et al., 2014), and enterovirus (Li et al., 2015).

4.2.7 GUDUCHI (TINOSPORA CORDIFOLIA)

Tinospora cordifolia is an Indian native medicinal plant belonging to the family Menispermaceae, also known as giloya. It is one of the important

TABLE 4.3 Antiviral Activity of Organosulfur Compounds of *A. sativum*

Organsulfur Compound	Assessment Method	Virus Species	Mechanism of Antiviral Action	References
Allicin	Direct preinfection incubation and plaque reduction assay	HSV-1 HSV-2 Parainfluenza virus Vaccinia virus Vesicular stomatitis virus	Disruption of viral envelope and cell membrane	Weber et al. (1992)
Allin	Anti-inflammatory assay	Dengue virus	Inhibition of inflammation via reduction of oxidative stress	Hall et al. (2017)
Joene	Anti-HIV activity	HIV-1	Prevention of induced destructions of CD+ cells	Weber et al. (1992)
	HIV infected platelet aggregation and fusion assays	HIV	Inhibition of adhesive bonds and fusion of leukocytes	Tatarintsev et al. (1992)
	HIV induced cellular toxicity assay	HIV-1	Inhibition of viral reverse transcriptase and cell attachment	Kaul, Middleton et al. (1985)
Allyl methyl thiosulfinate	Direct preinfection and plaque reduction assay	HSV-1 HSV-2 Parainfluenza virus Vaccinia virus Vesicular stomatitis virus	Disruption of viral envelope and cell membrane	Weber et al. (1992)
Diallyl trisulfinade	Plaque reduction assay	human cytomegalovirus IAV-H1N1	Inhibit viral DNA synthesis through inhibition of HCMV immediate early antigen expression	Feng et al. (1999)
Diallyl sulfide and Diallyl disulfide	Oxidative stress and anti-inflammatory assay	Dengue virus	Reduction of oxidative stress	Hall et al. (2017)

Source: Adapted and modified from Perera et al. (2021). Open access journal.

immunomodulatory ingredients of Ayurvedic medicine. The aqueous extract of *Tinospora cordifolia* is found to boost immunity in children. Many recent studies have investigated the anti-SARS-CoV-2 activity of *Tinospora cordifolia* (Chowdhury, 2021; Sagar and Kumar, 2020).

4.3 CONCLUDING REMARKS

Globally, viral infections remain the leading cause of morbidity and mortality. The constantly mutating nature of viruses, combined with the lack of access to effective antiviral treatments, compounds the challenge of treating these infections. Throughout history, plant extracts, as well as various common herbs and spices, have been used as immune boosters and natural home remedies for various ailments. Many plant secondary metabolites and essential oils, along with their nanoformulations, have demonstrated strong potential in combating viral infections. This chapter focuses on discussing the role of nanoformulations of herbs and spices as antiviral agents. It is important to note that most studies in this area are still in the preliminary stages. Therefore, it is crucial to encourage scientists to explore the vast potential of different plant metabolites, elucidate the mechanisms of the antiviral action of these natural products, and conduct more *in vivo* studies to evaluate their immunomodulatory effects. Additionally, further research is needed to explore the effectiveness of a combination of herbal and spice-based formulations.

KEYWORDS

- **antivirals**
- **herbs**
- **influenza virus**
- **nanotechnology**
- **phytochemicals**
- **phytopharmaceuticals**
- **spices**
- **therapeutics**

REFERENCES

Aḥmad, I., Aqil, F., & Owais, M. (2006). *Modern Phytomedicine: Turning Medical Plants into Drugs*. Wiley-VCH.

Ahmadi, R., Salari, S., Sharifi, M. D., Reihani, H., Rostamiani, M. B., Behmadi, M., Taherzadeh, Z., et al. (2021). Oral nano-curcumin formulation efficacy in the management of mild to moderate outpatient COVID-19: A randomized triple-blind placebo-controlled clinical trial. *Food Science & Nutrition*, *9*(8), 4068–4075. https://doi.org/10.1002/fsn3.2226 (accessed on 4th July 2024).

Alhajj, M. S., Qasem, M. A., & Al-Mufarrej, S. I. (2020). Inhibitory activity of *Illicium verum* extracts against avian viruses. *Advances in Virology*, *2020*(January), 1–8. https://doi.org/10.1155/2020/4594635 (accessed on 4th July 2024).

Ali, A., & Banerjea, A. C. (2016). Curcumin inhibits HIV-1 by promoting Tat protein degradation. *Scientific Reports*, *6*(1), 27539. https://doi.org/10.1038/srep27539 (accessed on 4th July 2024).

Almehmady, A. M., & Ali, S. A. (2021). Transdermal film loaded with garlic oil-acyclovir nano emulsion to overcome barriers for its use in alleviating cold sore conditions. *Pharmaceutics*, *13*(5), 669. https://doi.org/10.3390/pharmaceutics13050669 (accessed on 4th July 2024).

Al-Sanea, M. M., Abelyan, N., Abdelgawad, M. A., Musa, A., Ghoneim, M. M., Al-Warhi, T., Aljaeed, N., et al. (2021). Strawberry and ginger silver nanoparticles as potential inhibitors for SARS-CoV-2 assisted by *in silico* modeling and metabolic profiling. *Antibiotics*, *10*(7), 824. https://doi.org/10.3390/antibiotics10070824 (accessed on 4th July 2024).

Andleeb, R., Ashraf, A., Muzammil, S., Naz, S., Asad, F., Ali, T., Rafi, R., et al. (2020). Analysis of bioactive composites and antiviral activity of *Iresine herbstii* extracts against Newcastle disease virus in ovo. *Saudi Journal of Biological Sciences*, *27*(1), 335–340. https://doi.org/10.1016/j.sjbs.2019.10.002 (accessed on 4th July 2024).

Anggakusuma, Colpitts, C. C., Schang, L. M., Rachmawati, H., Frentzen, A., Pfaender, S., Behrendt, P., et al. (2014). Turmeric curcumin inhibits entry of all hepatitis C virus genotypes into human liver cells. *Gut*, *63*(7), 1137–1149. https://doi.org/10.1136/gutjnl-2012-304299 (accessed on 4th July 2024).

Balasubramanyam, K., Varier, R. A., Altaf, M., Swaminathan, V., Siddappa, N. B., Ranga, U., & Kundu, T. K. (2004). Curcumin, a novel p300/CREB-binding protein-specific inhibitor of acetyltransferase, represses the acetylation of histone/nonhistone proteins and histone acetyltransferase-dependent chromatin transcription. *Journal of Biological Chemistry*, *279*(49), 51163–51171. https://doi.org/10.1074/jbc.M409024200 (accessed on 4th July 2024).

Benassi-Zanqueta, É., Marques, C. F., Valone, L. M., Pellegrini, B. L., Bauermeister, A., Ferreira, I. C. P., Lopes, N. P., et al. (2019). Evaluation of anti-HSV-1 activity and toxicity of hydroethanolic extract of *Tanacetum parthenium* (L.) Sch.Bip. (Asteraceae). *Phytomedicine*, *55*(March), 249–254. https://doi.org/10.1016/j.phymed.2018.06.040 (accessed on 4th July 2024).

Ben-Shabat, S., Yarmolinsky, L., Porat, D., & Dahan, A. (2020). Antiviral effect of phytochemicals from medicinal plants: Applications and drug delivery strategies. *Drug*

Delivery and Translational Research, *10*(2), 354–367. https://doi.org/10.1007/s13346-019-00691-6 (accessed on 4th July 2024).

Bhuiyan, F. R., Howlader, S., Raihan, T., & Hasan, M. (2020). Plants metabolites: Possibility of natural therapeutics against the COVID-19 pandemic. *Frontiers in Medicine*, *7*(August), 444. https://doi.org/10.3389/fmed.2020.00444 (accessed on 4th July 2024).

Cao, Y., Hao, Y., Li, Z., Liu, S., & Wang, L. (2016). Antiviral activity of polysaccharide extract from *Laminaria japonica* against respiratory syncytial virus. *Biomedicine & Pharmacotherapy*, *84*(December), 1705–1710. https://doi.org/10.1016/j.biopha.2016.10.082 (accessed on 4th July 2024).

Castillo-Maldonado, I., Moreno-Altamirano, M. M. B., & Serrano-Gallardo, L. B. (2017). Anti-dengue serotype-2 activity effect of *Sambucus nigra* leaves-and flowers-derived compounds. *Virology: Research and Reviews*, *1*(3). https://doi.org/10.15761/VRR.1000117 (accessed on 4th July 2024).

Chang, J. S., Wang, K. C., Yeh, C. F., Shieh, D. E., & Chiang, L. C. (2013). Fresh ginger (*Zingiber officinale*) has anti-viral activity against human respiratory syncytial virus in human respiratory tract cell lines. *Journal of Ethnopharmacology*, *145*(1), 146–151. https://doi.org/10.1016/j.jep.2012.10.043 (accessed on 4th July 2024).

Chavan, R. D., Shinde, P., Girkar, K., Madage, R., & Chowdhary, A. (2016). Assessment of anti-influenza activity and hemagglutination inhibition of *Plumbago indica* and *Allium sativum* extracts. *Pharmacognosy Research*, *8*(2), 105. https://doi.org/10.4103/0974-8490.172562 (accessed on 4th July 2024).

Chen, C., Zuckerman, D. M., Brantley, S., Sharpe, M., Childress, K., Hoiczyk, E., & Pendleton, A. R. (2014). *Sambucus nigra* extracts inhibit infectious bronchitis virus at an early point during replication. *BMC Veterinary Research*, *10*(1), 24. https://doi.org/10.1186/1746-6148-10-24 (accessed on 4th July 2024).

Chen, D. Y., Shien, J. H., Tiley, L., Chiou, S. S., Wang, S. Y., Chang, T. J., Lee, Y. J., Chan, K. W., & Hsu, W. L. (2010). Curcumin inhibits influenza virus infection and hemagglutination activity. *Food Chemistry*, *119*(4), 1346–1351. https://doi.org/10.1016/j.foodchem.2009.09.011 (accessed on 4th July 2024).

Chen, F., Yang, L., Huang, Y., Chen, Y., Sang, H., Duan, W., & Yang, J. (2020). Isocorilagin, isolated from *Canarium album* (Lour.) Raeusch, as a potent neuraminidase inhibitor against influenza A virus. *Biochemical and Biophysical Research Communications*, *523*(1), 183–189. https://doi.org/10.1016/j.bbrc.2019.12.043 (accessed on 4th July 2024).

Chen, T. Y., Chen, D. Y., Wen, H. W., Ou, J. L., Chiou, S. S., Chen, J. M., Wong, M. L., & Hsu, W. L. (2013). Inhibition of enveloped viruses' infectivity by curcumin. *PLoS ONE*, *8*(5), e62482. https://doi.org/10.1371/journal.pone.0062482 (accessed on 4th July 2024).

Chiu, C. M., Zhu, W., & Ooi, V. E. C. (2004). A polysaccharide fraction from medicinal herb *Prunella vulgaris* downregulates the expression of herpes simplex virus antigen in Vero cells. *Journal of Ethnopharmacology*, *93*(1), 63–68. https://doi.org/10.1016/j.jep.2004.03.024 (accessed on 4th July 2024).

Cho, W. K., Kim, H., Choi, Y. J., Yim, N. H., Yang, H. J., & Ma, J. Y. (2012). *Epimedium koreanum* Nakai water extract exhibits antiviral activity against porcine epidemic diarrhea virus *in vitro* and *in vivo*. *Evidence-Based Complementary and Alternative Medicine*, *2012*, 1–10. https://doi.org/10.1155/2012/985151 (accessed on 4th July 2024).

Choi, J. G., Jin, Y. H., Lee, H., Oh, T. W., Yim, N. H., Cho, W. K., & Ma, J. Y. (2017). Protective effect of *Panax notoginseng* root water extract against influenza A virus infection by enhancing antiviral interferon-mediated immune responses and natural killer cell activity. *Frontiers in Immunology*, *8*(November), 1542. https://doi.org/10.3389/fimmu.2017.01542 (accessed on 4th July 2024).

Chowdhury, P. (2021). *In silico* investigation of phytoconstituents from Indian medicinal herb *Tinospora cordifolia* (Giloy) against SARS-CoV-2 (COVID-19) by molecular dynamics approach. *Journal of Biomolecular Structure and Dynamics*, *39*(17), 6792–6809. https://doi.org/10.1080/07391102.2020.1803968 (accessed on 4th July 2024).

Churqui, M. P., Lind, L., Thörn, K., Svensson, A., Savolainen, O., Terrazas Aranda, K., & Eriksson, K. (2018). Extracts of *Equisetum giganteum* L and *Copaifera reticulata* Ducke show strong antiviral activity against the sexually transmitted pathogen herpes simplex virus type 2. *Journal of Ethnopharmacology*, *210*(January), 192–197. https://doi.org/10.1016/j.jep.2017.08.010 (accessed on 4th July 2024).

Dai, J., Gu, L., Su, Y., Wang, Q., Zhao, Y., Chen, X., Deng, H., Li, W., Wang, G., & Li, K. (2018). Inhibition of curcumin on influenza A virus infection and influenzal pneumonia via oxidative stress, TLR2/4, P38/JNK MAPK and NF-κB pathways. *International Immunopharmacology*, *54*(January), 177–187. https://doi.org/10.1016/j.intimp.2017.11.009 (accessed on 4th July 2024).

Derksen, A., Kühn, J., Hafezi, W., Sendker, J., Ehrhardt, C., Ludwig, S., & Hensel, A. (2016). Antiviral activity of hydroalcoholic extract from *Eupatorium perfoliatum* L. against the attachment of influenza A virus. *Journal of Ethnopharmacology*, *188*(July), 144–152. https://doi.org/10.1016/j.jep.2016.05.016 (accessed on 4th July 2024).

Ding, Y., Dou, J., Teng, Z., Yu, J., Wang, T., Lu, N., Wang, H., & Zhou, C. (2014). Antiviral activity of baicalin against influenza A (H1N1/H3N2) virus in cell culture and in mice and its inhibition of neuraminidase. *Archives of Virology*, *159*(12), 3269–3278. https://doi.org/10.1007/s00705-014-2192-2 (accessed on 4th July 2024).

Długosz, O., Ochnik, M., Sochocka, M., Franz, D., Orzechowska, B., Chmielowiec-Korzeniowska, A., Drabik, A., & Banach, M. (2022). Antimicrobial and antiviral activity of selenium sulphide nanoparticles synthesized in extracts from spices in natural deep eutectic solvents (NDES). *Sustainable Materials and Technologies*, *32*(July), e00433. https://doi.org/10.1016/j.susmat.2022.e00433 (accessed on 4th July 2024).

Donalisio, M., Cagno, V., Civra, A., Gibellini, D., Musumeci, G., Rittà, M., Ghosh, M., & Lembo, D. (2018). The traditional use of *Vachellia nilotica* for sexually transmitted diseases is substantiated by the antiviral activity of its bark extract against sexually transmitted viruses. *Journal of Ethnopharmacology*, *213*(March), 403–408. https://doi.org/10.1016/j.jep.2017.11.039 (accessed on 4th July 2024).

Fatima, M., Zaidi, N. S. S., Amraiz, D., & Afzal, F. (2016). *In vitro* antiviral activity of *Cinnamomum cassia* and its nanoparticles against H7N3 influenza A virus. *Journal of Microbiology and Biotechnology*, *26*(1), 151–159. https://doi.org/10.4014/jmb.1508.08024 (accessed on 4th July 2024).

Feng, F., Hong, L., Wen, C., & Yongsui, D. (1999). Treatment of hepatitis caused by cytomegalovirus with allitridin injection—An experimental study. *Journal of Tongji Medical University*, *19*(4), 271–274. https://doi.org/10.1007/BF02886960 (accessed on 4th July 2024).

Ferreira, V. H., Nazli, A., Dizzell, S. E., Mueller, K., & Kaushic, C. (2015). The anti-inflammatory activity of curcumin protects the genital mucosal epithelial barrier from disruption and blocks replication of HIV-1 and HSV-2. *PLOS ONE, 10*(4), e0124903. https://doi.org/10.1371/journal.pone.0124903 (accessed on 4th July 2024).

Gasparini, R., Amicizia, D., Lai, P. L., & Panatto, D. (2012). Clinical and socioeconomic impact of seasonal and pandemic influenza in adults and the elderly. *Human Vaccines & Immunotherapeutics*, *8*(1), 21–28. https://doi.org/10.4161/hv.8.1.17622 (accessed on 4th July 2024).

Ghoke, S. S., Sood, R., Kumar, N., Pateriya, A. K., Bhatia, S., Mishra, A., Dixit, R., et al. (2018). Evaluation of antiviral activity of *Ocimum sanctum* and *Acacia arabica* leaves extracts against H9N2 virus using embryonated chicken egg model. *BMC Complementary and Alternative Medicine*, *18*(1), 174. https://doi.org/10.1186/s12906-018-2238-1 (accessed on 4th July 2024).

Ghosh, M., Civra, A., Rittà, M., Cagno, V., Mavuduru, S. G., Awasthi, P., Lembo, D., & Donalisio, M. (2016). *Ficus religiosa* L. bark extracts inhibit infection by herpes simplex virus type 2 *in vitro*. *Archives of Virology*, *161*(12), 3509–3514. https://doi.org/10.1007/s00705-016-3032-3 (accessed on 4th July 2024).

Gonçalves, J. L. S., Lopes, R. C., Oliveira, D. B., Costa, S. S., Miranda, M. M. F. S., Romanos, M. T. V., Santos, N. S. O., & Wigg, M. D. (2005). *In vitro* anti-rotavirus activity of some medicinal plants used in Brazil against diarrhea. *Journal of Ethnopharmacology*, *99*(3), 403–407. https://doi.org/10.1016/j.jep.2005.01.032 (accessed on 4th July 2024).

Gyuris, A., Szlávik, L., Minárovits, J., Vasas, A., Molnár, J., & Hohmann, J. (2009). Antiviral activities of extracts of *Euphorbia hirta* L. against HIV-1, HIV-2 and SIVmac251. *In Vivo (Athens, Greece)*, *23*(3), 429–432.

Hafez Ghoran, S., Calcaterra, A., Abbasi, M., Taktaz, F., Nieselt, K., & Babaei, E. (2022). Curcumin-based nanoformulations: A promising adjuvant towards cancer treatment. *Molecules*, *27*(16), 5236. https://doi.org/10.3390/molecules27165236 (accessed on 4th July 2024).

Hajimonfarednejad, M., Ostovar, M., Raee, M. J., Hashempur, M. H., Mayer, J. G., & Heydari, M. (2019). Cinnamon: A systematic review of adverse events. *Clinical Nutrition*, *38*(2), 594–602. https://doi.org/10.1016/j.clnu.2018.03.013 (accessed on 4th July 2024).

Hall, A., Troupin, A., Londono-Renteria, B., & Colpitts, T. (2017). Garlic organosulfur compounds reduce inflammation and oxidative stress during dengue virus infection. *Viruses*, *9*(7), 159. https://doi.org/10.3390/v9070159 (accessed on 4th July 2024).

Han, Y. A., Song, C. W., Koh, W. S., Yon, G. H., Kim, Y. S., Ryu, S. Y., Kwon, H. J., & Lee, K. H. (2013). Anti-inflammatory effects of the *Zingiber officinale* Roscoe constituent 12-dehydrogingerdione in lipopolysaccharide-stimulated RAW 264.7 cells: Anti-inflammatory effect of 12-dehydrogingerdione. *Phytotherapy Research*, *27*(8), 1200–1205. https://doi.org/10.1002/ptr.4847 (accessed on 4th July 2024).

Hayati, R. F., Better, C. D., Denis, D., Komarudin, A. G., Bowolaksono, A., Yohan, B., & Sasmono, R. T. (2021). [6]-Gingerol inhibits Chikungunya virus infection by suppressing viral replication. *BioMed Research International*, *2021*(March), 1–7. https://doi.org/10.1155/2021/6623400 (accessed on 4th July 2024).

Ho, T., Wu, S., Chen, J., Li, C., & Hsiang, C. (2007). Emodin blocks the SARS coronavirus spike protein and angiotensin-converting enzyme 2 interaction. *Antiviral Research*,

74(2), 92–101. https://doi.org/10.1016/j.antiviral.2006.04.014 (accessed on 4th July 2024).

Hsieh, C. F., Chen, Y. L., Lin, C. F., Ho, J. Y., Huang, C. H., Chiu, C. H., Hsieh, P. W., & Horng, J. T. (2016). An extract from *Taxodium distichum* targets hemagglutinin- and neuraminidase-related activities of influenza virus *in vitro*. *Scientific Reports*, *6*(1), 36015. https://doi.org/10.1038/srep36015 (accessed on 4th July 2024).

Imanishi, N., Andoh, T., Mantani, N., Sakai, S., Terasawa, K., Shimada, Y., Sato, M., Katada, Y., Ueda, K., & Ochiai, H. (2006). Macrophage-mediated inhibitory effect of *Zingiber officinale* Rosc, a traditional oriental herbal medicine, on the growth of influenza A/Aichi/2/68 virus. *The American Journal of Chinese Medicine*, *34*(1), 157–169. https://doi.org/10.1142/S0192415X06003722 (accessed on 4th July 2024).

Jiang, C., Luo, P., Zhao, Y., Hong, J., Morris-Natschke, S. L., Xu, J., Chen, C. H., Lee, K. H., & Gu, Q. (2016). Carolignans from the aerial parts of *Euphorbia sikkimensis* and their anti-HIV activity. *Journal of Natural Products*, *79*(3), 578–583. https://doi.org/10.1021/acs.jnatprod.5b01012 (accessed on 4th July 2024).

Kaul, T. N., Middleton, E., & Ogra, P. L. (1985). Antiviral effect of flavonoids on human viruses. *Journal of Medical Virology*, *15*(1), 71–79. https://doi.org/10.1002/jmv.1890150110 (accessed on 4th July 2024).

Kaushik, S., Jangra, G., Kundu, V., Yadav, J. P., & Kaushik, S. (2020). Anti-viral activity of *Zingiber officinale* (ginger) ingredients against the Chikungunya virus. *VirusDisease*, *31*(3), 270–276. https://doi.org/10.1007/s13337-020-00584-0 (accessed on 4th July 2024).

Kim, D. W., Seo, K. H., Curtis-Long, M. J., Oh, K. Y., Oh, J. W., Cho, J. K., Lee, K. H., & Park, K. H. (2014). Phenolic phytochemical displaying SARS-CoV papain-like protease inhibition from the seeds of *Psoralea corylifolia*. *Journal of Enzyme Inhibition and Medicinal Chemistry*, *29*(1), 59–63. https://doi.org/10.3109/14756366.2012.753591 (accessed on 4th July 2024).

Kim, H. B., Lee, C. Y., Kim, S. J., Han, J. H., & Choi, K. H. (2015). Medicinal herb extracts ameliorate impaired growth performance and intestinal lesion of newborn piglets challenged with the virulent porcine epidemic diarrhea virus. *Journal of Animal Science and Technology*, *57*(1), 33. https://doi.org/10.1186/s40781-015-0065-1 (accessed on 4th July 2024).

Kutluay, S. B., Doroghazi, J., Roemer, M. E., & Triezenberg, S. J. (2008). Curcumin inhibits herpes simplex virus immediate-early gene expression by a mechanism independent of p300/CBP histone acetyltransferase activity. *Virology*, *373*(2), 239–247. https://doi.org/10.1016/j.virol.2007.11.028 (accessed on 4th July 2024).

Lani, R., Hassandarvish, P., Chiam, C. W., Moghaddam, E., Chu, J. J. H., Rausalu, K., Merits, A., et al. (2015). Antiviral activity of silymarin against Chikungunya virus. *Scientific Reports*, *5*(1), 11421. https://doi.org/10.1038/srep11421 (accessed on 4th July 2024).

Lavoie, S., Côté, I., Pichette, A., Gauthier, C., Ouellet, M., Nagau-Lavoie, F., Mshvildadze, V., & Legault, J. (2017). Chemical composition and anti-herpes simplex virus type 1 (HSV-1) activity of extracts from *Cornus canadensis*. *BMC Complementary and Alternative Medicine*, *17*(1), 123. https://doi.org/10.1186/s12906-017-1618-2 (accessed on 4th July 2024).

Lee, J. S., Ko, E. J., Hwang, H. S., Lee, Y. N., Kwon, Y. M., Kim, M. C., & Kang, S. M. (2014). Antiviral activity of ginseng extract against respiratory syncytial virus infection. *International Journal of Molecular Medicine*, *34*(1), 183–190. https://doi.org/10.3892/ijmm.2014.1750 (accessed on 4th July 2024).

Lee, M. H., Lee, B. H., Jung, J. Y., Cheon, D. S., Kim, K. T., & Choi, C. S. (2011). Antiviral effect of Korean red ginseng extract and ginsenosides on murine norovirus and feline calicivirus as surrogates for human norovirus. *Journal of Ginseng Research*, *35*(4), 429–435. https://doi.org/10.5142/jgr.2011.35.4.429 (accessed on 4th July 2024).

Li, B. Q., Fu, T., Yan, Y. D., Baylor, N. W., Ruscetti, F. W., & Kung, H. F. (1993). Inhibition of HIV infection by baicalin—a flavonoid compound purified from Chinese herbal medicine. *Cellular & Molecular Biology Research*, *39*(2), 119–124.

Li, S., Chen, C., Zhang, H., Guo, H., Wang, H., Wang, L., Zhang, X., Hua, S., Yu, J., & Xiao, P. (2005). Identification of natural compounds with antiviral activities against SARS-associated coronavirus. *Antiviral Research*, *67*(1), 18–23. https://doi.org/10.1016/j.antiviral.2005.02.007 (accessed on 4th July 2024).

Li, X., Liu, Y., Wu, T., Jin, Y., Cheng, J., Wan, C., Qian, W., Xing, F., & Shi, W. (2015). The antiviral effect of baicalin on Enterovirus 71 *in vitro*. *Viruses*, *7*(8), 4756–4771. https://doi.org/10.3390/v7082841 (accessed on 4th July 2024).

Ling, A. P. K., Khoo, B. F., Seah, C. H., Foo, K. Y., Cheah, R. K., Chye, S. M., & Koh, R. Y. (2014). Inhibitory activities of methanol extracts of *Andrographis paniculata* and *Ocimum sanctum* against Dengue-1 virus. In *International Conference on Biological, Environment and Food Engineering (BEFE-2014), August 4–5, 2014, Bali (Indonesia)*. International Institute of Chemical, Biological & Environmental Engineering. https://doi.org/10.15242/IICBE.C814013 (accessed on 4th July 2024).

Liu, H., Ye, F., Sun, Q., Liang, H., Li, C., Li, S., Lu, R., Huang, B., Tan, W., & Lai, L. (2021). *Scutellaria baicalensis* extract and baicalein inhibit replication of SARS-CoV-2 and its 3C-like protease *in vitro*. *Journal of Enzyme Inhibition and Medicinal Chemistry*, *36*(1), 497–503. https://doi.org/10.1080/14756366.2021.1873977 (accessed on 4th July 2024).

Luo, W., Su, X., Gong, S., Qin, Y., Liu, W., Li, J., Yu, H., & Xu, Q. (2009). Anti-SARS coronavirus 3C-like protease effects of *Rheum palmatum* L. extracts. *Bioscience Trends*, *3*(4), 124–126.

Ma, F. W., Kong, S. Y., Tan, H. S., Wu, R., Xia, B., Zhou, Y., & Xu, H. X. (2016). Structural characterization and antiviral effect of a novel polysaccharide PSP-2B from *Prunellae spica*. *Carbohydrate Polymers*, *152*(November), 699–709. https://doi.org/10.1016/j.carbpol.2016.07.062 (accessed on 4th July 2024).

Maher, D. M., Bell, M. C., O'Donnell, E. A., Gupta, B. K., Jaggi, M., & Chauhan, S. C. (2011). Curcumin suppresses human papillomavirus oncoproteins, restores p53, Rb, and PTPN13 proteins and inhibits benzo[a]pyrene-induced upregulation of HPV E7. *Molecular Carcinogenesis*, *50*(1), 47–57. https://doi.org/10.1002/mc.20695 (accessed on 4th July 2024).

Maregesi, S. M., Pieters, L., Ngassapa, O. D., Apers, S., Vingerhoets, R., Cos, P., Vanden Berghe, D. A., & Vlietinck, A. J. (2008). Screening of some Tanzanian medicinal plants from Bunda district for antibacterial, antifungal and antiviral activities. *Journal of Ethnopharmacology*, *119*(1), 58–66. https://doi.org/10.1016/j.jep.2008.05.033 (accessed on 4th July 2024).

Mishra, A. (2015). Curcumin modulates cellular AP-1, NF-kB, and HPV16 E6 proteins in oral cancer. *Ecancermedicalscience*, *9*(April). https://doi.org/10.3332/ecancer.2015.525 (accessed on 4th July 2024).

Modi, M., Nutan, Pancholi, B., Kulshrestha, S., Rawat, A. K. S., Malhotra, S., & Gupta, S. K. (2013). Anti-HIV-1 activity, protease inhibition and safety profile of extracts prepared from *Rhus parviflora*. *BMC Complementary and Alternative Medicine*, *13*(1), 158. https://doi.org/10.1186/1472-6882-13-158 (accessed on 4th July 2024).

Mohajer Shojai, T., Langeroudi, A. G., Karimi, V., Barin, A., & Sadri, N. (2016). The effect of *Allium sativum* (garlic) extract on infectious bronchitis virus in specific pathogen free embryonic egg. *Avicenna Journal of Phytomedicine*, *6*(4), 458–467.

Mouler Rechtman, M., Har-Noy, O., Bar-Yishay, I., Fishman, S., Adamovich, Y., Shaul, Y., Halpern, Z., & Shlomai, A. (2010). Curcumin inhibits hepatitis B virus via down-regulation of the metabolic coactivator PGC-1α. *FEBS Letters*, *584*(11), 2485–2490. https://doi.org/10.1016/j.febslet.2010.04.067 (accessed on 4th July 2024).

Mounce, B. C., Cesaro, T., Carrau, L., Vallet, T., & Vignuzzi, M. (2017). Curcumin inhibits Zika and Chikungunya virus infection by inhibiting cell binding. *Antiviral Research*, *142*(June), 148–157. https://doi.org/10.1016/j.antiviral.2017.03.014 (accessed on 4th July 2024).

Mushi, N. F., Mbwambo, Z. H., Innocent, E., & Tewtrakul, S. (2012). Antibacterial, anti-HIV-1 protease and cytotoxic activities of aqueous ethanolic extracts from *Combretum adenogonium* Steud. ex A. Rich (Combretaceae). *BMC Complementary and Alternative Medicine*, *12*(1), 163. https://doi.org/10.1186/1472-6882-12-163 (accessed on 4th July 2024).

Namazi, R., Zabihollahi, R., Behbahani, M., & Rezaei, A. (2013). Inhibitory activity of *Avicennia marina*, a medicinal plant in Persian folk medicine, against HIV and HSV. *Iranian Journal of Pharmaceutical Research: IJPR*, *12*(2), 435–443.

Narayan, V., Ravindra, K. C., Chiaro, C., Cary, D., Aggarwal, B. B., Henderson, A. J., & Prabhu, K. S. (2011). Celastrol inhibits Tat-mediated human immunodeficiency virus (HIV) transcription and replication. *Journal of Molecular Biology*, *410*(5), 972–983. https://doi.org/10.1016/j.jmb.2011.04.013 (accessed on 4th July 2024).

Nocchi, S., Companhoni, M., de Mello, J., Dias Filho, B., Nakamura, C., Carollo, C., Silva, D., & Ueda-Nakamura, T. (2016). Antiviral activity of crude hydroethanolic extract from *Schinus terebinthifolia* against herpes simplex virus type 1. *Planta Medica*, *83*(06), 509–518. https://doi.org/10.1055/s-0042-117774 (accessed on 4th July 2024).

Nutan, Modi, M., Dezzutti, C. S., Kulshreshtha, S., Rawat, A. K. S., Srivastava, S. K., Malhotra, S., Verma, A., Ranga, U., & Gupta, S. K. (2013). Extracts from *Acacia catechu* suppress HIV-1 replication by inhibiting the activities of the viral protease and Tat. *Virology Journal*, *10*(1), 309. https://doi.org/10.1186/1743-422X-10-309 (accessed on 4th July 2024).

Perera, W. P. R. T., Liyanage, J. A., Dissanayake, K. G. C., Gunathilaka, H., Weerakoon, W. M. T. D. N., Wanigasekara, D. N., Fernando, W. S. K., Rajapaksha, R. M. H., Liyanage, R. P., & Perera, B. T. (2021). Antiviral potential of selected medicinal herbs and their isolated natural products. *BioMed Research International*, *2021*(December), 1–18. https://doi.org/10.1155/2021/7872406 (accessed on 4th July 2024).

Prasad, S., & Tyagi, A. K. (2015). Curcumin and its analogues: A potential natural compound against HIV infection and AIDS. *Food & Function, 6*(11), 3412–3419. https://doi.org/10.1039/C5FO00485C (accessed on 4th July 2024).

Pratheeba, T., Taranath, V., Sai Gopal, D., & Natarajan, D. (2019). Antidengue potential of leaf extracts of *Pavetta tomentosa* and *Tarenna asiatica* (Rubiaceae) against dengue virus and its vector *Aedes aegypti* (Diptera: Culicidae). *Heliyon, 5*(11), e02732. https://doi.org/10.1016/j.heliyon.2019.e02732 (accessed on 4th July 2024).

Rafieian-Kopaei, M., Saeedi, M., Asgari, S., Karimi, A., & Moradi, M. T. (2013). Antiviral activity of *Quercus persica* L.: High efficacy and low toxicity. *Advanced Biomedical Research, 2*(1), 36. https://doi.org/10.4103/2277-9175.109722 (accessed on 4th July 2024).

Ravikumar, Y. S., Ray, U., Nandhitha, M., Perween, A., Naika, H. R., Khanna, N., & Das, S. (2011). Inhibition of hepatitis C virus replication by herbal extract: *Phyllanthus amarus* as potent natural source. *Virus Research, 158*(1, 2), 89–97. https://doi.org/10.1016/j.virusres.2011.03.014 (accessed on 4th July 2024).

Rebensburg, S., Helfer, M., Schneider, M., Koppensteiner, H., Eberle, J., Schindler, M., Gürtler, L., & Brack-Werner, R. (2016). Potent *in vitro* antiviral activity of *Cistus incanus* extract against HIV and filoviruses targets viral envelope proteins. *Scientific Reports, 6*(1), 20394. https://doi.org/10.1038/srep20394 (accessed on 4th July 2024).

Rehman, S., Ijaz, B., Fatima, N., Muhammad, S. A., & Riazuddin, S. (2016). Therapeutic potential of *Taraxacum officinale* against HCV NS5B polymerase: *In-vitro* and *in silico* study. *Biomedicine & Pharmacotherapy, 83*(October), 881–891. https://doi.org/10.1016/j.biopha.2016.08.002 (accessed on 4th July 2024).

Reichling, J., Neuner, A., Sharaf, M., Harkenthal, M., & Schnitzler, P. (2009). Antiviral activity of *Rhus aromatica* (fragrant sumac) extract against two types of herpes simplex viruses in cell culture. *Die Pharmazie, 64*(8), 538–541.

Rhein, C. von, Weidner, T., Henß, L., Martin, J., Weber, C., Sliva, K., & Schnierle, B. S. (2016). Curcumin and *Boswellia serrata* gum resin extract inhibits Chikungunya and vesicular stomatitis virus infections *in vitro*. *Antiviral Research, 125*(January), 51–57. https://doi.org/10.1016/j.antiviral.2015.11.007 (accessed on 4th July 2024).

Rittà, M., Marengo, A., Civra, A., Lembo, D., Cagliero, C., Kant, K., Lal, U. R., Rubiolo, P., Ghosh, M., & Donalisio, M. (2020). Antiviral activity of a *Arisaema tortuosum* leaf extract and some of its constituents against herpes simplex virus type 2. *Planta Medica, 86*(04), 267–275. https://doi.org/10.1055/a-1087-8303 (accessed on 4th July 2024).

Rothan, H. A., Zulqarnain, M., Ammar, Y. A., Tan, E. C., Rahman, N. A., & Yusof, R. (2014). Screening of antiviral activities in medicinal plants extracts against dengue virus using dengue NS2B-NS3 protease assay. *Tropical Biomedicine, 31*(2), 286–296.

Ryu, Y. B., Jeong, H. J., Kim, J. H., Kim, Y. M., Park, J. Y., Kim, D., Naguyen, T. T. H., Park, S. J., Chang, J. S., & Park, K. H. (2010). Biflavonoids from *Torreya nucifera* displaying SARS-CoV 3CLpro inhibition. *Bioorganic & Medicinal Chemistry, 18*(22), 7940–7947. https://doi.org/10.1016/j.bmc.2010.09.035 (accessed on 4th July 2024).

Saber-Moghaddam, N., Salari, S., Hejazi, S., Amini, M., Taherzadeh, Z., Eslami, S., Rezayat, S. M., Jaafari, M. R., & Elyasi, S. (2021). Oral nano-curcumin formulation efficacy in management of mild to moderate hospitalized coronavirus disease-19 patients: An open label nonrandomized clinical trial. *Phytotherapy Research, 35*(5), 2616–2623. https://doi.org/10.1002/ptr.7004 (accessed on 4th July 2024).

Sagar, V., & Kumar, A. H. S. (2020). Efficacy of natural compounds from *Tinospora cordifolia* against SARS-CoV-2 protease, surface glycoprotein and RNA polymerase. *Preprint. In Review*. https://doi.org/10.21203/rs.3.rs-27375/v1 (accessed on 4th July 2024).

Shi, H., Ren, K., Lv, B., Zhang, W., Zhao, Y., Tan, R. X., & Li, E. (2016). Baicalin from *Scutellaria baicalensis* blocks respiratory syncytial virus (RSV) infection and reduces inflammatory cell infiltration and lung injury in mice. *Scientific Reports*, *6*(1), 35851. https://doi.org/10.1038/srep35851 (accessed on 4th July 2024).

Shi, Y., Wang, Y., Shao, C., Huang, J., Gan, J., Huang, X., Bucci, E., Piacentini, M., Ippolito, G., & Melino, G. (2020). COVID-19 infection: The perspectives on immune responses. *Cell Death & Differentiation*, *27*(5), 1451–1454. https://doi.org/10.1038/s41418-020-0530-3 (accessed on 4th July 2024).

Shin, W. J., Lee, K. H., Park, M. H., & Seong, B. L. (2010). Broad-spectrum antiviral effect of *Agrimonia pilosa* extract on influenza viruses. *Microbiology and Immunology*, *54*(1), 11–19. https://doi.org/10.1111/j.1348-0421.2009.00173.x (accessed on 4th July 2024).

Shoji, M., Woo, S. Y., Masuda, A., Win, N. N., Ngwe, H., Takahashi, E., Kido, H., Morita, H., Ito, T., & Kuzuhara, T. (2017). Anti-influenza virus activity of extracts from the stems of *Jatropha multifida* Linn. collected in Myanmar. *BMC Complementary and Alternative Medicine*, *17*(1), 96. https://doi.org/10.1186/s12906-017-1612-8 (accessed on 4th July 2024).

Singh, N. A., Kumar, P., Jyoti, & Kumar, N. (2021). Spices and herbs: Potential antiviral preventives and immunity boosters during COVID-19. *Phytotherapy Research*, *35*(5), 2745–2757. https://doi.org/10.1002/ptr.7019 (accessed on 4th July 2024).

Siow, Y. L., Gong, Y., Au-Yeung, K. K. W., Woo, C. W. H., Choy, P. C., & O, K. (2005). Emerging issues in traditional Chinese medicine. *Canadian Journal of Physiology and Pharmacology*, *83*(4), 321–334. https://doi.org/10.1139/y05-029 (accessed on 4th July 2024).

Soltan, M. M., & Zaki, A. K. (2009). Antiviral screening of forty-two Egyptian medicinal plants. *Journal of Ethnopharmacology*, *126*(1), 102–107. https://doi.org/10.1016/j.jep.2009.08.001 (accessed on 4th July 2024).

Sood, R., Raut, R., Tyagi, P., Pareek, P. K., Barman, T. K., Singhal, S., Shirumalla, R. K., et al. (2015). *Cissampelos pareira* Linn: Natural source of potent antiviral activity against all four dengue virus serotypes. *PLOS Neglected Tropical Diseases*, *9*(12), e0004255. https://doi.org/10.1371/journal.pntd.0004255 (accessed on 4th July 2024).

Su, M., Li, Y., Leung, K. T., Cen, Y., Li, T., Chen, R., & Ooi, V. E. C. (2006). Antiviral activity and constituent of *Ardisia chinensis* Benth against Coxsackie B3 virus. *Phytotherapy Research*, *20*(8), 634–639. https://doi.org/10.1002/ptr.1912 (accessed on 4th July 2024).

Šudomová, M., & Hassan, S. T. S. (2021). Nutraceutical curcumin with promising protection against herpesvirus infections and their associated inflammation: Mechanisms and pathways. *Microorganisms*, *9*(2), 292. https://doi.org/10.3390/microorganisms9020292 (accessed on 4th July 2024).

Sui, Z., Salto, R., Li, J., Craik, C., & Ortiz de Montellano, P. R. (1993). Inhibition of the HIV-1 and HIV-2 proteases by curcumin and curcumin boron complexes. *Bioorganic & Medicinal Chemistry*, *1*(6), 415–422. https://doi.org/10.1016/S0968-0896(00)82152-5 (accessed on 4th July 2024).

Tahmasebi, S., El-Esawi, M. A., Mahmoud, Z. H., Timoshin, A., Valizadeh, H., Roshangar, L., Varshoch, M., et al. (2021). Immunomodulatory effects of nanocurcumin on Th17 cell responses in mild and severe COVID-19 patients. *Journal of Cellular Physiology, 236*(7), 5325–5338. https://doi.org/10.1002/jcp.30233 (accessed on 4th July 2024).

Tatarintsev, A. V., Vrzhets, P. V., Ershov, D. E., Shchegolev, A. A., Turgiev, A. S., Karamov, E. V., Kornilaeva, G. V., Makarova, T. V., Fedorov, N. A., & Varfolomeev, S. D. (1992). [The ajoene blockade of integrin-dependent processes in an HIV-infected cell system]. *Vestnik Rossiiskoi Akademii Meditsinskikh Nauk*, (11, 12), 6–10.

Tolo, F. M., Rukunga, G. M., Muli, F. W., Njagi, E. N. M., Njue, W., Kumon, K., Mungai, G. M., et al. (2006). Anti-viral activity of the extracts of a Kenyan medicinal plant *Carissa edulis* against herpes simplex virus. *Journal of Ethnopharmacology, 104*(1, 2), 92–99. https://doi.org/10.1016/j.jep.2005.08.053 (accessed on 4th July 2024).

Tsai, Y. C., Hohmann, J., El-Shazly, M., Chang, L. K., Dankó, B., Kúsz, N., Hsieh, C. T., Hunyadi, A., & Chang, F. R. (2020). Bioactive constituents of *Lindernia crustacea* and its anti-EBV effect via Rta expression inhibition in the viral lytic cycle. *Journal of Ethnopharmacology, 250*(March), 112493. https://doi.org/10.1016/j.jep.2019.112493 (accessed on 4th July 2024).

Ulasli, M., Gurses, S. A., Bayraktar, R., Yumrutas, O., Oztuzcu, S., Igci, M., Igci, Y. Z., Cakmak, E. A., & Arslan, A. (2014). The effects of *Nigella sativa* (Ns), *Anthemis hyalina* (Ah) and *Citrus sinensis* (Cs) extracts on the replication of coronavirus and the expression of TRP genes family. *Molecular Biology Reports, 41*(3), 1703–1711. https://doi.org/10.1007/s11033-014-3019-7 (accessed on 4th July 2024).

Valizadeh, H., Abdolmohammadi-Vahid, S., Danshina, S., Gencer, M. Z., Ammari, A., Sadeghi, A., Roshangar, L., et al. (2020). Nano-curcumin therapy, a promising method in modulating inflammatory cytokines in COVID-19 patients. *International Immunopharmacology, 89*(December), 107088. https://doi.org/10.1016/j.intimp.2020.107088 (accessed on 4th July 2024).

Visintini Jaime, M. F., Redko, F., Muschietti, L. V., Campos, R. H., Martino, V. S., & Cavallaro, L. V. (2013). *In vitro* antiviral activity of plant extracts from *Asteraceae* medicinal plants. *Virology Journal, 10*(1), 245. https://doi.org/10.1186/1743-422X-10-245 (accessed on 4th July 2024).

Weber, N., Andersen, D., North, J., Murray, B., Lawson, L., & Hughes, B. (1992). *In vitro* virucidal effects of *Allium sativum* (garlic) extract and compounds. *Planta Medica, 58*(05), 417–423. https://doi.org/10.1055/s-2006-961504 (accessed on 4th July 2024).

Wei, Z. Q., Zhang, Y. H., Ke, C. Z., Chen, H. X., Ren, P., He, Y. L., Hu, P., Ma, D. Q., Luo, J., & Meng, Z. J. (2017). Curcumin inhibits hepatitis B virus infection by down-regulating cccDNA-bound histone acetylation. *World Journal of Gastroenterology, 23*(34), 6252. https://doi.org/10.3748/wjg.v23.i34.6252 (accessed on 4th July 2024).

Wen, C. C., Kuo, Y. H., Jan, J. T., Liang, P. H., Wang, S. Y., Liu, H. G., Lee, C. K., et al. (2007). Specific plant terpenoids and lignoids possess potent antiviral activities against severe acute respiratory syndrome coronavirus. *Journal of Medicinal Chemistry, 50*(17), 4087–4095. https://doi.org/10.1021/jm070295s (accessed on 4th July 2024).

Wen, C. C., Shyur, L. F., Jan, J. T., Liang, P. H., Kuo, C. J., Arulselvan, P., Wu, J. B., Kuo, S. C., & Yang, N. S. (2011). Traditional Chinese medicine herbal extracts of *Cibotium barometz, Gentiana scabra, Dioscorea batatas, Cassia tora,* and *Taxillus chinensis* inhibit SARS-CoV replication. *Journal of Traditional and Complementary Medicine,*

1(1), 41–50. https://doi.org/10.1016/S2225-4110(16)30055-4 (accessed on 4th July 2024).

Xu, H. B., Ma, Y. B., Huang, X. Y., Geng, C. A., Wang, H., Zhao, Y., Yang, T. H., et al. (2015). Bioactivity-guided isolation of anti-hepatitis B virus active sesquiterpenoids from the traditional Chinese medicine: Rhizomes of *Cyperus rotundus*. *Journal of Ethnopharmacology, 171*(August), 131–140. https://doi.org/10.1016/j.jep.2015.05.040 (accessed on 4th July 2024).

Yang, M., Lee, G., Si, J., Lee, S. J., You, H., & Ko, G. (2016). Curcumin shows antiviral properties against norovirus. *Molecules, 21*(10), 1401. https://doi.org/10.3390/molecules21101401 (accessed on 4th July 2024).

Zandi, K., Lim, T. H., Rahim, N. A., Shu, M. H., Teoh, B. T., Sam, S. S., Danlami, M. B., Tan, K. K., & Abubakar, S. (2013). Extract of *Scutellaria baicalensis* inhibits dengue virus replication. *BMC Complementary and Alternative Medicine, 13*(1), 91. https://doi.org/10.1186/1472-6882-13-91 (accessed on 4th July 2024).

Zeng, N., Chen, X., & Liu, Z. (2022). Natural products and nanotechnology against coronavirus disease 2019. *Frontiers in Chemistry, 10*(February), 819969. https://doi.org/10.3389/fchem.2022.819969 (accessed on 4th July 2024).

CHAPTER 5

Nanocarriers for Targeted Antiviral Drug Delivery

RASHMI SAREEN* and NITIN JAIN

DSEU Dwarka Campus (formerly Integrated Institute of Technology), New Delhi, India

*Corresponding author

ABSTRACT

Development of antiviral therapy is highly challenging due to the replication of the virus inside host cells. In the last decade, several new technologies have been explored to counter viral infections. Nanocarriers have emerged as a potential therapy to overcome the limitations of traditional antiviral drugs. The primary aim of nanocarriers is to deliver the drug to specific sites at specific rates, limiting the dose of the drug and its associated side effects. Additionally, these carriers offer improved selectivity of the drug toward viral cells compared to host cells. This chapter focuses on various nanocarriers as promising drug delivery systems for antiviral drugs. It includes nanoliposomes, nanoemulsions, solid lipid nanoparticles, nanostructured lipid carriers, nanoparticles, nanogels, hybrid nanoparticles, nanocrystals, self-nanoemulsifying drug delivery systems, dendrimers, gold nanoparticles, silver nanoparticles, nanobubbles, nanofibers, nanodiamonds, nanotraps, and nanorobots. The authors also present the role and applications of nanocarriers in targeted antiviral therapy.

Nanotechnological Management of Viral Infections.
Radhakrishnan EK, Shiji Mathew, and Riya Alex (Eds.)

DOI: 10.1201/9781779640895-5

5.1 INTRODUCTION

Today, viral infections are considered a major global problem, resulting in a higher number of morbidities and mortalities, which pose sustained unfavorable social and economic impacts. The estimated annual deaths due to viruses are around 2 million (Colpitts, 2015; Rivera, 2015). These viruses can invade the human body through various routes, such as the eyes, mouth, skin, and nose (Breitbart, 2005). A higher number of mortalities and morbidities are associated with the hepatitis virus, human immunodeficiency virus (HIV), human papillomavirus (HPV), norovirus, herpes simplex virus (HSV), and coronaviruses.

There are new challenges in drug discovery and drug delivery due to the increasing viral infections, developing drug resistance, and the emergence of new viruses. Over the past few decades, researchers have emphasized the development of new antiviral agents against several viral infections. Until 1990, only five antiviral drugs had been licensed (Milroy, 2002). However, by 2010, more than 40 antiviral drugs had entered the market. Most of these antiviral drugs were used for the treatment of HIV infection, and some were used against varicella-zoster virus (VZV), hepatitis B virus, hepatitis C virus, human cytomegalovirus (HCMV), herpes virus, influenza A and influenza B virus.

A virus is an intracellular parasite, made up of either DNA or RNA and a coat of protein (capsid). Some viruses also possess an outer bilayer membrane of lipid, known as the outer envelope. The replication of the nucleic acid codes of viruses depends on the host's biosynthetic pathway. The main obstacle for the development of an antiviral drug is determining the biosynthetic pathway in the replication of viruses, which is distinct for the virus and not used for normal cells. The different events in viral diseases include attachment and penetration of the virus followed by uncoating, reverse transcriptase/RNA-directed RNA synthesis, and then discharge of the virion.

Regarding the route of administration of antiviral drugs, most of these drugs are administered orally, while some are delivered parenterally, such as intravenously, subcutaneously, intravitreally, or topically. However, there are major problems with antiviral drugs, including their short half-life, limited solubility, and incomplete absorption, leading to a reduction in their efficacy. Therefore, frequent administration and high doses are needed, which can negatively impact patient compliance.

Most antiviral drugs, when taken orally, show less bioavailability, and for sufficient bioavailability, good solubility and permeability are considered essential requirements. Based on their solubility and permeability using the Biopharmaceutics Classification System (BCS), Amidon et al. (1995) classified all orally administered drugs into four classes (class I, II, III, IV). In addition to solubility and permeability, other factors such as efflux transport, intestinal metabolizing enzymes' actions, and food also affect the oral bioavailability of antiviral drugs.

To improve the efficacy and decrease the toxicity of antiviral drugs, novel approaches to modify conventional dosage forms can be adopted. These modifications can help overcome the challenges associated with antiviral agents. Numerous researchers and pharmaceutical companies have explored various modified drug delivery systems for antiviral drugs, such as depot formulations, sustained-release tablets, and topical and transdermal delivery systems. The goal of these modified systems is to deliver the drug to a specific site at a controlled rate, thereby reducing the required drug dosage and mitigating associated side effects. Currently, there is a growing focus on the nano-delivery of antiviral agents to enhance therapeutic efficacy and counteract drug toxicity and other potential side effects.

5.2 NANOTECHNOLOGY

The term "nanotechnology" implies methods and applications for the development of particles in the range of nanometers, usually 1–100 nm in diameter. The interlink between nanotechnology and biological science is termed as nanobiotechnology. The area that deals with nano-structured materials used to diagnose, treat, and prevent diseases is called nanomedicine.

Nanosystems were initially introduced in drug delivery primarily to improve the bioavailability of poorly absorbed drugs. Nanoparticles can exert their antiviral action by different mechanisms. The small particle size of nanoparticles provides the delivery of the drug to anatomically privileged sites. The large surface area of nanosystems also provides a higher payload of the drug, which can be entrapped inside the system. Moreover, tunable surface charge helps in the entry of nanoparticles inside the negatively charged cell membrane. Biomimetic properties of nanoparticles also induce some type of intrinsic antiviral activity. For example, dendrimers and silver nanoparticles can exhibit these properties. Additionally, structure modification with PEG can lead to optimized and targeted drug delivery. So, nanoparticles with suitable structure modification lead to cell specificity and improved drug delivery to the target cell and tissue. Other limitations with conventional drug delivery systems include crossing highly specific barriers like the blood-brain barrier and blood-testis barrier, which can be easily overcome using nanoparticulate drug delivery systems.

5.3 ROLE AND APPLICATION OF NANOCARRIERS FOR TARGETED ANTIVIRAL DRUG DELIVERY

Various types of nanoparticle delivery systems can be developed using food-grade or pharmaceutical-grade ingredients, such as nanoliposomes, biopolymer nanoparticles, microemulsions, solid lipid nanoparticles, nanoemulsions, and biopolymer nanogels. These nanoparticles can generally be fabricated using two main methods: 1. Top-down methods that employ mechanical devices like sonicators, homogenizers, or other size-reducing devices to decrease the size of large particles to smaller ones. 2. Bottom-up methods that utilize phase separation and coacervation techniques, emulsification techniques, or the addition of non-solvent techniques (Joye, 2013). These approaches can be combined to fabricate nanoparticle delivery systems with improved properties and efficacy. For instance, the homogenization technique can be employed to prepare nanoemulsions, which can then be entrapped by polymers using electrostatic precipitation or deposition techniques (McClements, 2010). The application of nanoparticles as a delivery system for antiviral drugs has been demonstrated by numerous researchers in the past (Table 5.1). The small size and surface characteristics of nanoparticles make them an attractive option for delivering antiviral drugs to specific sites (Li et al., 2019; Patra et al., 2018). For example, the release of an antiviral drug from a nanoparticle delivery system can lead to the binding of the drug to the viral receptor of the host cell or the release of the drug inside the cell, thereby interfering with the replication of the virus (Cojocaru, 2020; Maginnis, 2018) (Figure 5.1).

TABLE 5.1 Nanoparticulate Delivery System for Antiviral

Sl. No.	Nanoparticulate Delivery System	Fabrication Method	Advantage of Delivery System
1.	Solid lipid nanoparticles	High pressure hot homogenisation technique	High entrapment efficiency and comparatively high loading capacity and controlled release profile of Acyclovir
2.	Chitosan nanoparticles	Ionic gelation technique	Chitosan nanoparticles loaded with Saquinavir resulted in enhanced control of viral proliferation as studied on two different viral strain NL4-3 and Indie-Cl.
3.	Nanoemulsion	High pressure homogenisation technique	Nanoemulsion loaded with Indinavirand and lactoferrin showed improved brain penetration, which can be utilized as higher antiviral potential against HIV.
4.	Solid lipid nanoparticles	Solvent diffusion method	Solid lipid nanoparticles loaded with Adefovir dipivoxil resulted in enhanced inhibitory effect against hepatitis B surface antigen, hepatitis B e antigen and hepatitis B virus DNA levels in *in-vitro* studies.
5.	β-cyclodextrin nanoparticle	Crosslinking technique	Nanoparticle showed higher concentration of drug in CSF, which may be very effective in the treatment of HIV
6.	Nanoliposomes	Film method and sonication	Higher entrapment efficiency of Santolina insularis essential oil in nanoliposomes. This developed formulation showed antiviral activity against HSV-1.
7.	Nanoliposomes	Film hydration method	Acyclovir nanoliposomes showed prolonged contact time between drug and nasal cavity, which resulted in higher absorption from nasal mucosa.
8.	Dextran and stearic acid nanoparticles	Double emulsion solvent evaporation method	Hybrid nanoparticles resulted in improved delivery of drug and higher cellular internalization of Zidovudine.
9.	Gel nanoemulsion	Low energy method	Gel nanoemulsion loaded with Acyclovir showed 2.8 fold more permeation of drug; this can be useful for topical treatment of viral ophthalmic infection.
10.	Nanoliposomes	Film method and sonication	Nanoliposomes exhibited improved antiherpetic activity *in vitro*.
11.	Alginate nanoparticles	Emulsion solvent evaporation method	Nanoparticles showed higher cellular internalization of drug.

TABLE 5.1 *(Continued)*

Sl. No.	Nanoparticulate Delivery System	Fabrication Method	Advantage of Delivery System
12.	Solid lipid nanoparticles	Solvent evaporation and double emulsification method	Formulation showed high entrapment efficiency and enhanced antiviral activity.
13.	Nanoliposomes	Rapid extrusion	Nanoliposomes exhibited synergistic antiviral activity against HIV.
14.	PVP/Stearic acid-PEG nanoparticles	Emulsion solvent evaporation method	Improved cellular internalization.
15.	Chitosan-g-HPβCD nanoparticles	Ionic gelation method	Developed nanoparticles formulation exhibited sustained release of Efavirenz and showed higher permeability as compared to free drug.

Source: Delshadi (2021).

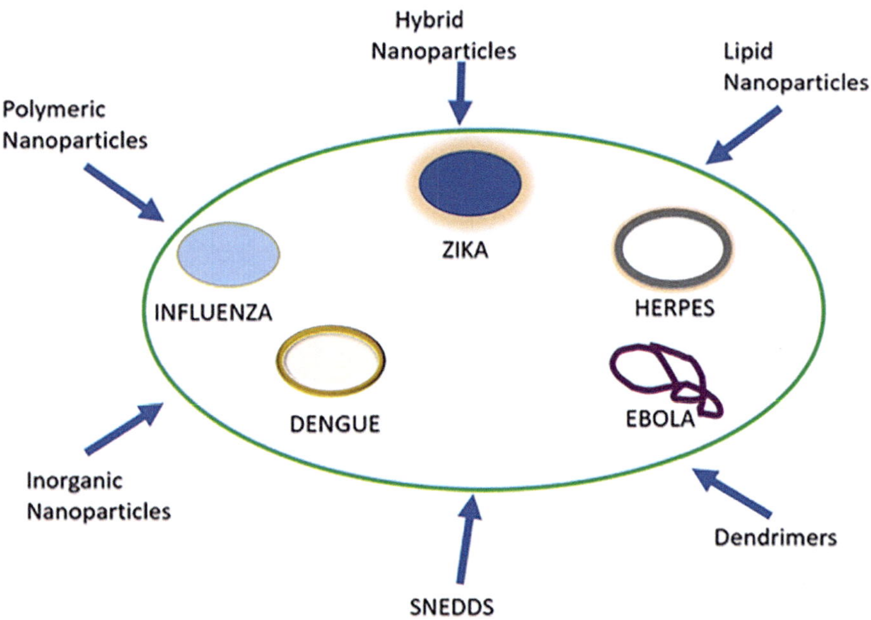

FIGURE 5.1 Nanocarriers in antiviral drug delivery.

5.3.1 MICELLES AND MICROEMULSIONS

Micelles represent a promising delivery system for antiviral drugs that require controlled drug delivery, cell selectivity, and prolonged circulation in the blood. Micelles are colloidal particles that are amphiphilic in nature, with a particle size ranging from 5–100 nm. Composed of two completely different molecules with different affinities for water, micelles require an optimum temperature condition and concentration of amphiphilic molecules for their formation. The inner part of a micelle is termed the core, formed by the hydrophobic part of the amphiphilic molecule, while the outer part is termed the shell, made of the hydrophilic portion of the amphiphilic molecules. Concentration of the amphiphilic molecules plays a vital role in the formation of micelles. At low concentrations, the micellar amphiphile molecule is present separately in an aqueous vehicle. When the concentration of the micellar molecule increases, the aggregation of amphiphilic molecules occurs in a narrow concentration range. The concentration at which the aggregation of monomers of the micellar amphiphile takes place is called the critical micelle concentration, and the temperature at which micellization occurs is called the critical micellization temperature. The formation of micelles from amphiphilic molecules involves the removal of the hydrophobic portion of amphiphilic molecules from the aqueous vehicle and the re-establishment of hydrogen bonding in water, which also reduces the free energy of micelles. Micelles are advantageous as drug delivery systems as they can carry both hydrophilic and hydrophobic drugs. Lipophilic drugs may be contained inside the core, while hydrophilic drugs may attach to the micelle's surface. Polymeric micelles can be fabricated with enhanced solubility, absorption, and stability compared to conventional micelles. To target the viral reservoirs, micelles formed by surface modification of PEG-polylactide copolymer can be achieved by attaching galactose, as galactose may interact with lectins.

5.3.2 NANOLIPOSOMES

Another widely used nanoparticle delivery system for the entrapment of antiviral drugs is nanoliposomes. Nanoliposomes differ from liposomes in their small size ($d < 200$ nm). Based on their internal structure, they are classified into unilamellar (single-ring) and multilamellar (onion-ring structure) vesicles. Various fabrication methods are employed for the preparation of nanoliposomes, such as the solvent evaporation method commonly used in the laboratory, and for large-scale production, other methods like homogenization, sonication, or microfluidization are utilized. The encapsulation of antivirals can be done either after the formation of liposomes or before the formation of nanoliposomes. Due to the presence of phospholipid heads (polar) and phospholipid tails (non-polar) in the bilayer structures of nanoliposomes, both hydrophilic and lipophilic antivirals can be delivered through them. Nanoliposomes are suitable for all routes of administration due to the presence of phospholipids used to prepare them. Ligands can be attached to nanoliposome surfaces to target the antiviral to specific sites. However, their low physicochemical stability and relatively high cost restrict their widespread application.

5.3.3 NANOEMULSIONS

Nanoemulsions, another type of colloidal system, have the capability for the protection, encapsulation, and delivery of antivirals. They contain water, oil, surfactants, and co-surfactants and exist in a single phase. The size of nanoemulsions varies between 20 and 500 nm, based on the composition and relative amount of surface-active agents, mechanical energy, and entrapped drug particle size. Nanoemulsions are classified based on the structural organization of water (W) and oil (O) phases. The first is water on oil (W/O), in which water is dispersed as minute globules into oil as the continuous phase. The next one is oil and water (O/W), in which oil is dispersed in the continuous water phase. The microdomains of water and oil are other bicontinuous nanoemulsions like water-in-oil-in-water (W/O/W) and oil-in-water-in-oil (O/W/O) nanoemulsions. Surfactants, also known as surface-active agents, are one of the constituents of nanoemulsions, comprising hydrophobic tails and hydrophilic heads. Nanoemulsions are further classified into three parts based on surfactants – cationic O/W nanoemulsions, anionic O/W nanoemulsions, and neutral O/W nanoemulsions. Various mechanical devices are used for the formation of nanoemulsions, such as microfluidizers, sonicators, and high-pressure valve homogenizers. The selection of emulsifier and a suitable homogenization method is a critical step in the formation of stable nanoemulsions. As compared to conventional emulsions, nanoemulsions offer advantages such as increased loading capacity, enhanced aqueous solubility, lymphatic uptake, residence time in the gastrointestinal tract, increased absorption, and bioavailability. Nanoemulsions can be utilized for delivering antiviral agents. Their very small particle size leads to increased solubility and dissolution of both lipophilic and hydrophilic drugs. Their small size also facilitates penetration from the epithelial layer compared to conventional topical antiviral delivery, resulting in increased absorption of the drug.

5.3.4 SOLID LIPID NANOPARTICLES (SLNs)

Solid lipid nanoparticles (SLNs) constitute a different drug delivery system than traditional colloidal nanoparticles. The objective of SLNs is to integrate the benefits of traditional nanocarriers while removing some of their drawbacks. For example, the commercial production of polymeric nanoparticles is a main obstacle that restricts their use in drug delivery, whereas manufacturing SLNs is not only cost-effective but also comparatively simple (e.g., performing high-pressure homogenization, microemulsion techniques) (Mueller, 2000). Further benefits of using SLNs include enhanced availability, stability, and safety, and decreased harmful effects, with a better drug-release pattern than synthetic polymer nanoparticles (Gupta, 2010; Patel, 2011; Xie et al., 2014).

5.3.5 SOLID LIPID NANOPARTICLES (SLNS) AND NANOSTRUCTURED LIPID CARRIERS (NLCS)

The structure of SLNs and NLCs in many ways resembles O/W nanoemulsions. The only difference is that the lipid phase of the nanoparticle is solid instead of liquid. In SLNs, the lipid phase is entirely solidified into a uniform crystal lattice, whereas the lipid phase of NLCs is incompletely solidified and has an irregular crystal lattice arrangement. SLNs are prepared from pure lipids and have a sharp melting point, while NLCs melt at a broad range of temperatures because they are prepared from a lipid mixture. Hydrophobic bioactive agents are incorporated in the solidified lipid mesh networks of NLCs and SLNs. The solidified lipid phase slows down molecular diffusion, hindering the discharge of the bioactive ingredients. However, due to particle morphological changes, the uniform crystalline phase in SLNs can result in the discharge of bioactives or particle clumping (Weiss, 2008). These complications are reduced by using NLCs because their irregular crystal arrangement can accommodate more bioactive compounds (Müller, 2002). NLCs and SLNs are used for the entrapment and release of many antiviral agents. For example, SLNs ($d = 167$ nm) are used to deliver a protease inhibitor, atazanavir, to the brain by employing a cell culture model of the BBB (blood-brain barrier) (Chattopadhyay, 2008). Entrapping the antiviral agents raises the quantity aggregating in endothelial cells, resulting in an enhancement in its capability to handle HIV-encephalitis. SLNs and NLCs were explored to increase their ocular bioavailability for acyclovir (Seyfoddin, 2013). The NLCs were proved to have a better encapsulation tendency and efficacy compared to SLNs due to their irregular pattern of crystal arrangement. SLNs are also refined for topical delivery systems by successful encapsulation. For example, an *ex-vivo* experiment with an antiviral aromatic essential oil, *Artemisia arborescence*, and pig skin demonstrated that the nanoemulsions improved the aggregation of the antiviral agent on the epidermis of the skin but, in fact, decreased its penetration into the skin compared to a pure oil formulation (Lai, 2007). It was proven that *in vitro* activity of the antiviral agent was not severely affected by entrapment against HSV-1. SLNs were proved to be a good formulation of the antiviral agents for skin applications. Encapsulation of ritonavir in SLNs was shown to possess sustained release as well as antiviral activity by employing an *in vitro* anti-HIV-1 model (Javan, 2017). El-Gizawy and El-Maghraby et al. designed an SLN-based system for acyclovir targeting the brain (El-Gizawy, 2019). The formulation of SLNs includes a wide range of lipids and surfactants, and to make the nanoparticles cationic, they were coated with chitosan. It was proven that the acyclovir-loaded SLNs could make the antiviral agent cross the BBB, and the drug remains in the bloodstream for a prolonged time. This improved efficacy was partially due to the efficiency of the surfactants (Pluronic®F68 and Tween 80) not only to restrict the P-glycoprotein efflux system but also to enable them to cross the BBB. SLNs have cationic chitosan on their surface that has improved their transport across the BBB by interacting with anionic moieties present on the endothelial cells of the brain.

5.3.6 BIOPOLYMER PARTICLES: NANOPARTICLES AND NANOGELS

Proteins, polysaccharides, and their complexes produce several biopolymer-based nanocarriers (Matalanis, 2011). These colloidal dispersions comprise small fragments that consist of a complex of cross-linked biopolymers. These biopolymers are called nanoparticles, whereas when made up of a solvent, they are called nanogels. Biopolymer fragments can be manufactured by several bottom-up and top-down techniques, comprising emulsion-templating, injection-gelation, fragmentation, anti-solvent precipitation, thermodynamic incompatibility, molding, and coacervation methods (McClements 2017, 2018). The chemical and physical characteristics of the biopolymer particles are regulated by selecting proper ingredients along with fabrication methods. Chitosan nanoparticles are among the popular biopolymer-based nanoparticles for target-specific release of antivirals, as they promote improved encapsulation, extended release, and decreased cell toxicity. A nanogel is a nanoparticle composed of hydrogel which can be used for retroviral drug delivery. Hydrogel has a 3D cross-linked polymeric arrangement that has distinctive characteristics, making them swell. They consist of 95% water (at this point called a superabsorbent) not dissolving in an aqueous medium. A nanogel can be manufactured by natural, synthetic, or by blending both polymers. A nanogel shows the properties of both solid and fluid in combination and depends on the participation of both the components. The liquid segment prevents the nanogel from forming a dense insoluble clump, whereas the solid segment prevents the free flow of the liquid. Cross-linked polymers are formed by heterogeneous polymerization reactions accompanied by bifunctional or multifunctional cross-linkers. This consists of the living radical polymerization methods forms the nanogels with different configurations, size, along with core-shell and hollow nanogel constituents. Addition of functional initiators and macroinitiators adds more properties on the periphery or inside nanogels. Their dimensions, charge, permeability, amphiphilicity, pliability, and degradability are improved by changing the composition of the nanogel (Soni, 2016). This varying composition allows the nanogel to have several properties in antiviral drug delivery, such as improved encapsulation efficiency and prevention of active agent from degeneracy. The hydrophilic nature of nanogels makes them highly biocompatible, and an increased quantity of nano drugs can be loaded. They have improved stability and are also multifunctional. So, they can be employed for diagnosis and therapy of viral exposure. Nanogels can be modified for selective targets, actively in combination with a target ligand or passively. They are responsive to internal and external stimuli such as temperature, pH, enzyme, amount of enzyme, magnetic field, and redox potential. The stimulation will change the conformation or structure of the nanogel that can be seen as swelling or deswelling of the nanogel mass, resulting in the release of encapsulated antiviral. This property makes the nanogel in formulating effective antivirals. So, a pH-sensitive nanogel can be used as a target at a viral reservoir where it can release the drug at low pH. It was also found that PVCL nanogels prepared by thermal precipitation are heat-sensitive in an aqueous medium through free radical polymerization. PVCL804 NG (nanogel) showed antiviral activity against the HIV-1 infection by evaluating the enzymatic activity of luciferase (Macchione, 2019), when administered through the vagina. Introducing a coating of PEG on the exterior of the nanogel enables it to have hydrophilicity and sheath-like property. The sheath carries some charge as the interior of the gel because of the nanoparticles present, which eliminates the chances of interactions with plasma proteins. Some points to be taken care of before commercial use of nanogels for antiviral drug delivery are the maintenance of stimuli reaction delivery rate, biocompatibility, and stability (Chakravarty, 2020).

5.3.7 HYBRID NANOPARTICLES

Hybrid nanoparticles are used to make antiviral delivery complexes, which integrate the useful features of discrete nanoparticles. For example, hybrid nanoparticles may be manufactured by closing in smaller fragments into a larger fragment or by preparing core-shell compositions that can result in improved entrapping, protecting, or releasing characteristics (Chan, 2009; Zhang, 2008). Alginate and stearic acid-polyethylene glycol (SA-PEG) are utilized in preparing a nanoparticle delivery approach for zidovudine (Joshy, 2017). Zidovudine and alginate are employed as core materials, but SA-PEG is used on the surface. This blend results in a dendritic structure with inner voids and networks. An *in vitro* investigation proved that the hybrid nanoparticles were safe, compatible with blood, and could efficiently deliver the antiviral drug to model brain ganglia. These hybrid nanoparticles can be useful for treating HIV infections.

5.3.8 NANOCRYSTALS

Approximately 40% of newly formed drugs are imperfectly soluble in the aqueous phase. The main objective in drug delivery studies is to discover biomaterials which allow proper dissolution of the drug having solid efficacy. Whereas immediate-release-based systems of cyclodextrin prove themselves as favorable vehicles, nanocrystals have recently proven themselves as an equally useful solution. They came into being in the late 1990s, and their size ranges between 100 and 1000 nm. Nanocrystals are not accepted as carriers as they are only composed of the pure drug administered, and very few surfactants are added for stability. After processing, they can be easily changed physically to existing drug delivery systems such as tablets (Gao, 2008). To form nanocrystals by precipitation, several features are reviewed that directly affect the characteristics of the outcome, such as the stirring rate, the ratio of anti-solvent to solvent, drug content, and temperature. When the stirring rate is increased, the particle size decreases, and hence the tablet will be homogenous. When the anti-solvent to solvent ratio is high, the solution will be more concentrated. The amount and characteristics of the drug under investigation determine flow properties and homogeneity. Lower temperature creates crystals of smaller size between 100 and 1000 nm. Nanocrystals can be manufactured by milling techniques, where properties are determined by the content of the drug, pearl number involved in milling, milling velocity, duration, and temperature. Increasing the drug content and milling duration will increase clumping in the finished product. An increase in the number of milling pearls and velocity may result in clumping. However, lots of pearls moving too fast will lead to weight loading issues. Aggregation is also improved by increasing the milling speed and temperature. These multiple methods help in the production of different nanocrystals with different properties. Several varying properties are beneficial for their application in potential antiviral therapies.

5.3.9 SELF-NANOEMULSIFYING DRUG DELIVERY SYSTEMS (SNEDDS)

The SNEDDS is a part of nanoemulsions. They are prepared by the emulsification of water and oil with the addition of surfactants, followed by gentle stirring. They are a lipid-based monotropic system and have the capability to dissolve a hydrophobic drug in the oil phase. Many antiviral drugs, such as Lauroglycol 90, Capryol 90, and Capmul MCM, can be given by this system. An increase in the released dosage was found when an HIV antiviral (Nevirapine) was given in the form of a self-nanoemulsifying drug delivery system, that is, in the aqueous part of the GIT, the drug release was found to be 98.9% (Selvam, 2014).

5.3.10 DENDRIMERS

Dendrimers are radially nano-sized structures. They have multiple branches that arise from a central element by branching units that form a 3D tree-like structure. Interactions with the functional environment are governed by the last group. They are highly functional, as they can entrap many chemical constituents and inner layers and have a multivalent surface property. They have three major domains: core, inner portion, and peripheral shell. All these domains possess varying characteristics, such as solubility or bonding with ligands. Their size is lower than 100 nm, and they can chain with different ligands, which enables them to be appreciable for drug delivery. Proper biological and physicochemical properties can be obtained by using different sorts of polymers as well as functional groups. A single dendrimer gets incorporated with several drugs or ligands. They are used for releasing DNA, siRNA, and many antiviral therapeutics. The most popular dendrimer for antiviral remedy is VivaGel, manufactured as mucoadhesive gel. It is the earliest topical nanomicrobicide prepared from the divalent benzhydrylamine amide of l-lysine and has 32 sodium 1-(carboxymethoxy) naphthalene-3,6-disulfonate as the last negatively charged functional group, which allows prolonged antiviral activity. Dendrimers are used successfully in antiviral therapy and gene therapy, also as a vehicle of transportation all over the body. Dendrimers are multiple-branched polymers constituting a central core, a repetitive monomer called a dendron, and surface groups. Some examples of dendrimers are the PAMAM that own 4 and 5 nm diameters, respectively. Mostly, the diameter ranges from 2 nm^{-10} nm and are monodisperse in expression of their molecular structure. The surface groups add functional groups that alter the chemical constitution of the carrier. The central core is hydrophobic and charged; they possess comparatively high-water solubility and attract lipophilic drugs more efficiently. It is possible to change the pharmacokinetic rates of the lipophilic drugs by maintaining the constitution of the innermost hydrophobic moiety. Several antiviral uses of this system include remedies for the influenza virus, human immunodeficiency virus, and respiratory syncytial virus. The effectiveness of this treatment is due to the result of varying functional groups on the periphery that restrict the entry of the virus into the cell. However, being highly effective in the initial stages of viral infection, efficiency declines dramatically once the virus moves into the cell (Rabiee et al., 2020).

5.4 INORGANIC-BASED NANOFORMULATIONS

Inorganic compounds were utilized for medicinal preparations in Ancient Greece and Rome. Silver, for instance, was used to store food and prevent degradation and decomposition. Hippocrates suggested that silver compounds could block infections and enhance healing while treating ulcers. Researchers began incorporating more inorganic constituents to treat and identify various diseases (Konop, 2016). Gold, silver, CuO, TiO_2, CeO_2, and SiO nanoparticles have shown high efficacy against many viruses, including non-retro and retro viruses. These compounds link with proteins on the virus capsid through Kazimir interactions and van der Waals forces, inactivating the virus due to their similar size and shape (Lembo, 2010). Metals and oxides with functionally active surfaces show improved interaction with biomolecules that allow viruses to enter the host cell. However, the use of inorganic nanoparticles is limited due to toxicity concerns (Chakravarty, 2020).

5.4.1 GOLD NANOPARTICLES (GNPs)

Gold nanoparticles (GNPs) are commercially used as nanocarriers due to their remarkable conductivity, surface flexibility, biocompatibility, and simple manufacturing methods. Gold has unique physicochemical properties, including the gold core, light-sensitive properties that can promote proper drug release at target sites, and variation of functionalization through thiol conjugation. They can be manufactured in different sizes (1–2 nm, 1.5–5 nm, or 10–150 nm based on application) using simple methods.

Gold nanoparticles (AuNPs) are colloids used for structured nano-treatments against viruses. AuNPs have special optical characteristics caused by the spinning of non-bonding electrons, which determine the functionality of the nanoparticles. Studies have shown that AuNPs can enter cells used by HIV for duplication, such as lymphocytes, macrophages, and micro-endothelial ganglia in the brain. Scientists incorporated a thiol group as a linker between the antiviral drug Raltegravir and AuNP. When this complex enters infected peripheral blood mononuclear cells (PBMCs), it inhibits HIV duplication. In contrast, free AuNP (control) allowed to enter infected cells did not show any antiviral activity (Liu et al., 2011). AuNPs combined with siRNA target specific viral genes and were found to have improved stability relative to free siRNA, reducing viral RNA duplication of dengue. These conjugates also inhibit the growth of pathogenic dengue virions. GNPs can cause viral deformation, eliminating metabolic functions. By attaching linkers that mimic heparin sulfate proteoglycans (HSPG) to the exterior surface of AuNPs, these particles can bind to viral ligands, releasing strong forces to deform them. These particles are neutral to cells and effective against several virus strains such as HSV, HPV, RSV, and dengue. Gold particles stabilized by gallic acid produce monodisperse, spherical AuNPs with a diameter of 7–8 nm. These nanoparticles effectively hinder viruses with an enhanced safety profile compared to other drugs on the market, acting by inhibiting viral attachment and penetration (Cagno et al., 2018).

5.4.2 SILVER NANOPARTICLES (AgNPs)

Silver nanoparticles (AgNPs) are the most efficient metallic nanoparticles against microorganisms. Silver not only has bacteriostatic and bactericidal properties but also exhibits good conductivity, catalytic qualities, and chemical stability. Silver nanoparticles promote the release of silver ions, resulting in antimicrobial activity, plasma membrane degradation, and DNA degeneration.

AgNPs are widely used as antiviral agents due to their inherent antimicrobial activity. They conjugate with the respiratory tree, electron transport system enzymes, and prokaryotic DNA. Despite their small size, they have a large surface area, which results in rapid dissolution.

Silver nanoparticles possess several favorable characteristics that make them suitable antiviral agents, such as chemical stability, good conductivity, and restricted plasma resonance. Due to their different targets, they have fewer chances of developing drug resistance (Lee, 2019). Scientists primarily targeted the activity of silver nanoparticles against HIV-1. Galdiero was the first company to investigate and demonstrate the antiviral activity of AgNPs against HIV-1. The nanoparticles were studied under three surface phenomena with glycerol as a reducing factor, and AgNPs linked with BSA. The theory showed that the conjugation between the BSA-conjugated particles and HIV virions depended on the size. Only AgNPs in the size range of 1–10 nm bound with the virions. After binding, they inhibited infectious stages post-viral introduction by competing with the sulfur and oxygen atoms connected to the thiol or phosphate groups on nucleotides or amino acids. These conjugations caused a reduction in the reverse transcription speed of HIV-1. When AgNPs were coated with oseltamivir, a medicine used to treat H1N1, the AgNP absorbed with oseltamivir prevented H1N1 attachment to host cells. This disruption of the reactive oxygen species (ROS)-mediated signaling pathway demonstrates the antimicrobial activities of nanoparticles.

5.5 FUTURE NANO SYSTEMS FOR ANTIVIRAL DRUG DELIVERY

5.5.1 NANOBUBBLES

Nanobubbles are capable of generating and reflecting sound waves, with an oxygen core allowing them to carry drugs. Leveraging their echogenic nature, they are used for site-specific drug delivery, utilizing ultrasound technology. The core may also contain other gases such as perfluoropentane and decafluoropentane. Their shell comprises a lipid polymer conjugated with a surfactant, providing stability, an appropriate half-life, and proper sound parameters for drug release at the target organ. Ultrasound for active targeting is non-invasive and provides higher stability compared to other targeting methods. Nanobubbles can be surface-altered for theragnostic properties, featuring an adaptable structure that can be conjugated with various molecules for diagnosis, treatment, and infection mitigation. Their echogenic nature allows real-time ultrasound visualization of the target organ and drug application (Alheshibri, 2016).

5.5.2 NANOFIBERS

Nanofibers are produced using the electrospinning method with polymers such as polyvinyl alcohol, chitosan, polyethylene oxide, and cellulite acetate. The drug can be distinctly conjugated with the nanofiber in its pure form or nanoparticulate form. Initially, drug delivery is crucial, but maintaining a core-sheath complex reduces the risk (Xue, 2017). Nanofibers possess a large surface area, high porosity with small pore size, and high tensile strength. Their surface can be modified to enable controlled release of hydrophilic anti-HIV drugs, such as raltegravir and maraviroc. These fibers were twisted and blended with biodegradable polymers such as PCL and PLGA. Altering the polymer ratios results in perfect sustained release (Carson, 2016).

5.5.3 NANODIAMONDS

Nanodiamonds are safe carbon-derived materials with a stable sp3 carbon core, while the surfaces have many sides to form coordination with neighboring water molecules. They effectively solubilize lipid-soluble drugs. Furthermore, they are manufactured at elevated temperatures and pressure or by the detonation method. They possess desirable properties such as a stable structure, safety, better ADME, biocompatibility, loading capacity, and prolonged circulation time. Their surface can be altered for target-specific delivery and modified with growth factors (Laan, 2018).

5.5.4 NANOTRAPS

Nanotraps are homogenous hydrogels used for capturing viruses, identified by their charge and highly associated aromatic centers adjoining a polymerized shell. The hydrophobic and electrostatic conjugation is governed by the hydrogel derivative and surface charge, respectively. The outer shell captures the virus, and the inner hydrogel keeps the virus trapped. Nanotraps can be physicochemically altered for varying needs. Nanotraps capture the virus through the sieving shell, preserving the trapped virus in the lipophilic interior. Nanotraps prevent the trapped virus through the action of proteases. They are used to trap HIV-1 from patients; an example of this is Cibacron Blue (Shi, 2020). Their polymer shells are composed of N-isopropyl acrylamide, N, N-dimethylene bis-acrylamide, allyl amine, methacrylate, and vinyl sulfonic acid. Other ingredients to prepare nanotraps include acrylic acid, Acid Black 48, and red pigment. Nanotraps are employed to trap RSV, rift valley fever virus (RVFV), Venezuelan equine encephalitis virus (VEEV), and intact foot-and-mouth disease virus (FMDV). They are used to trap viruses and formulate vaccines. Other uses include the clearance of viruses like FMDV. Nanotrap particles can identify the molecular size of the virus, increasing spotting and capture efficiency. Their magnetic characteristics keep the viruses at definite temperatures for proper storage, including VEEV, which requires a temperature of around 40°C. Nanotraps are employed to treat severe sepsis using telodendrimer nanotraps (TDNTs). TDNTs capture biomolecules in contact with sepsis through multivalent, hybrid, and synergistic connections. It was proven that nanotraps in combination with typical antibiotic therapy provide 100% survivability in septic mice test subjects, effectively checking hyperinflammation. Nanotraps are highly efficient in investigating viral diseases, trapping viruses, and their genetic material for studies.

5.5.5 NANOROBOTS

Nanorobots are devices composed of inorganic, polymeric, and biomimetic components that can move through the circulation. This method is used for visualizing and treating cancer and diabetes, as well as various neural and cardiovascular diseases. These nanomachines can perform many functions to deliver APIs to target areas of the body through circulation. They are miniature circuits consisting of a power source, detectors, levers, minicomputers, pumps, mechanical support sections for drug delivery, and cameras for accurately locating the site. Nanorobots have not been used for antiviral therapy to date. Collectively, nanorobots present themselves as a highly innovative means for the future of antiviral target drug delivery.

5.6 CONCLUSION

Nanoparticle drug delivery systems play a vital role in addressing the challenges associated with traditional delivery systems and have proven to be effective in treating viral infections. Nanomaterials are tailored to integrate traditional antiviral properties with distinctive qualifications specific to nanosystems. This approach represents a promising tool for biomedical research and clinical applications. Recent advancements in nanotechnology offer greater therapeutic potential compared to traditional approaches. These innovations help overcome common limitations associated with nanoparticles in biomedical applications, such as enhanced cell membrane penetration, specific uptake, and reduced toxicity. Additionally, the integration of lipid-soluble and unstable drugs with nanoparticles enhances water solubility and stability under normal conditions.

Future research should explore the potential for:

- Multi-functionalization to achieve simultaneous drug delivery and imaging for locating specific *in vitro* targets; and
- Multiplexing to broaden the spectrum of treatable diseases in diverse populations through simple, efficient, and cost-effective methods. Upgrading pharmacokinetics and reducing toxicity of current antivirals should be investigated using advanced nanotechnology.

The advancement of nanotechnology in infectious disease treatment presents numerous opportunities to improve mechanisms of action or develop new drug therapeutics. Nano drug delivery systems can be tailored to enhance the efficacy of many antiviral drugs by overcoming physical, chemical, and biological barriers. Despite the many advantages of these nanoparticles, further research on their toxicities and potential harmful effects is necessary. Microbial expansion leading to drug resistance remains a major concern. Therefore, the development of technology to harness the robust and versatile nature of nanomedicine is crucial for the effective treatment of infectious pathogens.

It is anticipated that the use of nanomedicine will yield promising effects in the treatment and eradication of infectious pathogens. Nanoparticles can enhance the efficiency of antiviral agents and reduce drug toxicity. These properties of nanoparticles are particularly beneficial in antiviral medication, where large doses are often required and the drugs are generally expensive. The use of nanoparticulates can reduce the frequency of drug administration and the duration of medication, improve the efficacy of the antiviral agents, and overcome their disadvantages, such as poor absorption.

The primary focus of future research on antiviral drugs will be the development of new methods for classifying nanomaterials, the improvement of biologically acceptable and degradable nano-carrier approaches with no cellular toxicity, and the design of nanocarriers that are specific to viral infections. Nanoparticle design should play a pivotal role in drug delivery while possessing inherent antiviral properties.

Addressing the challenge of treating or enhancing the treatment efficacy for viral infections represents a significant endeavor. The continued exploration and advancement of nanotechnology in antiviral treatment development foster high expectations for future therapeutic innovations in treating and curing viral infections. Presently, numerous nano-platforms, including nanoparticles, liposomes, micelles, microemulsions, nanoliposomes, nanoemulsions, solid lipid nanoparticles, and biopolymer nanoparticles, have been investigated as potential carriers for antiviral drug delivery. Each drug delivery system has its distinct characteristics and limitations for specific applications, necessitating careful selection and modification of the most suitable formulation. These methodologies are critical for standardizing techniques to effectively evaluate antiviral drugs against specific viruses using different delivery approaches. These efforts are crucial for comparing the advantages of various systems.

These systems present different factors that address the current limitations of therapy. However, the clinical use of nano-carrier antiviral preparations, based on our current understanding, is limited, with only a few approved or undergoing clinical trials of nano preparations, such as vaccines, following 22 years of continuous research. It is expected that in the coming years, part of this "success preclinical story" will be refined, translated, and utilized to achieve better outcomes, use, and approach for patients.

KEYWORDS

- **antiviral**
- **drug delivery**
- **nanocarriers**
- **nanocrystals**
- **nanoemulsions**
- **nanoliposomes**
- **nanorobots**
- **nanotechnology**
- **solid lipid nanoparticles**

REFERENCES

Akbarzadeh, A., Rezaei-Sadabady, R., Davaran, S., Joo, S. W., Zarghami, N., Hanifehpour, Y., Samiei, M., Kouhi, M., & Nejati-Koshki, K. (2013). Liposome: Classification, preparation, and applications. *Nanoscale Research Letters, 8*(1), 102.

Alexis, F., Pridgen, E., Molnar, L. K. I., & Farokhzad, O. C. (2008). Factors affecting the clearance and biodistribution of polymeric nanoparticles. *Molecular Pharmaceutics, 5*, 505–515.

Alheshibri, M., Qian, J., Jehannin, M., & Craig, V. S. J. (2016). A history of nanobubbles. *Langmuir, 32*(43), 11086–11100.

Amidon, G. L., Lennernas, H., Shah, V. P., & Crison, J. R. (1995). A theoretical basis for a biopharmaceutic drug classification: The correlation of *in vitro* drug product dissolution and *in vivo* bioavailability. *Pharmaceutical Research, 12*, 413–420.

Bowman, M. C., Ballard, T. E., Ackerson, C. J., Feldheim, D. L., & Margolis, D. M. (2008). Inhibition of HIV fusion with multivalent gold nanoparticles. *Journal of the American Chemical Society, 130*, 6896–6897.

Breitbart, M., & Rohwer, F. (2005). Here a virus, there a virus, everywhere the same virus? *Trends in Microbiology, 13*(6), 278–284.

Cagno, V., Andreozzi, P., Alicarnasso, M. D., Silva, P. J., Mueller, M., Galloux, M., Le Goffic, R., Jones, S. T., Vallino, M., Hodek, J., Weber, J., Sen, S., Janecek, E. R., Bekdemir, A., Sanavio, B., Martinelli, C., & Donalisio, M. (2018). Broad-spectrum non-toxic antiviral nanoparticles with a virucidal inhibition mechanism. *Nature Materials, 17*(2), 195–203.

Calderón, L., Harris, R., Córdoba-Díaz, M., Elorza, M., Elorza, B., Lenoir, J., Adriaens, E., Remon, J., Heras, A., & Córdoba-Díaz, D. (2013). Nano and microparticulate chitosan-based systems for antiviral topical delivery. *European Journal of Pharmaceutical Sciences, 48*(1, 2), 216–222.

Caron, J., Reddy, L. H., Lepetre-Mouelhi, S., Wack, S., Clayette, P., Rogez-Kreuz, C., Yousfi, R., Couvreur, P., & Desmaele, D. (2010). Squalenoyl nucleoside monophosphate nanoassemblies: New prodrug strategy for the delivery of nucleotide analogues. *Bioorganic & Medicinal Chemistry Letters, 20*, 2761–2764.

Carson, D., Jiang, Y., & Woodrow, K. A. (2016). Tunable release of multiclass anti-HIV drugs that are water-soluble and loaded at high drug content in polyester blended electro spun fibers. *Pharmaceutical Research, 33*(1), 125–136.

Chakravarty, M., & Vora, A. (2020). Nanotechnology-based antiviral therapeutics. *Drug Delivery and Translational Research*, 1–40.

Chan, J. M., Zhang, L., Yuet, K. P., Liao, G., Rhee, J. W., Langer, R., & Farokhzad, O. C. (2009). PLGA–lecithin–PEG core–shell nanoparticles for controlled drug delivery. *Biomaterials, 30*(8), 1627–1634.

Chattopadhyay, N., Zastre, J., Wong, H. L., Wu, X. Y., & Bendayan, R. (2008). Solid lipid nanoparticles enhance the delivery of the HIV protease inhibitor, atazanavir, by a human brain endothelial cell line. *Pharmaceutical Research, 25*(10), 2262–2271.

Cojocaru, F. D., Botezat, D., Gardikiotis, I., Uritu, C. M., Dodi, G., Trandafir, L., Rezus, C., Rezus, E., Tamba, B. I., & Mihai, C. T. (2020). Nanomaterials designed for antiviral drug delivery transport across biological barriers. *Pharmaceutics, 12*(2), 171.

Colpitts, C. C., Verrier, E. R., & Baumert, T. F. (2015). Targeting viral entry for treatment of hepatitis B and C virus infections. *ACS Infectious Diseases, 1*(9), 420–427.

De Oliveira, M. P., Garcion, E., Venisse, N., Benoit, J. P., Couet, W., & Olivier. (2005). Tissue distribution of indinavir administered as solid lipid Nano capsule formulation in mdr1a (+/+) and mdr1a (−/−) CF-1 mice. *Pharmaceutical Research, 22*, 1898–1905.

Delshadi, R., Bahrami, A., McClements, D. J., Moore, M. D., & Williams, L. (2021). Development of nanoparticle-delivery systems for antiviral agents: A review. *Journal of Controlled Release, 331*, 30–44.

Demirci, M., Caglar, M. Y., Cakir, B., & Gulseren, I. (2017). Encapsulation by nanoliposomes. In *Nano capsulation Technologies for the Food and Nutraceutical Industries* (pp. 74–113).

El-Gizawy, S. A., El-Maghraby, G. M., & Hedaya, A. A. (2019). Formulation of acyclovir-loaded solid lipid nanoparticles: Design, optimization, and *in-vitro* characterization. *Pharmaceutical Development and Technology, 24*(10), 1287–1298.

Emery, V. C. (2001). Progress in understanding cytomegalovirus drug resistance. *Journal of Clinical Virology, 21*, 223–228.

Fridland, A., Connelly, M. C., & Robbins, B. L. (2000). Cellular factors for resistance against antiretroviral agents. *Antiviral Therapy, 5*, 181–185.

Gagliardi, M. (2017). Biomimetic and bioinspired nanoparticles for targeted drug delivery. *Therapeutic Delivery, 8*, 289–299.

Gao, L., Zhang, D., & Chen, M. (2008). Drug nanocrystals for the formulation of poorly soluble drugs and its application as a potential drug delivery system. *Journal of Nanoparticle Research, 10*(5), 845–862.

Gupta, U., & Jain, N. K. (2010). Non-polymeric nano-carriers in HIV/AIDS drug delivery and targeting. *Advanced Drug Delivery Reviews, 62*, 478–490.

Javan, F., Vatanara, A., Azadmanesh, K., Nabi-Meibodi, M., & Shakouri, M. (2017). Encapsulation of ritonavir in solid lipid nanoparticles: *In-vitro* anti-HIV-1 activity using lentiviral particles. *Journal of Pharmacy and Pharmacology, 69*(8), 1002–1009.

Joshy, K., George, A., Jose, J., Kalarikkal, N., Pothen, L. A., & Thomas, S. (2017). Novel dendritic structure of alginate hybrid nanoparticles for effective anti-viral drug delivery. *International Journal of Biological Macromolecules, 103*, 1265–1275.

Joye, I. J., & McClements, D. J. (2013). Production of nanoparticles by anti-solvent precipitation for use in food systems. *Trends in Food Science and Technology, 34*(2), 109–123.

Khorasani, S., Danaei, M., & Mozafari, M. R. (2018). Nanoliposome technology for the food and nutraceutical industries. *Trends in Food Science and Technology, 79*, 106–115.

Konop, M., Damps, T., Misicka, A., & Rudnicka, L. (2016). Certain aspects of silver and silver nanoparticles in wound care: A minireview. *Journal of Nanomaterials, 2016*, 7614753.

Kumar, A., Ma, H., Zhang, X., Huang, K., Jin, S., Liu, J., Wei, T., Cao, W., Zou, G., & Liang, X. J. (2012). Gold nanoparticles functionalized with therapeutic and targeted peptides for cancer treatment. *Biomaterials, 33*, 1180–1189.

Laan, K. V. D., Hasani, M., Zheng, T., & Schirhagl, R. (2018). Nanodiamonds for *in vivo* applications. *Small, 14*(13), 1703838.

Lai, F., Sinico, C., De Logu, A., Zaru, M., Müller, R., & Fadda, A. M. (2007). SLN as a topical delivery system for *Artemisia arborescens* essential oil: *In vitro* antiviral activity and skin permeation study. *International Journal of Nanomedicine, 2*(3), 419–425.

Lara, H. H., Ayala-Nuñez, N. V., Ixtepan-Turrent, L., & Padilla, C. R. (2010). Mode of antiviral action of silver nanoparticles against HIV-1. *Journal of Nanobiotechnology, 8*, 1.

Lee, S. H. J. B. H. (2019). Silver nanoparticles: Synthesis and application for nanomedicine. *International Journal of Molecular Sciences, 20*, 865.

Lembo, D., & Cavalli, R. (2010). Nanoparticulate delivery systems for antiviral drugs. *Antiviral Chemistry and Chemotherapy, 21*(2), 53–70.

Lembo, D., Donalisio, M., Civra, A., Argenziano, M., & Cavalli, R. (2018). Nanomedicine formulations for the delivery of antiviral drugs: A promising solution for the treatment of viral infections. *Expert Opinion on Drug Delivery, 15*(1), 93–114.

Li, C., Wang, J., Wang, Y., Gao, H., Wei, G., Huang, Y., Yu, H., Gan, Y., Wang, Y., & Mei, L. (2019). Recent progress in drug delivery. *Acta Pharmaceutica Sinica B, 9*(6), 1145–1162.

Liaw, Y. F. (2005). The current management of HBV drug resistance. *Journal of Clinical Virology, 34*(Suppl 1), S143–S146.

Liu, F., Lovejoy, D. B., Hassani, A. A., He, Y., Herold, J. M., Chen, X., Yates, C. M., Frye, S. V., Brown, P. J., Huang, J., Vedadi, M., Arrowsmith, C. H., & Jin, J. (2011). Optimization of cellular activity of G9a inhibitors 7-aminoalkoxy-quinazolines. *Journal of Medicinal Chemistry, 54*(17), 6139–6150.

Macchione, M. A., Beltran, C. G., Rosso, A. P., Euti, E. M., Martinelli, M., Strumia, M. C., & Fernandez, M. A. M. (2019). Poly(N-vinylcaprolactam) nanogels with antiviral behavior against HIV-1 infection. *Scientific Reports, 9*(1), 5732.

Maginnis, M. S. (2018). Virus–receptor interactions: The key to cellular invasion. *Journal of Molecular Biology, 430*(17), 2590–2611.

Mallipeddi, R., & Rohan, L. S. (2010). Progress in antiretroviral drug delivery using nanotechnology. *International Journal of Nanomedicine, 5*, 533–547.

Matalanis, A., Jones, O. G., & McClements, D. J. (2011). Structured biopolymer-based delivery systems for encapsulation, protection, and release of lipophilic compounds. *Food Hydrocolloids, 25*(8), 1865–1880.

McClements, D. J. (2010). Design of nano-laminated coatings to control bioavailability of lipophilic food components. *Journal of Food Science, 75*(1), R30–R42.

McClements, D. J. (2011). Edible Nano emulsions: Fabrication, properties, and functional performance. *Soft Matter, 7*(6), 2297–2316.

McClements, D. J. (2017). Designing biopolymer microgels to encapsulate, protect and deliver bioactive components: Physicochemical aspects. *Advances in Colloid and Interface Science, 240*, 31–59.

McClements, D. J. (2018). Encapsulation, protection, and delivery of bioactive proteins and peptides using nanoparticle and microparticle systems: A review. *Advances in Colloid and Interface Science, 253*, 1–22.

McNeil, S. E. (2011). Unique benefits of nanotechnology to drug delivery and diagnostics. *Methods in Molecular Biology, 697*, 3–8.

Medepalli, K. K. (2008). *Advanced Nanomaterials for Biomedical Applications*. Cambridge: ProQuest.

Milroy, D., & Featherstone, J. (2002). Antiviral market overview. *Nature Reviews Drug Discovery, 1*, 11–12.

Mozafari, M. R., Johnson, C., Hatziantoniou, S., & Demetzos, C. (2008). Nanoliposomes and their applications in food nanotechnology. *Journal of Liposome Research, 18*(4), 309–327.

Mozafari, M. R., Khosravi-Darani, K., Borazan, G. G., Cui, J., Pardakhty, A., & Yurdugul, S. (2008). Encapsulation of food ingredients using nanoliposome technology. *International Journal of Food Properties, 11*(4), 833–844.

Mueller, R. H., Maeder, K., & Gohla, S. (2000). Solid lipid nanoparticles (SLN) for controlled drug delivery—a review of the state of the art. *European Journal of Pharmaceutics and Biopharmaceutics, 50*, 161–177.

Müller, R., Radtke, M., & Wissing, S. (2002). Nanostructured lipid matrices for improved microencapsulation of drugs. *International Journal of Pharmaceutics, 242*(1, 2), 121–128.

Muthu, M. S., & Singh, S. (2009). Targeted nanomedicines: Effective treatment modalities for cancer, AIDS and brain disorders. *Nanomedicine (London), 4*, 105–118.

Nalwa, H. S. (1999). *Handbook of Nanostructured Materials and Nanotechnology* (Vol. 1). San Diego, CA: Academic Press.

Niemeyer, C. M., & Mirkin, C. A. (2004). *Nanobiotechnology: Concepts, Applications and Perspectives* (Vol. 1). Weinheim: John Wiley & Sons.

Parboosing, R., Maguire, G. E., Govender, P., & Kruger, H. G. (2012). Nanotechnology and the treatment of HIV infection. *Viruses, 4*, 488–520.

Patel, P. A., & Patravale, V. B. (2011). AmbiOnp: Solid lipid nanoparticles of amphotericin B for oral administration. *Journal of Biomedical Nanotechnology, 7*, 632–639.

Patra, J. K., Das, G., Fraceto, L. F., Campos, E. V. R., Rodriguez-Torres, M. P., Acosta-Torres, L. S., Diaz-Torres, L. A., Grillo, R., Swamy, M. K., & Sharma, S. (2018). Nano based drug delivery systems: Recent developments and future prospects. *Journal of Nanobiotechnology, 16*(1), 71.

Petros, R. A., & Desimone, J. M. (2010). Strategies in the design of nanoparticles for therapeutic applications. *Nature Reviews Drug Discovery, 9*, 615–627.

Rabiee, N., Ahmadvand, S., Ahmadi, S., Fatahi, Y., Dinarvand, R., Bagherzadeh, M., Rabiee, M., Tahiri, M., Tayebi, L., & Hamblin, M. R. (2020). Carbosilane dendrimers: Drug and gene delivery applications. *Journal of Drug Delivery Science and Technology, 59*, 101879.

Rivera, A., & Messaoudi, I. (2015). Pathophysiology of Ebola virus infection: Current challenges and future hopes. *ACS Infectious Diseases, 1*(5), 186–197.

Sanvicens, N., & Marco, M. P. (2008). Multifunctional nanoparticles—properties and prospects for their use in human medicine. *Trends in Biotechnology, 26*, 425–433.

Scheller, F. W., Bier, F. F., & Pfeiffer, D. (1995). Biosensoren: Grundlagen und Anwendungen. *TM-Technisches Messen, 62*, 213–219.

Selvam, R., & Kulkarni, P. (2014). Design and evaluation of self-nanoemulsifying systems for poorly water-soluble HIV drug. *Journal of Pharmaceutical Science and Technology, 4*, 23–28.

Seyfoddin, A., & Al-Kassas, R. (2013). Development of solid lipid nanoparticles and nanostructured lipid carriers for improving ocular delivery of acyclovir. *Drug Development and Industrial Pharmacy, 39*(4), 508–519.

Shi, C., Wang, X., Wang, L., Meng, Q., Guo, D., Chen, L., Dai, M., Wang, G., Cooney, R., & Luo, J. (2020). A nano trap improves survival in severe sepsis by attenuating hyperinflammation. *Nature Communications, 11*(1), 3384.

Soni, K. S., Desale, S. S., & Bronich, T. K. (2016). Nanogels: An overview of properties, biomedical applications and obstacles to clinical translation. *Journal of Controlled Release, 240*, 109–126.

Sun, R. W., Chen, R., Chung, N. P., Ho, C. M., Lin, C. L. S., & Che, C. M. (2005). Silver nanoparticles fabricated in HEPES buffer exhibit cytoprotective activities toward HIV-1 infected cells. *Chemical Communications (Cambridge), 2005*, 5059–5061.

Sutradhar, K. B., & Amin, M. L. (2013). Nano emulsions: Increasing possibilities in drug delivery. *European Journal of Nanomedicine, 5*(2), 97.

Toub, N., Malvy, C., Fattal, E. I., & Couvreur, P. (2006). Innovative nanotechnologies for the delivery of oligonucleotides and siRNA. *Biomedicine & Pharmacotherapy, 60*, 607–620.

Wang, W., Guo, Z., Chen, Y., Liu, T., & Jiang, L. (2006). Influence of generation 2–5 of PAMAM dendrimer on the inhibition of Tat peptide/TAR RNA binding in HIV-1 transcription. *Chemical Biology and Drug Design, 68*, 314–318.

Weiss, J., Decker, E. A., McClements, D. J., Kristbergsson, K., Helgason, T., & Awad, T. (2008). Solid lipid nanoparticles as delivery systems for bioactive food components. *Food Biophysics, 3*(2), 146–154.

Xie, S., Tao, Y., Pan, Y., Qu, W., Cheng, G., Huang, L., Chen, D., Wang, X., Zhenli, L., & Yuan, Z. (2014). Biodegradable nanoparticles for intracellular delivery of antimicrobial agents. *Journal of Controlled Release, 187*, 101–117.

Xue, J., Xie, J., Liu, W., & Xia, Y. (2017). Electro spun nanofibers: New concepts, materials, and applications. *Accounts of Chemical Research, 50*(8), 1976–1987.

Zhang, L., Chan, J. M., Gu, F. X., Rhee, J. W., Wang, A. Z., Radovic-Moreno, A. F., Alexis, F., Langer, R., & Farokhzad, O. C. (2008). Self-assembled lipid polymer hybrid nanoparticles: A robust drug delivery platform. *ACS Nano, 2*(8), 1696–1702.

CHAPTER 6

Nano-Based Theragnostics for Virus-Induced Cancer

BINELKA SIRIWARDANA, SENURI HASARA, SANDALI FERNANDO, SHANALI DE SILVA, RAVINDU KAVEESHA, and GOBIKA THIRIPURANATHAR*

College of Chemical Sciences, Institute of Chemistry Ceylon, Welikada, Rajagiriya, Sri Lanka

*Corresponding author

ABSTRACT

Viral infections are categorized as a cancer etiology, known to cause 17% of human cancers. There are seven oncolytic viruses currently known: Merkel Cell Polyomavirus, Papillomavirus, Hepatitis viruses (HBV), T-cell leukemia virus-type 1 (HTLV-1), Herpesvirus-8 (HHV-8), Epstein Barr Virus (EBV), and Hepatitis C viruses. Even though various diagnostic and therapeutic measures are currently being employed to treat these viral-induced cancers, certain limitations need to be addressed in order to ensure the early detection and successful elimination of these tumors. Recent advances in nanotechnology have introduced a variety of nanoparticles such as liposomes, dendrimers, micelles, polymeric nanoparticles, metallic nanoparticles, carbon nanomaterials, quantum dots, and so forth. Owing to the unique properties of these nanoparticle formulations, such as a high surface-to-volume ratio, super paramagnetic property, enhanced electrical conductivity, unique fluorescence properties, increased permeability, and improved biocompatibility, they have been widely studied for their potential use in cancer nano-theragnostics. This chapter focuses on the application of nanotechnology for the diagnosis and treatment of viral-induced cancers.

Nanotechnological Management of Viral Infections.
Radhakrishnan EK, Shiji Mathew, and Riya Alex (Eds.)

DOI: 10.1201/9781779640895-6

6.1 INTRODUCTION

Infectious agents, including bacteria, viruses, and parasites, are linked to 20% of the global cancer burden (zur Hausen, 2009). Among infectious agents, oncoviruses stand as leading causative factors for cancers observed worldwide (Parkin, 2006), and 17% of human cancers are caused by viral infections (Tempera and Lieberman, 2021). A considerable proportion of the world's population carries at least one oncovirus; however, progression to cancer happens only in a limited number of cases. The complex interactions that take place between the host and the virus lead to the creation of a microenvironment inducing oncogenesis (Mui et al., 2017), and the involvement of one or more requirements among immunosuppression, chronic inflammation, and environmental carcinogens is essential to develop cancer (zur Hausen, 2009).

HHV-8, HBV, EBV, HPV, HCV, MCPyV, and HTLV-1 are the seven human oncogenic viruses currently known (Mui et al., 2017). Infectious cancer agents have been categorized as direct and indirect carcinogens, considering their contribution to cancer cell transformation. Direct carcinogens contribute directly to cancer cell transformation, whereas indirect carcinogens induce mechanisms of chronic infection and inflammation, which lead to carcinogenic mutations in host cells (Moore and Chang, 2010).

Modern cancer therapeutics and diagnostics have undergone significant developments over the years, which has caused fatalities to decrease. Current conventional cancer treatment methods include chemotherapy, surgery, radiotherapy, and immunotherapy. However, these approaches entail several limitations, including invasive procedures, systemic toxicity, drug resistance, severe long-term side effects, and limited efficacy. Even when treatment is carried out aiming for full recovery, the possibility of recurrence remains. Various approaches have been employed for the diagnosis of tumors so that effective therapeutic regimens can be proposed accordingly. Imaging modalities, including conventional X-rays, magnetic resonance imaging (MRI), computed tomography (CT), positron emission tomography (PET), single-photon emission computed tomography (SPECT), and ultrasound (US), are most frequently used to determine response to therapies. Despite the numerous techniques reported for the diagnosis of tumors, several limitations with regard to the lack of significant cancer biomarkers, early diagnosis, efficient mass screening strategies, and cancer awareness remain to be addressed for accurate and early detection of cancer. Theragnostics, which is the combination of diagnostic and therapeutic approaches, allowing the simultaneous detection of targets, monitoring of drug distribution, and the evaluation of therapeutic response to achieve personalized medicine, has been reported to increase the survival rate of cancer patients, with nano-theragnostics being investigated as an emerging solution for this deadly disease (Kelkar and Reineke, 2011).

6.2 ONCOGENIC VIRUSES

Oncogenic viruses can be classified into four broad categories: oncogenic retroviruses (RNA viruses that reverse transcribe their genome into DNA before integrating it into a host cell chromosome), RNA tumor viruses, small DNA tumor viruses, and large DNA tumor viruses (Chang et al., 2017). Further, seven human viruses have been reported to induce the development of certain cancers, which are RNA viruses (Table 6.1).

TABLE 6.1 Viruses Associated with Human Cancer

Virus Category	Oncogenic Virus	Malignancies
Retrovirus	Human T-lymphotropic virus type I	Adult T cell leukemia
RNA tumor viruses	Hepatitis C	Hepatocellular carcinoma
Small DNA tumor virus	Hepatitis B	Hepatocellular carcinoma
	Merkel cell polyomavirus	Merkel cell carcinoma
	Human papillomavirus	Cervical, anal, vulvar, vaginal, penile, and oropharyngeal cancers
Large DNA tumor virus	Epstein–Barr virus	Hodgkin's lymphoma, non-Hodgkin's lymphoma, leiomyosarcomas, nasopharyngeal carcinoma, and gastric carcinoma
	Human herpesvirus-8	Kaposi's sarcoma, primary effusion lymphoma, and multicentric Castleman's disease

6.2.1 HUMAN T-LYMPHOTROPIC VIRUS TYPE I (HTLV-1)

Human T-lymphotrophic virus (HTLV) belongs to the Retroviridae family and Delta retrovirus genus. The virus is round-shaped and has an approximate diameter of 100 nm. The virion is surrounded by an envelope made up of a proteolipid bilayer, which has the origin of the host cell membrane, along with viral transmembrane and surface proteins. Viral RNA and the functional protease, reverse transcriptase, and integrase, which are organized together with the nucleocapsid into a ribonucleoprotein complex, are surrounded by the icosahedral capsid (Ohtsuki et al., 1982). HTLV contains a single-stranded RNA as its genome, which will be converted into double-stranded DNA and get inserted into host cell DNA (Gallo, 2005). The retrovirus, which is now called the provirus, initiates infections, infecting the $CD4^{+}$ T cells preferentially, but $CD8^{+}$ T cells are also used as an important reservoir for HTLV (Jones et al., 2006).

There are two types of HTLV, HTLV-1 and HTLV-2. HTLV-1 is responsible for tropical spastic paraparesis (TSP). HTLV-2 causes a rare form of human hairy cell leukemia. HTLV retroviruses require transactivators, viral gene products that are crucial for increasing viral gene expression, in order to replicate. Tax is a transactivator that is encoded by HTLV-1 and -2, which promotes the replication of these retroviruses (Bex and Gaynor, 1998). The significance of HTLV-1 infected individuals is the spontaneous proliferation of peripheral blood mononuclear cells without the aid of exogenous antigens and stimulants, but by the tax protein, encoded by HTLV-1 (Of and Of, 2007).

In ATL, the provirus gets integrated into the $CD4^{+}$ post-thymic T cells and causes the malignancy by inducing abnormal growth of infected T cells by different pathways, which is carried by the regulatory protein tax. T cells can accumulate DNA mutations and result in transformation and monoclonal outgrowth of a highly malignant cell in this situation while undergoing epigenetic changes such as DNA methylation, which plays an important role in leukaemogenesis (Taylor and Matsuoka, 2005). HAM/TSP disease shows chronic inflammation in the white and gray matter of the spinal cord. Mononuclear cells, especially T cells, cause the perivascular cuffing and infiltrate the parenchyma. The condition worsens over time, becoming less cellular and atrophic, and primarily harming the lower thoracic spinal cord's white matter, which is consistent with the spastic paraparesis of the lower limbs.

The lesions in the spinal cord and in the brain can be observed with many changes and damages occurring to the Central Nervous System (Aye et al., 2000).

6.2.2 HEPATITIS B AND C VIRUSES (HBV AND HCV)

HBV and HCV viruses are capable of infecting hepatocytes present in the liver, hence causing chronic hepatitis. Epidemiological and clinical studies have concluded that the major etiologies for hepatocellular carcinoma (HCC) are chronic HBV and HCV infections (Beasley et al., 1981; Beasley, 1988; Kiyosawa et al., 1984; Yu and Chen, 1994).

HBV, a species of the genus Orthohepadnavirus belonging to Hepadnaviridae, is a partially double-stranded and enveloped DNA virus, and it replicates via an RNA intermediate and reverse transcription. It is capable of encoding seven proteins, one of which, protein X (HBx), has been reported to participate in oncogenic progression (Ringehan et al., 2017; Vousden and Farrell, 1994). The primary pathogenesis for oncogenesis in HBV is attributed to the integration of the hepatitis B virus genome into the host (Wang et al., 1990). Chronic hepatitis can lead to fibrosis and cirrhosis that develop to a cancerous state due to the inflammation that induces hepatocyte DNA damage and mutations. Furthermore, HBV favors progression of HCC even without cirrhosis (Llovet et al., 2021).

HCV is an RNA virus belonging to Flaviviridae and is single stranded with 11 major genotypes and 15 different subtypes. This oncogenic virus of humans is unique due to its positive stranded RNA nature. Chronic HCV infection can cause active inflammation with subsequent fibrosis, necrosis, and regeneration, which contributes to tumor development. Unlike HBV, HCV does not get integrated into the genome of the host and, hence, the threat of HCC here could be mainly to those having cirrhosis or related conditions. Even though HCV primarily targets hepatocytes, it also shows lymphotropism and is capable of replicating in the lymphocytes. Hence, apart from HCC, HCV infections have also been reported to increase the risk of lymphoproliferative disorders including non-Hodgkin's lymphoma (NHL) and mixed cryoglobulinemia (Couronné et al., 2018; Kayali et al., 2002; Khaled et al., 2017; Matsuo et al., 2004).

6.2.3 MERKEL CELL POLYOMAVIRUS (MCPyV OR MCV)

Merkel cell polyomavirus (MCPyV or MCV) belongs to the family Polyomaviridae, and research of the Polyomaviridae family has resulted in substantial discoveries in viral oncogenesis, general cell biology, and cancer molecular biology. 22 different species of polyomaviruses belong to three genera, and they have an icosahedral shape with a non-enveloped nature and a genome of double-stranded DNA in circular form (Buck, 2013). There are nine known polyomaviruses that infect humans (Buck et al., 2012), yet MCPyV is the first polyomavirus that was detected as linked directly with Merkel Cell Carcinoma (MCC) (Chang and Moore, 2013). MCC is a skin cancer that is rare yet extremely malignant. Friedrich S. Merkel first described the Merkel cell, which is the cell of origin, as "clear cells" located at the epidermal layer of the skin. Merkel nerve endings, which form a cluster in glabrous skin, were called "touch corpuscles," and they are the mechanoreceptors of the human skin (Halata et al., 2003). MCPyV was initially isolated from tissue samples of MCC (Feng et al., 2009). MCC has the appearance of a cyst or a nodule, and it appears as a painless subcutaneous mass. Sometimes it can have a plaque-like appearance that may be surrounded by satellite lesions. The lesions may appear in various colors such as red, blue, or skin color (Heath et al., 2008).

6.2.4 HUMAN PAPILLOMAVIRUS (HPV)

Papillomaviruses belong to the family Papillomaviridae and have a size range of approximately ~50 nm. The papillomavirus family contains a wide range of distinct kinds that infect practically all vertebrate species while exhibiting a high level of species specificity, with over 100 species infecting either the cutaneous or the mucosal tissues (De Villiers et al., 2004). 30–40 types are identified as infecting the genital tract, and these are identified as the most common sexually transmitted agents (Stanley et al., 2007).

Warts and anogenital dysplasias typically contain HPVs, though infections are frequently still asymptomatic. Anogenital HPVs are divided into "low-risk" and "high-risk" varieties depending on whether they are linked to benign, pre-cancerous, or malignant lesions (zur Hausen, 2009). High-risk HPVs, especially like HPV 16 and HPV 18, are identified as the causative agents for cervical cancer, which is the second most common cancer diagnosed in women worldwide (Bosch et al., 2002; Hoory et al., 2008). Anal and other genital neoplasia have also been linked to high-risk HPV strains, particularly HPV-16 (Gillison et al., 2000). The anogenital and upper aerodigestive tract epithelia can become infected by mucosal HPV strains. Despite the fact that HPV infections are very frequent, the majority are asymptomatic and clear up in 6–12 months due to a robust immune response, where a small subset of infections finally result in neoplasia (Bosch et al., 2002). People with HIV and other immunosuppressed conditions have an increased threat of developing non-melanoma skin malignancies, particularly at sun-exposed locations when infected with HPV (Nindl and Rösl, 2008). Additionally, other genital neoplasia, such as vulvovaginal and penile malignancies, have also been associated with HPV (Partridge and Koutsky, 2006). Being immunosuppressed, smoking, high parity, oral contraceptive use, pregnancy, transplant recipients, and the number of sexual partners are among the main factors that increase the risk of HPV carcinogenesis (Bosch et al., 2002; Nindl and Rösl, 2008).

6.2.5 EPSTEIN-BARR VIRUS (EBV)

EBV, or the species *Human gammahepesvirus 4*, is the first human cancer-causing virus discovered (Epstein et al., 1963), which is classified under the Herpesviridae family, Gammaherpesvirinae subfamily, and under genus Lymphocryptovirus (Gequelin et al., 2011). EBV has a linear, double-stranded DNA as its genome (Baer et al., 1984). There are two main types of EBV strains, which are called EBV-1 and EBV-2 (Rowe et al., 1989). The difference between the two types is identified by the difference between the two genes which code for the nuclear antigens (Sample et al., 1990).

The British surgeon, Denis Burkitt, identified and described a malignant tumor which had started widely spreading among children of equatorial African countries in 1958, which was subsequently termed Burkitt's Lymphoma (BL). The tumor was mainly identified as a sarcoma involving the jaws of African children (Burkitt, 1972). Originally, after focusing on the epidemiology of the disease, it was hypothesized that the disease was affected by climate factors and that the infectious agent was transmitted by a mosquito, which automatically directed attention to the potential of the infectious agent to be a virus (Dicke, 1962). The virus particles were observed under the electron microscope, and it was detected that the shape of the virus particles was similar to herpes simplex virus particles, and later it was classified as EBV (Epstein et al., 1965). After identifying the relationship between BL and EBV with the increased antibodies to antigens of EBV with patients' sera, it was determined that the patients with infectious mononucleosis (IM) also showed the elevation of antibodies to EBV, and it was decided that this virus or a close member of the virus group is the cause for IM (Griffin, 1998). After identifying the relationship between EBV and IM, it was reported that EBV also causes diseases such as Hodgkin's Lymphoma (HL), NHL, BL, Post-transplant lymphoproliferative disease (PTLD), and Nasopharyngeal carcinoma (NPC).

6.2.6 HUMAN HERPES VIRUS (HHV-8)

HHV-8, which is also called the Kaposi's sarcoma-associated Herpesvirus (KSHV), is a double-stranded DNA herpesvirus, and it belongs to the gamma herpesevirinae subfamily (Wen and Damania, 2010). Recent studies show that this is the Herpesvirus type mostly observed in the samples obtained from the lesions of patients who are affected with immunodeficiency syndrome-associated Kaposi's Sarcoma (Chang et al., 1994). HHV-8, or the KSHV, causes several human cancers, including Kaposi sarcoma (KS) (Chang et al., 1994; U and Fleckenstein, 1999), primary effusion lymphoma (PEL) (Press, 2018), and Multicentric Castleman Disease (MCD) (Hao-wei Wang et al., 2017).

Kaposi sarcoma initiates with lesions that appear in the skin and in lymphatic nodes containing irregular vascular spaces lined by plump endothelial cells. Then, the lesions undergo neovascularization, accumulation of collagen, and inflammatory cells with the proliferation of abnormal endothelial cells around a core composed of a morphologically and phenotypically normal capillary, venule, or arteriole. With the further proliferation of the abnormal endothelial cells, solid chords are produced, and in response to the tumor, vascular cores also proliferate, resulting in a highly vascular tumor (Beckstead and Wood, 1984; Hsei-wei Wang et al., 2004). PEL was identified as an aggressive large B-cell lymphoma associated with the HHV-8 infection by the World Health Organization, and it was classified under the tumors of hematopoietic and lymphoid tissues in the 2016 revision (Campo et al., 2014). In 1995, PEL was discovered to be an HHV8-driven body cavity lymphoma in HIV-positive patients (Chang et al., 1994). PEL typically manifests as a serous effusion without a distinguishable tumor mass, but with time, the presence of an extracavitary mass will be experienced by the patients (Pan et al., 2012). Castleman's disease (CD) is a rare disease that shows a massive lymphoid tissue growth. MCD is a type of CD associated with HHV-8 and is a systemic disease that involves infecting multiple regions of lymph nodes, unlike unicentric CD, which involves infecting lymph nodes in only one region of the body (Bowne et al., 1999).

6.3 CURRENT THERAGNOSTICS AVAILABLE TO BATTLE VIRUS-INDUCED CANCER

6.3.1 CONVENTIONAL CANCER DIAGNOSIS AND IMAGING

Over the years, both invasive and non-invasive techniques have been employed for the diagnosis of cancers. Early detection is critical for the timely elimination of malignancies. Different non-invasive modalities have been employed, such as SPECT, MRI, PET, US, photoacoustic imaging (PAI), and optical imaging (OI) (Table 6.2). Despite their high spatial resolution at μm range, conventional widefield microscope-based optical imaging techniques are not suitable for imaging thick tissue and are often limited to open surface or exposed areas of the body, such as eyes and skin, owing to the limited depth penetration of light into tissues and unclear background signals. MRI, on the other hand, generates high-definition images of an entire organism with deep penetration and detailed anatomical information under a magnetic field, without releasing any ionizing radiation. However, even though MRI is capable of differentiating between tissues, limitations still exist in the detection of diseased states. Therefore, to increase the resolution of images, contrast agents are used, which can readily detect primary and metastatic diseases. Currently, MRI is the most accurate technique for staging cervical carcinomas. However, the use of MRI contrast agents for the early detection of cancer is limited due to the low specificity of the probe and fast clearance from the body. In US imaging, high-frequency sound waves are applied to the body, and reflected sound waves are detected by a transducer to create images.

Even though it is a relatively inexpensive technique, attenuation from tissue or gas, or vice versa, can reduce the resolution of the image. CT is a tomographic X-ray imaging modality that has the highest resolution of the imaging techniques, with the capacity to obtain three-dimensional and cross-sectional images. In certain cancers, it can be employed to gather information on staging, metastases, and planning of treatment. Noninvasive nuclear imaging modalities are frequently used to obtain accurate images after administration of radiopharmaceuticals to patients. Three-dimensional images can be obtained using SPECT by rotating cameras around the patient. PET offers substantial benefits over anatomic imaging modalities as it can often be used to differentiate between benign and malignant lesions. Molecular changes in cancer-like receptors or antigens can be specifically detected with integrated imaging techniques such as PET/CT. PET/CT can also differentiate tumors from other lesions such as inflammation or necrosis following radiotherapy.

Biopsy is an invasive technique that involves the removal of tissue samples from a tumor while being guided by imaging methods such as CT or MRI, and its pathological investigation (Table 6.2). It has been deemed useful in distinguishing between benign and malignant lesions. Liquid biopsies enable sequential sampling, which is needed to monitor HCC and to organize the study of resistance and tumor clonal composition at a molecular level. Furthermore, various tests such as the Papanicolau test for women to identify cervical cancer, Prostate Specific Antigen (PSA) level detection in blood samples in order to identify prostate cancer in men, performing Fecal Occult Blood Test (FOBT) to identify colon cancer, and endoscopy have also been employed (Zhang et al., 2019).

Even though imaging techniques have improved and help in early detection of certain virus-induced cancers such as HCC and cervical cancer, issues like expense, radiologic capacity, contrast exposure, and radiation limit their popularity. While semi-annual ultrasonography with and without α-fetoprotein is often recommended as a surveillance strategy for HCC, intensive protocols which involve the mix of cross-sectional imaging, USG scanning, and markers in serological samples are also being employed. Current imaging techniques are not always effective in early detection at a cellular or molecular level. Even though they are able to diagnose cancers at a stage when there are visible changes in the tissues, several tumor cells would already have undergone proliferation and even metastasis.

It is important to distinguish cancer from other lesions using proper imaging approaches with high sensitivity and specificity.

6.3.2 CURRENT THERAPEUTICS AVAILABLE FOR THE TREATMENT OF VIRALLY INDUCED CANCERS

Some of the most common therapeutics available for virus-induced cancers include chemotherapy, surgery, and radiation treatment. Chemotherapy works by halting or slowing the growth of cancer cells, which multiply rapidly. Cancer chemotherapy is the administration of cytotoxic chemicals, or chemicals with cell-killing properties, with the goal of eradicating the tumor or, at the very least, reducing the tumor burden and, thus, reducing tumor-related symptoms and possibly prolonging life. Chemotherapy helps to recuperate from types of advanced cancer like small cell lung cancer, choriocarcinoma, germ cell cancer, Hodgkin's and non–Hodgkin's lymphoma, and ovarian cancer. In pediatric patients, curable cancers include Wilms' tumor, embryonal rhabdomyosarcoma, acute leukemia, and Burkitt's lymphoma. Although treatment may not be entirely helpful for these cancers, there has been betterment in survival on the whole (Nygren, 2001).

Surgery increases cancer cell shedding into the blood circulation, allowing circulating cells to survive, suppresses anti-tumor immunity, recruits immune cells for trapping tumor cells, upregulates adhesion molecules in target organs, and induces changes in the target tissue and cancer cells themselves to enhance migration and invasion at the target site (Tohme et al., 2017). When compared to chemotherapy and radiotherapy, surgery, resection, or operation is thought to be one of the most promising and conventional treatments for many benign and malignant tumors as it causes the least damage to the surrounding tissues (Abbas and Rehman, 2018). To treat MCC, various surgical techniques such as complete circumferential and peripheral deep margin assessment, Mohs technique, local excision, wide local excision, and modified Mohs (Mohs technique with additional final margin for permanent section assessment) are used (Tai, 2013). In HCV and HBV associated diseases, postoperative complications are increased in patients with decompensated liver disease such as acute hepatic failure, sepsis, and bleeding. The degree of liver dysfunction, the type of surgery, especially liver transplantation, and the patient's preclinical status are used to predict surgical risk. The Childs-Pugh score is commonly used to stratify the risk of patients with liver disease (Asthana and Kneteman, 2009). ATL is treated with bone marrow transplantation or hematopoietic stem cell transplantation (Bazarbachi et al., 2011). HHV-8-associated Germinotrophic lymphoproliferative disorders (GLPD) in its current form, has a generally favorable prognosis after chemotherapy, and curettage is used to treat Kaposi Sarcoma, surgical removal with or without radiotherapy and surgery, including local excision or electrodesiccation (Guerrero et al., 2019).

When treating cancers using radiotherapy, a consequence of lethal DNA damage is induced by X-rays (Hall and Brenner, 1991). Since the radiation creates ions and stores energy in the cells of the tissues it travels through, it is known as ionizing radiation. This stored energy has the ability to harm cancer cells or alter their genetic makeup, resulting in eventual death of replicating cancer cells (Veness and Richards, 2003). Several radiotherapy techniques are used in treating cancers, such as Image-guided radiotherapy, fractionation, 3D conformal radiotherapy, stereotactic body radiation, and intensity modulated radiation therapy. Electrons, protons, and neutron beams are used in radiotherapy, and the cell death is caused by different mechanisms when using radiotherapy, which are apoptosis, necrosis, mitotic catastrophe, senescence, and autophagy (Jackson and Bartek, 2009).

As alternatives to conventional resectional surgery, numerous ablative methods are being suggested. These include laser ablation (LA), cryosurgery, high-intensity focused ultrasound therapy, microwave ablation, and radio-frequency ablation (Table 6.2). All of these methods promise to eradicate cancer while protecting healthy tissue (Schena et al., 2017). LA is carried out with the help of a laser and a medium that transports the laser light inside the tissue. The laser, which consists of a power source, a lasing medium, and reflecting mirrors, emits monochromatic light (light at a specific wavelength), the wavelength of which defines the laser's properties and interaction with biological tissue. Heat is produced when light is absorbed by tissue. Long-term exposure of tumor cells to temperatures ranging from 45°C–55°C, or short exposure to temperatures higher than 60°C, causes irreversible cell damage (Izzo, 2003). Cryosurgery uses liquid nitrogen or argon to produce extreme cold to destroy cancerous and dysfunctioning cells. It is a local intervention focused on a specific site in the body. Cryosurgery is used to treat skin tumors as well as some internal tumors (Theodorescu, 2004). In conjunction with MRI scans or diagnostic USG scans, high-intensity focused ultrasound (HIFU) is a safer technique for tumor treatment and has the potential to be a considerable option adjunct to present standard protocols such as surgery, chemotherapy, and radiotherapy. In biological tissues, ultrasound has both thermal and non-thermal effects. High-intensity ultrasound energy absorption causes elevated tissue temperatures and ablation at specific temperature thresholds. Mechanical tissue disruption can also be caused by non-thermal effects such as cavitation (the formation and collapse of gas-filled bubbles in an ultrasound field) or the generation of boiling bubbles (Maloney and Hwang, 2015). Radiofrequency ablation (RFA) is a modified electrocautery technique that has emerged as the leading option for local, minimally invasive tissue ablation. Radiofrequency electric fields cause resistive heating by driving ionic currents in tissue. Cells go through coagulation necrosis in 4–6 minutes at 50°C –52°C; at temperatures above 60°C, coagulation necrosis occurs instantly (Lin et al., 2014). In microwave ablation, in order to generate heat, dielectric hysteresis is used to treat cancer cells and tissues. Tissue destruction occurs when tissues are heated to lethal temperatures by an applied electromagnetic field, typically at frequencies ranging from 900–2500 MHz (Lubner et al., 2010).

Immunotherapy has the potential to benefit many virus-associated cancers as it can work in three stages: preventing viral infections, treating infections before they cause malignancy, and eradicating an established malignancy through selective recognition of virus-infected cells. Immunotherapy can be used to target viral gene products in infected cells that cause inflammation or uncontrolled cell proliferation once a viral infection has been established. Unlike traditional cancer treatments such as chemotherapy, radiotherapy, and surgery, cell-based immunotherapies can distinguish virus-infected cells from non-infected cells (Tashiro and Brenner, 2017). Immune-based interventions based on adoptive transfer of immunoactive cells and antibodies have emerged as potent solutions for virus-associated cancers. In immunocompromised individuals, T cells play a critical role in mediating the control of virus-associated cancers. Immunocompromised people are more likely to develop cancers caused by EBV and KSHV, Merkel cell polyomavirus (MCPyV), and HPV (Table 6.2). This increased susceptibility is a direct result of the immunosuppression used to prevent organ rejection, and it is associated with a lack of virus-specific T cell immunity. There are several techniques in immunotherapy to treat virally induced cancers, such as oncolytic immunotherapy, immune checkpoint inhibitors, small molecule inhibitors, monoclonal antibodies, cytokine therapy, vaccination, T-cell receptor mediated immunotherapies, and chimeric antigen receptor T cell therapy (Smith and Khanna, 2018).

TABLE 6.2 Current Diagnostic and Therapeutic Approaches Employed for Some Virus-Induced Cancers

Virus Induced Cancer	Diagnostic Approaches	Current Therapeutics Available
Hepatocellular carcinoma	Ultrasound; CT; MRI; PET; Alpha-fetoprotein tumor marker; Blood tests; Liver biopsy – Fine-needle aspiration biopsy, core needle biopsy, laparoscopy	Surgery – hepatic resection/liver transplantation; Transarterial embolization/chemoembolization; Ablation – radiofrequency ablation, cryoablation, microwave therapy, percutaneous ethanol injection, electroporation therapy; Targeted therapy – bevacizumab, cabozantinib, Lenvatinib, ramucirumab, regorafenib, sorafenib; Chemotherapy; Radiation therapy – Stereotactic body radiotherapy (SBRT), Conformal radiation therapy, Proton beam radiation therapy. Immune checkpoint inhibitor therapy using atezolizumab with the targeted therapy, bevacizumab, nivolumab with ipilimumab, pembrolizumab
Cervical cancer	Pelvic exam; Cervical cytology (Pap smear); HPV test; Endocervical curettage; Colposcopy; Lymph node biopsy; CT; PET; Cystoscopy; Laparoscopy; Chest x-ray; Ultrasonography; MRI	Surgery – cryosurgery, laser ablation, conization, hysterectomy, trachelectomy, pelvic lymph node dissection; Chemotherapy; Radiation therapy; Targeted therapy – monoclonal antibody therapy (Bevacizumab); Immunotherapy – PD-1 and PD-L1 inhibitor therapy
Adult T cell leukemia	Blood chemistry studies; Peripheral blood smear; Bone marrow aspiration; Lymph node biopsy; Cytogenetic analysis; Immunophenotyping; CT; MRI	Anti-viral therapy; Chemotherapy; Allogeneic stem cell transplantation; Immunotherapy – monoclonal antibody therapy; Interferon-α/zidovudine
Merkel cell carcinoma	Physical exam; CT; PET; Skin biopsy; Lymph node biopsy; Immunohistochemistry	Surgery – Wide local excision, lymph node dissection; Radiation therapy; Chemotherapy; Immunotherapy – PD-1 and PD-L1 inhibitor therapy, CTLA-4 inhibitor therapy
Hodgkin's lymphoma	Physical exam; Complete blood count; Blood chemistry studies; LDH test; PET/CT; MRI; Ultrasound; Lymph node biopsy	Chemotherapy; Radiation therapy – Proton beam radiation therapy, External radiation therapy; Targeted therapy; Immunotherapy – PD-1 and PD-L1 inhibitor therapy

TABLE 6.2 *(Continued)*

Virus Induced Cancer	Diagnostic Approaches	Current Therapeutics Available
Non-Hodgkin's lymphoma	MRI; Lumbar puncture; Bone marrow aspiration and biopsy; Lymph node biopsy	Radiation therapy; Chemotherapy; Immunotherapy; Targeted therapy; Plasmapheresis; Antibiotic therapy; Surgery; Stem cell transplant
Gastric carcinoma	Physical exam; Blood chemistry studies; Complete blood count; Barium swallow; CT; PET; MRI; Endoscopic ultrasound; Biopsy; Laparoscopy	Surgery – Subtotal gastrectomy, total gastrectomy; Endoscopic mucosal resection; Chemotherapy; Radiation therapy; Chemoradiation; Targeted therapy – Monoclonal antibody drugs (trastuzumab and ramucirumab), Multikinase inhibitors (regorafenib); Immunotherapy – PD-1 and PD-L1 inhibitor therapy
Kaposi's sarcoma	Physical exam; Chest x-ray; Biopsy – Excisional biopsy, Incisional biopsy, Core biopsy, Fine-needle aspiration (FNA) biopsy; Blood chemistry studies; CT; PET; CD34 lymphocyte count	Radiation therapy; Surgery – local excision, electrodesiccation and curettage; Cryosurgery; Chemotherapy; Immunotherapy – Interferon alfa and interleukin-12

Cancer treatment methods should be selected according to the cancer type and disease stage (e.g., malignant, benign, metastatic), and the most curative treatment type should be employed. Conventional treatment methods are not effective in all cases and may cause devastating side effects. To prevent and reduce the incidence of death, improved diagnostic methods and more effective and less toxic treatments are needed.

6.4 NANO-BASED APPROACHES FOR THE TREATMENT AND DIAGNOSIS OF VIRUS-INDUCED CANCER

Over the years, nanotechnology has provided promising methods for the treatment and diagnosis of cancers, addressing most of the challenges encountered in conventional treatment methods by exhibiting efficient entrapment of drugs incorporated in the nanocarriers, reducing the toxic effects of drugs, and targeting or delivery in the site of action, further improving the bioavailability of drugs. Nanomaterials possess several common characteristics such as a high surface to volume ratio, super paramagnetic property, enhanced electrical conductivity, unique fluorescence properties, and spectral shift of optical absorption. Moreover, the increased permeability which has enabled crossing through biological barriers and improved biocompatibility are also noticeable features. The high surface area to volume ratio of nanomaterials allows them to assemble with biomolecules or residues, which in turn enhances the specificity of chemical drug complex in targeted therapy. Thus, it enhances the efficacy of nanomaterial-based treatment while reducing its toxicity to normal cells (Song et al., 2010). Many nanomaterials have been examined for their applications in the cure, prophylaxis, and detection of viral induced cancers, including lipid-based, polymeric, carbon-based, metallic, and silica-based nanoparticles.

6.4.1 LIPOSOMES

Liposomes are artificially generated closed spherical vesicles prepared from naturally derived phospholipids. Different techniques and preparation methods have allowed scientists to form three types of liposomes. Unilamellar vesicles (SUV) are single phospholipid bilayer spheres having diameters of 40–80 nm, and the other multilamellar vesicles (MUV) and large unilamellar vesicles (LUV) with a size ranging greater than 60 nm, having a concentric structure (Frézard et al., 2005). Liposomes are efficient in drug delivery due to the fact that they are biologically compatible, have versatile characteristics that makes them available to both polar and non-polar surfaces, and are non-toxic in biological structures. Liposomes can carry both hydrophilic and hydrophobic drugs, such as chemotherapeutic drugs, phytochemicals, and immune-cytokines for treatment of cancer. The effectiveness of a cancer treatment is based on the ability to destroy cancer cells without damaging the normal cells with the application of limited amounts of drug. The ability to encapsulate the drugs within the liposomes and delivering them specifically to cancer cells by attaching antibodies to the surface increases the effectiveness of the treatments (Balzus et al., 2017; Gogoi et al., 2016; Maruyama et al., 1999; Olusanya et al., 2018). Site specific delivery can be attained using curated ligands against tumor cell receptors that can attach on the liposome (Sawant and Torchilin, 2012). Recently, they were used to deliver anti-cancer drugs, curcumin, and interleukin 2 (IL-2) to treat cancer in the cervix (Casagrande et al., 2013; Saengkrit et al., 2014; Sreekanth et al., 2011). However, this approach is limited to antigen-antibody specifications. To overcome this limitation, an additional targeting method has been developed that uses the release of the chemotherapeutic agent within the interstitium after accumulating on the tumor tissues (Olusanya et al., 2018).

The possibility to reconstruct proteins in the lipid membrane of liposomes has been heavily exploited in the design of biosensors to detect and study the interaction between small molecules and ligands with plasma membrane receptors. Liposomes were exploited as chemical vessels, which are designed to serve as nanoscale reaction vessels for remotely controlled reactions. The ultra-small reaction volume helps in rapid diffusional mixing between biological molecules inside lipid-enclosed environments, allowing rapid chemical kinetics and reaction dynamics imitating the working of cell membranes to be assessed and studied (Al-Jamal and Kostarelos, 2011). For diagnostic use of liposomes, they have to be incorporated with radionuclides. There are four general approaches to achieve this: passive encapsulation, membrane labeling, surface chelation, and remote loading (Petersen et al., 2012). In the passive encapsulation method, the radionuclides are introduced to the solution of liposome formation to ensure that the radionuclides are trapped inside the core (van der Geest et al., 2016), while in membrane labeling, an organic dye is introduced which can get into the lipid bilayer membrane of the liposomes (Mousseau et al., 2019). For surface chelation, the radionuclides or the dyes are attached to the outer membrane of the liposomes (Petersen et al., 2012), while in the remote loading process, the drug moves through the membrane bilayer inside the vesicular region, followed by an alteration of the drug, resisting membrane repermeation, and drug accumulation inside liposomes (Hood et al., 2014). Radiolabeled liposomes can be traced by imaging of photons emitted directly (SPECT) or following positron annihilation (PET) of the decaying radionuclide. For SPECT imaging, single photon emitting radionuclides are required, whereas positron emitting radionuclides are needed for PET imaging (Petersen et al., 2012). Some examples for the therapeutic uses of liposomes are: DC-Chol liposomes have been shown to overcome the observed nonresponse to hepatitis B vaccine. The combination of a cationic lipid (particularly dimethyldioctadecylammonium bromide, DDA) with an immunostimulatory agent (trehalose 6,6' dibehenate, TDB) has been shown to be a versatile adjuvant system which mediates protection against tuberculosis and has shown promising protective efficacy against other infectious diseases requiring different immunological profiles (Gregoriadis and Perrie, 2010). For Merkel cell carcinoma, an attractive option is the use of liposomal doxorubicin (DOX) combined with radio-chemotherapy, and it is well tolerated even in older patients with other illnesses and can be given on an outpatient basis. It is an attractive option for metastatic Merkel cell carcinoma (Wobser et al., 2009). It has been reported that the HVJ-liposome is effective for electroporation in killing EBNA-1 positive cells (Hirai et al., 1997). Polyunsaturated endoplasmic reticulum liposomes (PERLs) have a greater antiviral activity towards HCV, HBV, and HIV due to the lowering of virus-associated cholesterol and plasma membrane cholesterol content of cells (Pollock et al., 2010).

6.4.2 DENDRIMERS

Dendrimers are synthetic polymers with monodisperse systems having a defined structure consisting of tree-like arms or branches with internal cavities to carry drugs (Pearson et al., 2012). Dendrimers have the ability to combine small molecules by electrostatic or hydrophobic interactions and bind drugs on their surface by polar interchanges with amine and carboxyl groups. In some cases, the surface groups are covalently modified by added sugar and drugs; thus, dendrimers are used in medical and biotechnological applications due to their biocompatibility. According to Donalisio et al., dendrimers of peptides consist of surface functional units covalently bound (Donalisio et al., 2010). A series of linear peptides with basic nature has been evaluated, showing that the peptide dendrimer SB105-A10 was potent against genital HPV types with a 50% inhibitory concentration and has shown no evidence of cytotoxicity. The dendrimer molecule interacts with heparin derivatives exposed on the cell exterior, which restrains the binding of the virus to the cell exterior. Thus, it is a prospective component in topical products with microbicide effect on HPV (Donalisio et al., 2010). The disadvantage of dendrimers is that their immunogenicity causes allergic reactions. There is an importance for the use of dendrimers in the treatment of cervical cancer, and these systems allow the entry of nanocarriers in the tumor with enhanced effects and fewer unwanted effects.

Gadolinium-diethylenetriaminepentaacetic acid (Gd-DTPA) complexes can be used as MRI agents (Langereis et al., 2004), and the biocompatible polyamidoamine (PAMAM) dendrimers can be used in both FI (fluorescence imaging) and MRI (Talanov et al., 2006). A new method was developed to use dendrimer with lactobionic acid with gold nanoparticles (LA-Au DENPs) in CT imaging of HCC, with use as a nanoprobe for specific imaging of human HCC in lab conditions and the non-permanent grafted tumor model in the human body (Liu et al., 2014). PEG core dendrimers are showing greater potential in CT imaging (Fu et al., 2006).

6.4.3 POLYMERIC NANOPARTICLES (PNPS)

As drug carriers, PNPs achieve the sustained release to targeted cancerous sites. Drugs are encapsulated to the surface of nanoparticles (NPs) to form a nano-capsule. Use of non-biodegradable polymeric substances such as polystyrene, polymethyl methacrylate (PMMA), and polyacrylates to fabricate NPs (Shastri, 2003; Vijayan et al., 2013) has been limited in order to avoid toxicity and long-term allergic reactions. As a solution, to avoid the accumulation of these non-biodegradable polymer-based NPs in tissues to a toxic level and get them degraded or physically removed, biodegradable polymers have been fabricated. Thus, these biodegradable PNPs have reduced toxicity, improved drug release, and have better compatibility in biological systems. These polymers include polylactic acid (PLA), poly(lactic-co-glycolic acid) (PLGA), poly(amino acids) [29], poly(ε-caprolactone) (PCL), and natural polymers consist of chitosan, alginate, gelatin, and albumin (Elsabahy and Wooley, 2012). The properties and structures of these improved PNPs have special advantages. For volatile pharmaceutical agents, PNPs help in increasing stability. For chemical drugs, PNPs provide optional administration methods such as oral and intravenous and higher loading ability compared to free drugs. The ability that protects drugs from degradation helps minimize undesired toxicity to normal tissues; for instance, PNPs loaded with cisplatin such as dexamethasone or α-tocopheryl succinate have been employed in chemotherapy, which prevents cisplatin-induced ototoxicity (Martín-Saldaña et al., 2017).

Further, PNPs are used as an antibacterial and a chemotherapeutic in the treatment of cervical cancer. Various biomaterials have been used to form PNPs for drug delivery. Chitosan, a natural polysaccharide known to be an exceptional biomaterial due to its biodegradability, non-toxicity, and biocompatibility, was able to provide small interfering RNA against E6 and E7 into carcinoma in the cervical region (Yang et al., 2013). Silver NPs using aqueous dispersion of chitosan-graft-poly(acrylamide) as a reducing agent and polyethylene glycol (PEG) as a stabilizer. The synthesized NPs have shown significant cytotoxicity to human cervical cancer cells, and the inhibitory concentration at 50% cell death (IC 50) was found at 8 μg/mL (Banerjee et al., 2016). Polyethyleneiminechitosan shell/poly (methyl methacrylate) core NPs (CS-PEI) and Poly(lactide-co-glycolide) have been developed for siRNA targeting cervical cancer and to send paclitaxel to HeLa cells with better drug action, respectively (Saengkrit et al., 2012). Chitosan NPs prepared using TPP have proven to be more stable and do not require any stabilizing or external cross-linking agents. The therapeutic agent, curcumin, is encapsulated within the polymer matrix. The curcumin-loaded chitosan NPs are reported to be more effective under *in vitro* conditions with time due to greater cellular uptake, sustained intracellular drug retention, and enhanced anti-proliferative effect by inducing apoptosis (Khan et al., 2016). When managing HCC, AuNCs-CS-AS1411-based nano transporters, gold nanoclusters, and anti-nucleolin aptamer (AS1411) have proven effective. The anti-cancer drug (methotrexate-MTX) is encapsulated in the nanovehicle. MTX@AuNCs-CS–AS1411 demonstrates more intensive cytotoxicity and apoptosis-inducing activity against HepG2 cells than against normal LO2 cells. In this system, the tumor-targeting capability is enhanced by the presence of AS1411, and the drug, MTX, is released much faster with mildly acidic pH; therefore, the drug is selectively released at the tumor site (Zhang et al., 2021).

Hydrogels are 3D polymeric networks used for numerous biomedical applications, such as localized and targeted drug delivery applications. Characteristically, hydrogels are biodegradable, biocompatible, mechanically tunable, and non-toxic. Numerous polymers meet these criteria, including synthetic [polyvinyl alcohol (PVA), PEG, poly(acrylamide), etc.], and natural [chitosan (CS), HA, alginate, collagen, etc.]. As a new avenue, "smart" nano-theragnostic hydrogels are engineered to respond to stimuli, thus changing the drug-releasing behaviors (Hoque et al., 2019). This hydrogel has potential application for gene targeting, tissue engineering, imaging, diagnosis, biosensing, as well as targeted drug delivery.

SMANCS was synthesized by covalently uniting the anti-tumorous neocarzinostatin (NCS) to two substituted styrene polymer chains, developed by Maeda and co-workers, to treat liver cancer. Among the few anti-cancer agents existing to treat liver cancer, SMANCS has proven to be very effective; therefore, it is used for the treatment of advanced and recurrent HCC. The idea was to produce a polymeric derivative that was sufficiently hydrophobic to enable dispersion in the phase-contrast agent Lipiodol. This facilitated local administration through the hepatic artery to patients with liver cancer (Fang et al., 2004).

Amylose is an exceptional biopolymer that can act as a nanocarrier due to its biocompatibility and high transfection rate. When treating HCC, folate-functionalized cationic amylose NPs are loaded with survivin-siRNA. It has been reported that cationic amylose NPs can facilitate a specific and safe transport of these RNA with notable transfection capacities, giving rise to a sturdy survivin gene downregulation in HCC cells (Wu et al., 2017).

Poly(beta-amino ester) (PBAE) is a class of cationic polymers designed for non-viral gene delivery. PBAEs can be degraded by hydrolysis, releasing the nucleic acid cargo and reducing cytotoxicity. The selectivity can be increased by engineering properties of the polymeric NPs. Further, PBAE-based NPs formulations facilitate high and specific DNA delivery to varied HCC tumor cells, all the while protecting healthy cells (Zamboni et al., 2017).

When compared to cisplatin, carboplatin (CRB) has far fewer adverse reactions in the host and exhibits remarkable antineoplastic activity. The still-remaining negative consequences of CRB rising from unwanted tissue distributions, which hamper the therapeutic efficacy, can be solved by using folic acid-conjugated chitosan-coated PLGA NPs (FPCC), which are globe-shaped nanoparticles with a magnitude below 200 nm, have shown increased cellular uptake and controlled the release rate of CRB from the PNPs. The selectivity factor is achieved by the conjugation with folic acid (Ji et al., 2015).

Therapies for cervical cancer with HPV-positive status could lead to increased therapeutic efficacy if used in combinations. One treatment method—PDT—generally has low precision, and the early release of phototherapeutic drugs into the bloodstream creates toxic effects on normal cells. On the other hand, the CAP strategy has a high affinity for triggering cancer cell elimination. Ha and co-workers tried the PDT/CAP strategy to raise the curative efficacy on cervical cancer using the PPHE PNPs, in which cancer-targeting ligands (HA and EAE7) are deployed via the progressively layered self-arrangement process for the HER3/CD44 bispecific binding of cervical neoplastic cells. The PDT/CAP combinatory treatment more successfully cleared these cells by elevating ROS levels, which led to apoptosis in the cancer cells (Ha and Kim, 2021).

6.4.4 MICELLES

Polymeric micelles have a notable capacity in trafficking several drugs, with quick circulation and penetrability and EPR effect; therefore, polymeric micelles are considered to be exceptional drug carrier systems. Polymeric micelles are macromolecular structures formed by the aggregation of copolymers, having few synthetic blocks of copolymer with different hydrophobicity. The micelles have a two-phase structure with a spherical inner core consisting of hydrophobic blocks and an outer shell consisting of hydrophilic units. These nanostructures have varying sizes from 10–200 nm and are stable beyond the critical micellar concentration (Yokoyama, 2014). Different types of polymeric micelles can be developed, depending on the structure of the amphiphilic copolymer present and the blend parameters (solvent type, pH, ionic strength, temperature, solvent/co-solvent ratio, and others). When encapsulating drugs within the micelle, the important aspects to consider are the copolymer characteristics, the molecular weight, and the hydrophilic-lipophilic balance (HLB) of the micelle (Simões et al., 2015).

In targeted therapy of HCC, the utilization of dual-functionalized spray-dried casein micelles has been reported for delivering two phytochemicals, berberine (BRB) and diosmin (DSN). This strategy enabled efficient solubilization of the poorly soluble drug DSN within the hydrophobic core of casein micelles (CAS-MCs). And the dual functionalization of CAS–MCs by two targeting ligands, LA and folic acid (FA), enhanced their cytotoxicity against HepG2 cells. Overall, it has been confirmed that the dual-targeted LA/FA-CAS MCs have outstanding *in vivo* antitumor efficacy of combined delivery of BRB and DSN (Abdelmoneem et al., 2018).

Polymeric micelles have emerged as a potential vector for future cancer theragnostics due to their simple preparation and versatility in both structure and functionality. Liu and co-workers synthesized a tri-block polymer, poly (lactic acid)–poly (ethylene glycol)–poly(L-lysine), PLA–PEG–PLL. To improve target specificity, the polymeric micelle is functionalized with

AFP antibodies, which are overexpressed in HCC tumors even in the early stages, and the imaging agent, Gd-DTPA, is linked to the micelle through the amino groups of PLL. The anti-cancer drug paclitaxel (PTX) is hydrophobic and is encapsulated within the micelle to give it better solubility. This system has proven to be a highly effective nano-theragnostic for HCC (Liu et al., 2015).

EpCAM, or epithelial cell adhesion molecule, is a signature molecule of cancer stem cells (CSCs), which are mainly responsible for the reinitiation and spread of HCC. Han and co-workers have designed a PEGylated UCNPs-based micelle loaded with the anti-tumor drug and a photosensitizer, mitoxantrone (MX), and it showed antitumor effect, better simultaneous action in integrated MR/UCL imaging (Han et al., 2018).

Curcumin, which possesses wide anti-cancer activity, can be loaded into the micelles to produce effective anti-cancer therapeutics. Kumari and co-workers have synthesized transferrin (Tf) anchored methoxy-polyethylene glycol-poly (D, L-Lactide) polymeric micelles (Tf-PPC) to treat cervical cancer (Kumari et al., 2018). Tf was conjugated to the micelles for easy recognition by the overexpressed TfR in hepatic and cervical cancer cells. In this case, Tf has shown higher internalization compared to non-targeted micelles, and the curcumin-mediated cytotoxicity increased significantly following Tf-PPC treatment in both the tested cell lines (HepG2 and HeLa).

PEG-poly (lactic-co-glycolic acid) (PEG-PLGA) micelles loaded with indocyanine green (ICG), modified with TMTP1, a tumor metastasis targeting peptide, was utilized by Wei and co-workers to treat cervical cancer by targeting cancerous cells. This method simultaneously maps the primary tumor, metastasis, and metastatic sentinel lymph nodes (SLNs), providing real-time intraoperative guidance in cervical cancer (Wei et al., 2019).

6.4.5 METALLIC AND MAGNETIC NANOPARTICLES (MNPS)

Metallic NPs have been widely used in the field of biomedicine for the detection and treatment of cancer, based on the study of metallic NPs. Due to excellent properties, which include their small adaptable shape, good mono-dispersity, size, surface-chemistry, bio-inertness and low toxicity, high tissue permeability, and colloidal stability, AuNPs have been identified as a popular metallic NP for research (Gu et al., 2012). Further, AuNPs can be used to manage tumors by restraining angiogenesis and loading antitumor drugs. The application of AuNPs in immunotherapy has emerged as one of the most successful therapeutic methods for eradicating cancer by releasing antigens, oligonucleotides, adjuvants, and immune-stimulating agents into the body. When treating cancer, AuNPs have proven to be excellent nanocarriers of anti-cancer drugs (DOX, 6-mercaptopurine) (Ghorbani and Hamishehkar, 2018) and immuno-adjuvants (imiquimod (R837) (Zhou et al., 2018). SM5-1 is a humanized mouse monoclonal antibody, and it can be used for target therapy in HCC due to its ability to inhibit cell growth and induce apoptosis. However, SM5-1 has low efficacy, and studies have shown that AuNPs-conjugated antibodies can be used for increasing cytotoxicity and delivery efficacy in several cancer cells (Ghosh et al., 2008; Rana et al., 2012). Therefore, Ma and co-workers have designed a conjugate system by combining SM5-1 and AuNPs (Au-SM5-1 NPs). Both *in vitro* and in live organisms, results have shown that the above-mentioned conjugated system effectively inhibited the tumor growth rates in HCC, which over-expressed a membrane protein (p230) with 230-kDa (Ma et al., 2016).

Multifunctional theragnostic NPs is an emerging field with the potential to offer highly effective diagnosis and targeted cancer therapy. One framework like this is Lipid-AuNPs@PDA. This nanohybrid system AuNPs@polydopamine (PDA) functions as the inner core, while ICG, which is absorbed onto the surface of PDA, functions as the photothermal therapeutic agent. The outer surface is composed of lipids modified with gadolinium−1,4,7,10-tetraacetic acid and LA. LA acts as the targeting agent on the outer surface, which is able to selectively internalize the nanohybrid into the HepG2 cells. This theragnostic agent, which is referred to as LA-LAPNHs, is able to conduct simultaneous noninvasive MR/CT dual-modal imaging and targeted PTT of HCC (Zeng et al., 2014).

Paclitaxel (PAC) is a well-known anti-cancer drug used to treat HCC. Gao and co-workers have utilized mesoporous hollow alumina nanoparticles (MHA) as the carrier of the above-mentioned drug since the hollow structure of MHA is ideal for drug-delivery. To improve the targeting ability of the nanocarrier, hyaluronic acid (HA) was grafted with the amino group of MHAs to form PAC-HMHA. It was reported that this system caused cell apoptosis after being ingested by SMMC-7721 cells (Gao et al., 2019).

One of the reasons why conventional chemotherapy has proven to be unsuccessful when battling HCC is due to the fact that tumor-initiating cancer stem-like cells (CSLCs) are refractory to chemotherapy. To overcome the chemoresistance, Xia and colleagues have formed a nano-system by assembling Pt nanoclusters (Pt-NA) and incorporating a pH-sensitive polymer and HCC-targeting peptide in the cluster. Several advantageous features are exhibited by the system, such as Pt-NA being latent in peripheral blood and targeting tumor cells, including CLSC as the targeting peptide, and due to the presence of pH-sensitive polymers, in an acidic intracellular environment, Pt-NA disassembly is triggered, resulting in extremely small Pt nanoclusters with a large specific surface, accelerating the release of toxic Pt ions inside the cells for effective cancer treatment (Xia et al., 2016).

Precise detection and orderly management of small hepatocellular carcinoma is a big step forward when treating HCC, due to the difficulty in diagnosing liver cancers in the early stages. Mesoporous Fe_3O_4 containing glucose oxidase (GOD)-conjugated GPC3 peptide nanoparticles (FGP NPs) were designed by Deng and co-workers to enhance the accuracy of visualization of small liver tumors. In this system, Fe_3O_4 is used as a contrast agent for PAI. It not only enhances the accuracy of small HCC detection but also produces a Fenton-like reaction in the tumor microenvironment. The tumor environment contains high levels of glucose to support rapid tumor growth, and GOD catalyzes glucose into H_2O_2, which reacts with Fe_3O_4 to produce hydroxyl radicals and kill the tumor cells. In this study, due to the promoted HCC cell apoptosis, the survival of the model mice was significantly increased. This nano-system provides a starting point for the accurate detection and elimination of small HCCs in the complicated liver environment (Deng et al., 2022).

MNPs have increased in popularity and have emerged as an important biomedical functional nanomaterial due to their exceptional characteristics, biocompatibility, sizes, capability of biofunctionalization, responses to the external field, chemical stability, high saturation magnetization, lower toxicity, and workability at the molecular extent. MNPs can be employed for drug/gene delivery, diagnosis, phototherapy, imaging mechanisms, and chemotherapy due to their distinctive characteristics and in combinatorial approaches for theragnostics.

Theragnostic agents based on MRI could achieve not only sensitive and accurate diagnosis, but also accomplish *in vivo* real-time monitoring.

As a result, various MRI-based theragnostic systems have been developed. For example, to improve the detection ability of HCC, the usage of superparamagnetic iron oxide nanoparticles (SPIONs) as a contrast developer in T2-weighted MRI images was reported (Chen et al., 2014; Depalo et al., 2017). SPIONs are very effective for drug delivery as they can target certain sites in the body by use of a magnetizing field, with specificity being improved and reducing toxicity of the anti-cancer drugs. However, liver tissues actively absorb iron ions. Therefore, it is important to optimize the contrast agent. Yet the problem could be overcome through the formation of new MRI contrast nanocomposites and multifunctional composite nanomaterials. This improves the efficiency of magnetic carriers, imaging capabilities, and drug-delivery. For instance, functionalized porous kaolinite is not only a drug delivery complex for killing neoplastic cells but also as a structural scaffolding for FePt NPs and drugs such as DOX. Further, multifunctional FePt@Kao as a magnetic fluid hyperthermia (MFH) agent can also be used to concurrently perceive and kill HCC cancer cells (Chan et al., 2020). FePt@MMT-2 is another multifunctional nanocomposite formed by embedding FePt NPs in mesoporous silica nanospheres which exhibits ferromagnetic-like properties and could be applied as a contrast agent for MRI. Also, it increased the sensitivity of HeLa cells toward TPT (Lin et al., 2017). The nanocomposite, CMDP–OTPBA–SPION, which is a result of tethering dechlorinated cisplatin (CMDP) to maghemite NPs modified with 4-oxo-4-(3-(triethoxysilyl)propylamino) butanoic acid (OTPBA–SPION) through the surface carboxylate groups. The DNA binding ability of CMDP–OTPBA–SPION is prominent in acidic medium thus proving to be an effective anti-cancer nanomaterial. The results demonstrate that Pt drugs could be attached to Fe_2O_3 NPs to form anticancer theragnostic agents, in which NPs act as both drug carriers and T2-weighted MRI contrast agents (CAs) (Wang et al., 2013).

Gadolinium (Gd)-based MRI contrast agents are also adapted as theragnostics as their MRI properties alone are excellent. Gadolinium (III)-1,4,7,10-tetraazacyclododecane-1,4,7,10- tetraacetate (Gd-DOTA) complex and an anti-cancer drug camptothecin (CPT) modified with the targeting agent biotin is used to target HeLa cells. This system provides better spatial resolution and soft tissue contrast that could selectively target biotin-receptor overexpressed cancer cells with high uptake, effectively release CPT in reducing environments, and kill cancer cells (Yang et al., 2019).

6.4.6 CARBON NANOMATERIALS (CNMS)

The distinct physicochemical properties possessed by CNMs such as graphenes, fullerenes, carbon nanotubes (CNTs), carbon quantum dots (CQDs), and graphdiyne play a key role in their implication in various cancer therapeutic strategies such as cancer stem cell inhibition, immune-stimulation, anti-angiogenesis, anti-hypoxia, microenvironment-based stimuli-responsive drug delivery, and photodynamic and photothermal therapy (Saleem et al., 2018).

Graphene, which is a 2D material with a planar topography, possesses extraordinary physicochemical properties, such as a high surface-area-to-mass ratio, unique surface chemistry functions, and inherent optical properties, making them promising nanoplatforms for various biomedical applications. Nanographene has been investigated for its potential applications in photothermal therapy, PAI, PET imaging, drug delivery, and combined theragnostics (Cheng et al., 2020). However, various factors such as the zero-band width of graphene, pointed edges, the doping requirements, hydrophobicity, and poor solubility and agglomeration of nanosheets formed by graphene in solution caused by van der Waals forces and π–π stacking interactions significantly affect toxicity and hamper its fabrication, thus requiring effectuation of graphene for its application diversity. Numerous graphene originated byproducts – oxide of graphene (GO), reduced graphene oxide (rGO), quantum dots from graphene (GQDs), graphene nanoribbons (GNRs), and graphene nanoplatelets (GNPs) have been investigated for their potential biomedical applications particularly in cancer theragnostics (Liu et al., 2017; Orecchioni et al., 2015). Graphene-based biosensors coupled with field-effect transistors (FET), fluorescence, surface plasmon resonance (SPR), surface-enhanced Raman scattering (SERS), electrochemical and electro-chemiluminescent technologies have been widely investigated for the detection of cancer biomarkers (Pourmadadi et al., 2022). The unique planar π–π domains of graphene, the presence of carboxyl groups on the tips, and defects in the layers allow charge exchange reactions with biomolecules and help in developing GO as cellular photographing markers and biological sensing agents. Studies focusing on high-performance biosensing and electrochemical detection of HPV via nanosensors based on GO, rGO and GQDs have been reported (Mousavi et al., 2021). Furthermore, graphene-based electrochemical immunosensors also have several advantages such as short detection time, good selectivity, low detection limit, and wide detection range, when utilized for the detection of HCC biomarkers including alpha-fetoprotein (AFP), Golgi protein-73 (GP73), exosomes, and microRNA-122 (miR-122) (Liang et al., 2022).

GO exhibits excellent drug-loading capacity due to its high surface area, being able to form specific interactions with various drug molecules through covalent conjugation or noncovalent adsorption, serving as a good carrier owing to the high electron transfer of individual graphene sheets (Cheng et al., 2020). Furthermore, GO has been proven to set off apoptosis in cells of liver HepG2 causing cancer, thus allowing itself to be a promising nanocarrier material in the treatment of HCC (Lammel et al., 2013; Loutfy et al., 2017). Buskaran et al. reported the fabrication of a folic acid-coated GO-PEG nanocomposite loaded with protocatechuic acid and chlorogenic acid for the treatment of human HCC cells, which resulted in an observable decrease in cytotoxicity as dual drug piling and a slow-paced controlled liberation of the two phenolic compounds exhibiting anti-cancer action (Buskaran et al., 2021). Shen et al. synthesized a multifunctional nanocomposite based on GO functionalized with PEG, and folic acid as the targeting ligand, and modified with gadolinium-diethylenetriamine-pentaacetic acid-poly (diallyl dimethylammonium) chloride (Gd-DTPA-PDDA) as a magnetic MRI probe. The anti-cancer drug, DOX hydrochloride, was loaded via π-π stacking and hydrophobic interaction, which caused higher cytotoxic activity to HepG2 cells. The theragnostic approach, which was successfully investigated in this study, serves as a potential candidate for the specific and synergistic diagnosis and treatment of HCC (Shen et al., 2012).

Graphdiyne, a novel member of two-dimensional carbon nanomaterials, is formed by alternately connecting acetylene and benzene rings, with a high degree of π-π conjugation. It serves as a multifunctional platform when compared to traditional carbon nanomaterials owing to its wide scope of applications in targeted drug delivery, radiation protection, biosensing and bioimaging, and cancer therapy. A three-dimensional framework GDYO-CDDP/DOX@DSPE-PEG-MTX (GCDM), which comprises graphdiyne oxide (GDYO) loaded with anti-cancer drugs: cisplatin (CDDP), DOX, and methotrexate (MTX), was fabricated by Xing et al. as a multifunctional nanodrug which exhibited good biocompatibility, active targeting, long-term retention, sustained drug release, excellent fluorescence imaging capabilities, enhanced photothermal conversion efficiency (47%), and good photodynamic effects under NIR irradiation, thus proving its ability to act as a remarkable platform for integrated diagnosis and photo-chemo synergistic therapeutic effect on HeLa cells (Xing et al., 2021).

Fullerenes, another type of carbon allotropes, are hollow, cage-like structures that include pentagonal and hexagonal shapes, and the most common form being a truncated icosahedron containing 60 carbon atoms (C60). They can easily penetrate intracellularly, and their hollow interior can be used to load up biomedical payloads (Watson et al., 1997). Another research demonstrated that C60 nanofilms are capable of mimicking the extracellular matrix of liver cancer cells. Their mechanical signal ultimately creates an environment that affected the cell cycle and reduced cell proliferation, thus colonizing and limiting cell division without inducing toxicity (Sosnowska et al., 2019). Fullerenes can be modified through covalent surface functionalization to increase hydrophilicity. They can generate heat, up to their ignition temperature, when exposed to low-intensity near-infrared light (NIR), thus proving themselves to be a favorable candidate for the non-invasive treatment of cancer (Krishna et al., 2010). Moreover, they can efficiently generate reactive oxygen species (ROS) when exposed to visible light inducing cytotoxicity, leading to their application as a photosensitizer in PDT (Yamakoshi et al., 2003). The fabrication of NIR light-harvesting fullerene-based nanoparticles (DAF NPs) for photoacoustic (PA) imaging-guided photothermal and photodynamic therapy was reported by Shi et al. ROS and heat generated by DAF NPs under 730 nm laser illumination were capable of destroying HeLa cells effectively with excellent biocompatibility and low dark toxicity, while exhibiting *in vivo* and *in vitro* inhibition of tumor cell growth. The DAF NPs, which were synthesized by conjugating NIR-absorbing antenna with fullerene, were able to accumulate and generate PA signals around the tumor via the EPR effect (Shi et al., 2019). Moreover, water-soluble fullerene derivatives such as pyridinium and pyrrolidinium type fullerenes have been investigated for the treatment of primary effusion lymphoma (PEL) via suppressed cell proliferation and apoptosis (Kadota et al., 2022; Watanabe et al., 2014). Metallofullerenes, which usually consist of a lanthanide encapsulated within the fullerene cage, have gained wide attention as MRI contrast-enhancing agents due to the intra-fullerene electron movement from metal atom to the fullerene cage. Gadolinium-containing metallofullerenes act as excellent MRI contrast agents owing to relatively high spatiotemporal resolution (Chen et al., 2012; Mody et al., 2009).

In addition, mesoporous carbon nanoparticles (MCNs) have also been investigated as potential nano-theragnostic agents for the treatment and diagnosis of virus-induced cancers. A multifunctional nanoplatform based on oxidized MCNs and perfluoropentane (PFP), derived by Li et al., was reported to act as a NIR photoresponse carrier, which causes the heat-induced eradication of cancer cells and promotes liquid–gas phase change for gassing of PFP to generate microbubbles, thus enhancing the US and PAI signals in HeLa tumor cells. Furthermore, the NPs were capable of being employed for simultaneous *in vivo* PAI and PTT, thus serving as a potential candidate for imaging-guided precision cancer therapy, owing to good biocompatibility and high photothermal conversion efficiency (Li et al., 2020). Another study reported the fabrication of fluorescent hollow mesoporous carbon spheres (HMCSs) and the investigation of its synergistic photothermal and chemotherapeutic effect on nasopharyngeal carcinoma. The synthesized HMCSs showed excellent drug loading efficiency, having incorporated 10 different drugs, and low cytotoxicity as compared with typical carbon nanomaterials such as C60, MWCNTs, and rGO. Furthermore, high photothermal conversion efficiency was reported upon the combination of microwave and 980-nm laser irradiation, causing enhanced cell destruction and tumor growth inhibition (Gui et al., 2020).

6.4.7 QUANTUM DOTS (QDs)

Quantum dots (QDs) are spherical nanocrystals composed of semiconductor materials with diameters ranging from 2–10 nm. Countless interesting features, such as the exceptional optical properties, long-term stability, simultaneously detecting multiple signals, high brightness, and tunable emission spectrum, have made semiconducting NPs a vital diagnostic and therapeutic instrument. Most of the QDs fabricated had provided a versatile platform for drug delivery systems to treat different types of invasive and non-invasive cancers. QDs will either conjugate or adsorb anticancer drugs, which allow the delivery of such complex systems to the specific sites. Then, therapeutic moieties will be released or desorbed from the surface of the QD in response to biological conditions in the environment, such as pH, the presence of enzymes (Luo et al., 2012). The expansive optical properties of QD, which are acting as semiconductors, are well suited for optical encoding where a lot of different intensities are manipulated to encode thousands of different genes, proteins, or small molecule compounds (Han et al., 2001).

Various investigations have been underway to probe the ability of QDs to upgrade drug delivery. An approach to enhance the accumulation of the anticancer drug daunorubicin in leukemia K562 cells by combining with CdS QDs was reported. The CdS QDs readily facilitated the binding of daunorubicin molecules to cell membranes and promoted the uptake of drug in leukemia cancer cells (Li et al., 2006). *In situ* immobilization of CdSe QDs and temozolomide in pH- and temperature-responsive hydroxy-propylcellulose-poly (acrylic acid) (HPCPAA) nanogels integrated the functional building blocks for optical pH sensing, imaging cancer cells, and controlled drug liberation into a one-part NP system. This offered diverse chances for pH-triggered sustained release, combined diagnosis of drug molecules (Wu et al., 2010). Li et al. reported the fabrication of QD-aluminum phthalocyanine conjugates and for their potential application in PDT via fluorescence resonance energy transfer (FRET). The sulfonated aluminum phthalocyanines (AlPcSs) with amine-dihydrolipoic acid–coated QDs conjugated by electrostatic binding, effortlessly got into nasopharyngeal carcinoma cells and worked out FRET in cells, with nearly 80% efficiency. Under the effect of a 532 nm laser, the cellular AlPcS-QD conjugates destroyed cancer cells, proving the efficacy of this new PDT method (Li et al., 2012).

GQDs, nano-diamond, and CDs are three common carbon-based QDs, which are most commonly used in bioimaging. The characteristic surface suitability for molecular conjugation, superior biocompatibility, and rapid excretion of GQDs has made them considered as emerging nanomaterials in bio-sensing and cancer therapy. A specifically modified GQD which exhibited strong absorption (1070 nm) in the NIR-II region was prepared with uniform size distribution, tunable fluorescence, and high photothermal conversion efficacy (33.45%), which made it effective for ablating tumor cells and thus inhibited the growth of tumors under NIR-II irradiation, showing the potentiality of GQDs in PTT (Liu et al., 2020). Tang and co-workers described the use of direct surface coupling to prepare FRET-based carbon dot drug delivery systems (FRET-C-dots-DDS) for both cellular imaging and drug release monitoring. The FRET signal is based on the distance of separation between acceptor and donor, which was used to monitor the interactions between drugs and the fluorescent nanomaterial. This system has exhibited high drug release efficacy and had good-targeted delivery to the cancer cells (Tang et al., 2013).

Xu and co-workers developed a photo-responsive NO-releasing carbon dots that focused its aim at the mitochondria. The targeted release of NO from carbon dot-based nano-systems was prolonged to eight hours, which broke the half-life limit of exogenous NO. The action of this nano-system on HeLa, HepG2, and A549 cancerous cells showed higher cytotoxicity by specifically damaging their mitochondria (Xu et al., 2014). Compared to other carbon materials, investigation on carbon QDs is in its rising stage. Major barriers in clinical translation of QDs are the lack of a standard protocol in high-quality QD fabrication and their exact reaction mechanism and formation process. Another study reported the synthesis of trichrome-tryptophan-sorbitol CQDs (TC-WS-CQDs) from natural biofriendly tryptophan via the one-step autoclaving method to investigate its potential as an anticancer nano-theragnostic agent with the integration of diagnosis, targeting, and therapy for HCC. TC-WS-CQDs showed high affinity for targeting HCC cells via endocytosis instead of normal hepatocytes, which is detected as a green fluorescence upon imaging. These green-emitting TC-WS-CQDs were found to be capable of generating large amounts of ROS, furthering autophagy of HCC cells, and cause marked tumor annihilation by stimulating p53-AMPK pathway induced autophagy in photodynamic therapy (in laboratory conditions and living systems) with almost no systemic toxicity and excellent biocompatibility (Wang et al., 2022).

6.4.8 SILICA-BASED NANOMATERIALS

Due to their large surface area, tunable porous structure, biocompatibility, highly porous interior structure, and ease to alter functionality, medium pore sized porous silica nanoparticles (MSN) have shown exceptional suitability for the development of cancer-based theragnostics. Concerning therapeutic property, MSNP are very good nanocarriers for a diverse array of pharmaceuticals and biomolecules. MSNP have been shown to easily deliver ribonucleic acid molecules for gene knockdown, transfection, and many anticancer agents such as the hydrophobic drug CPT, paclitaxel, and DOX (Li et al., 2012; Slowing et al., 2008; Tang et al., 2012). These unique features endow MSNs with advantages to encapsulate a variety of therapeutic and bioimaging agents and implement the desired functions.

MSN characteristically possess two surfaces: external and the surface inside mesopores, which can in turn be functionalized to contain different active agents. This feature allows the formation of nano-theragnostic materials which can concurrently deliver multiple drugs and in turn makes MSN an effective anti-cancer agent. Multifunctional hybrid nanostructures of MSN that have both therapy and diagnosis abilities are highlighted in treatment against HCC, which is directly influenced by Hepatitis C or Hepatitis B infection. On account of the properties like penetrability and retention of the cancerous tissue, when the drug-carrier system is introduced to the body, it spontaneously accumulates in the extracellular medium of the cancer tissue. The EPR effect of nanomaterials in passive targeting depends on the particle size. Among different types of nanocarriers, MSN have been highlighted as an exceptional target-based drug carrier due to its tunable pore size and particle size, and it has been reported that 50 nm MSNs coated with PEI-PEG copolymer yield accumulation of about 12% of the total dose, which is significantly higher compared to 1% of 100 nm phosphonate-coated MSNs and 3% of 50 nm PEGylated MSNs (Meng et al., 2011). The specificity factor of the drug-carrier system is introduced by the ligands attached to the MSN. This paves the way for active cancer targeting by functionalizing the outer surface of the MSN. PEI functionalized MSN (Rosenholm et al., 2009), mannose-functionalized MSN (Brevet et al., 2009) has been reported.

The exterior and interior surfaces of MSNs can be fashioned differently to treat human cervical cancer. Due to the incorporation of phenanthridium (PAP) functionality, the MSNs are able to cross the plasma membrane of living cells. There are two types of MSNs utilized for this purpose: PAP-LP-MSN and AP-PAP-MSN that have the different average particle size (320 and 200 nm) and pore diameters (approx 2–6 nm). The large particle sizes of both materials prevent them from entering the nuclei of live mammalian cells; therefore, they are likely to be interacting only with cytoplasmic species. In the case of PAP-LP-MSN, the oligonucleotide intercalating PAP groups are located on the outer surface of MSN. In contrast, AP-PAP-MSN contains the same intercalator functionality inside of the mesopores, preventing any possibility of interaction with oligonucleotides that are too large in size to penetrate the 2.5 nm nanopores. It was reported that the PAP-LP-MSN NPs were able to adhere to small length nucleotides like messenger RNAs, resulting in impeding of growing cell. On the other hand, the cytotoxicity of AP-PAP-MSN, was markedly reduced upon the endocytosis from cervical cancer cells (Vivero-Escoto et al., 2010).

Fluorescent MSNs are used as a pre-screening method for cervical cancer. Infection with oncogenic HPV is the most severe hazard factor. In this case, the fluorescent dye is encapsulated within the MSN while the cancer-cell targeting ability is achieved through functionalizing the MSN with folic acid. It was reported that there was a substantial difference in movement of particle into normal and cancerous/precancerous cells after incubating for a short 15 minute time slots. Compared to HPV-DNA and cell pathology tests for pre-screening of cervical cancer, it was found out that the sensitivity was significantly better in this method (Palantavida et al., 2013).

Silica-based nanoframeworks (SNFs) have been broadly studied in the field of HCC theragnostics. The structure of the MSN can be modified by doping the skeleton with metal ions to give metal-doped MSNs. These novel SNFs have the ability to contribute to the diagnosis and treatment of HCC, while retaining their superior drug-carrier capabilities. Mn-doped MSN disintegrates in the reducing cytoplasmic environment to release $Mn2^{+}$, which could be used for the MRI diagnosis of HCC (Tang et al., 2019). SNFs can also be used as a radiotherapeutic. Au-mesoporous silica Janus nanoparticles (GSJNs), which consist of metal NPs hybridized with silica NPs to form a single carrier, have proven to be highly effective in treating HCC (Wang et al., 2017). These GSJNs have an asymmetrical nanostructure, which allows the NP to have an increased radiation efficiency and retain adequate space for filling anticancer agents. For radiosensitizers, Au is considerable, while the tumor-targeting capabilities are enhanced by conjugating FA with the GSJN. MSNs have also been employed in the field of immunotherapy. Pathogen-mimicking nano systems (MSP-DOX-SP-LPS) have been designed to recruit phagocytes when injected into the tumor site, thus simulating an infection (Dong et al., 2017). This system delivers a synergistic chemo-immunotherapy for HCC. Moreover, MSNs loaded with isoimperatorin encased within the membrane of lymphoma cells (cancer cell membranes-CCM) to construct a novel nano-targeted drug delivery system (CCM@MSNs-ISOIM) have been used. This nanocomplex, which possesses exceptional targeting ability of tumor cells, high drug loading rates, and low pH value sensitivity, is a highly effective and non-toxic treatment method for use against NHL (Zhao et al., 2021).

6.5 CONCLUSION

Various nanoparticle formulations, which possess intrinsic properties that influence their biodistribution, elimination, and target site accumulation, have been fabricated and evaluated for their application in the diagnosis and treatment of virus-induced cancers. Some viral gene products in cancer and premalignant cells are very enticing targets that may be exploited in new therapies that separate these cells from normal cells. Many promising nano-theragnostic approaches are yet to be executed in clinical practice. Some of the limitations that contribute to this hindrance, such as the difficulties in large-scale synthesis, sterility of nanoformulations, regulatory hurdles, nanotoxicity, and economy, need to be addressed at the earliest to ensure successful implementation. Successful confrontation of viral-induced cancers is possible when nano-theragnostic agents are capable of early-stage diagnosis guided by biomarkers at a molecular level and the integration of imaging techniques with therapeutic methods.

KEYWORDS

- **biocompatibility**
- **cancer therapy**
- **imaging**
- **nanoformulations**
- **nanoparticles**
- **nanotheragnostics**
- **oncolytic viruses**
- **quantum dots**
- **viral induced cancers**

REFERENCES

Abbas, Z., & Rehman, S. (2018). An overview of cancer treatment modalities. *Neoplasm, 1*, 139–157.

Asthana, S., & Kneteman, N. (2009). Operating on a patient with hepatitis C. *Canadian Journal of Surgery, 52*(4), 337.

Balzus, B., Sahle, F. F., Hönzke, S., Gerecke, C., Schumacher, F., Hedtrich, S., Kleuser, B., & Bodmeier, R. (2017). Formulation and *ex vivo* evaluation of polymeric nanoparticles for controlled delivery of corticosteroids to the skin and the corneal epithelium. *European Journal of Pharmaceutics and Biopharmaceutics, 115*, 122–130.

Banerjee, S. L., Khamrai, M., Sarkar, K., Singha, N. K., & Kundu, P. P. (2016). Modified chitosan encapsulated core-shell Ag NPs for superior antimicrobial and anticancer activity. *International Journal of Biological Macromolecules, 85*, 157–167.

Bazarbachi, A., Suarez, F., Fields, P., & Hermine, O. (2011). How I treat adult T-cell leukemia/lymphoma. *Blood, The Journal of the American Society of Hematology, 118*(7), 1736–1745.

Beasley, R. P. (1988). Hepatitis B virus. The major etiology of hepatocellular carcinoma. *Cancer, 61*(10), 1942–1956.

Beasley, R. P., Lin, C. C., Hwang, L. Y., & Chien, C. S. (1981). Hepatocellular carcinoma and hepatitis B virus: A prospective study of 22,707 men in Taiwan. *The Lancet, 318*(8256), 1129–1133.

Buskaran, K., Hussein, M. Z., Moklas, M. A. M., Masarudin, M. J., & Fakurazi, S. (2021). Graphene oxide loaded with protocatechuic acid and chlorogenic acid dual drug nano delivery system for human hepatocellular carcinoma therapeutic application. *International Journal of Molecular Sciences, 22*(11), 5786.

Casagrande, N., De Paoli, M., Celegato, M., Borghese, C., Mongiat, M., Colombatti, A., & Aldinucci, D. (2013). Preclinical evaluation of a new liposomal formulation of cisplatin, lipoplatin, to treat cisplatin-resistant cervical cancer. *Gynecologic Oncology, 131*(3), 744–752.

Chang, Y., Moore, P. S., & Weiss, R. A. (2017). *Human Oncogenic Viruses: Nature and Discovery*. The Royal Society.

Chen, Z., Ma, L., Liu, Y., & Chen, C. (2012). Applications of functionalized fullerenes in tumor theranostics. *Theranostics, 2*(3), 238.

Cheng, L., Wang, X., Gong, F., Liu, T., & Liu, Z. (2020). 2D nanomaterials for cancer theranostic applications. *Advanced Materials, 32*(13), 1902333.

Couronné, L., Bachy, E., Roulland, S., Nadel, B., Davi, F., Armand, M., Canioni, D., Michot, J. M., Visco, C., & Arcaini, L. (2018). From hepatitis C virus infection to B-cell lymphoma. *Annals of Oncology, 29*(1), 92–100.

Deng, H., Shang, W., Wang, K., Guo, K., Liu, Y., Tian, J., & Fang, C. (2022). Targeted-detection and sequential-treatment of small hepatocellular carcinoma in the complex liver environment by GPC-3-targeted nanoparticles. *Journal of Nanobiotechnology, 20*(1), 156. https://doi.org/10.1186/s12951-022-01378-w (accessed on 4th July 2025).

Depalo, N., Iacobazzi, R. M., Valente, G., Arduino, I., Villa, S., Canepa, F., Laquintana, V., et al. (2017). Sorafenib delivery nanoplatform based on superparamagnetic iron oxide nanoparticles magnetically targets hepatocellular carcinoma. *Nano Research, 10*(7), 2431–2448. https://doi.org/10.1007/s12274-017-1444-3 (accessed on 4th July 2025).

Dicke, R. H. (1962). © 1962 Nature Publishing Group. *Nature International Journal of Science, 196*, 1048–1050.

Donalisio, M., Rusnati, M., Civra, A., Bugatti, A., Allemand, D., Pirri, G., Giuliani, A., Landolfo, S., & Lembo, D. (2010). Identification of a dendrimeric heparan sulfate-binding peptide that inhibits infectivity of genital types of human papillomaviruses. *Antimicrobial Agents and Chemotherapy, 54*(10), 4290–4299.

Dong, K., Li, Z., Sun, H., Ju, E., Ren, J., & Qu, X. (2017). Pathogen-mimicking nanocomplexes: Self-stimulating oxidative stress in tumor microenvironment for chemo-immunotherapy. *Materials Today, 20*(7), 346–353. https://doi.org/10.1016/j.mattod.2017.06.003 (accessed on 4th July 2025).

Elsabahy, M., & Wooley, K. L. (2012). Design of polymeric nanoparticles for biomedical delivery applications. *Chemical Society Reviews, 41*(7), 2545–2561.

Epstein, M. A., Achong, B. G., Barr, Y. M., Nat, C., Morgan, H. M., Rose, M., Holden, M., Jones, E. P., Hummeler, K., Berkaloff, A., & Holt, S. (1963). Cancer Inst. Monogr. (in the press). *Exp. Med. 1954, 100*, 195. *J. J. Cell. Biol, 19*(cm), 337.

Epstein, M. A., Henle, G., Achong, B. G., & Barr, Y. M. (1965). Morphological and biological studies on a virus in cultured lymphoblasts from Burkitt's lymphoma. *The Journal of Experimental Medicine, 121*(11), 761–770. https://doi.org/10.1084/jem.121.5.761 (accessed on 4th July 2025).

Fang, J., Sawa, T., & Maeda, H. (2004). Factors and mechanism of 'EPR' effect and the enhanced antitumor effects of macromolecular drugs including SMANCS. In *Polymer Drugs in the Clinical Stage* (pp. 29–49). Boston: Kluwer Academic Publishers. https://doi.org/10.1007/0-306-47932-X_2 (accessed on 4th July 2025).

Feng, H., Chang, Y., Shuda, M., & Moore, P. S. (2009). *NIH Public Access, 319*(5866), 1096–1100. https://doi.org/10.1126/science.1152586.Clonal (accessed on 4th July 2025).

Frézard, F., Schettini, D. A., Rocha, O. G. F., & Demicheli, C. (2005). Liposomes: Physicochemical and pharmacological properties, applications in antimony-based chemotherapy. *Química Nova, 28*, 511–518.

Fu, Y., Nitecki, D. E., Maltby, D., Simon, G. H., Berejnoi, K., Raatschen, H. J., Yeh, B. M., Shames, D. M., & Brasch, R. C. (2006). Dendritic iodinated contrast agents with PEG-cores for CT imaging: Synthesis and preliminary characterization. *Bioconjugate Chemistry, 17*(4), 1043–1056. https://doi.org/10.1021/bc060019c (accessed on 4th July 2025).

Gallo, R. C. (2005). The discovery of the first human retrovirus: HTLV-1 and HTLV-2. *Retrovirology, 2*, 1–7. https://doi.org/10.1186/1742-4690-2-17 (accessed on 4th July 2025).

Gao, Y., Hu, L., Liu, Y., Xu, X., & Wu, C. (2019). Targeted delivery of paclitaxel in liver cancer using hyaluronic acid functionalized mesoporous hollow alumina nanoparticles. *BioMed Research International, 2019* (April), 1–10. https://doi.org/10.1155/2019/2928507 (accessed on 4th July 2025).

Geest, T. van der, Laverman, P., Metselaar, J. M., Storm, G., & Boerman, O. C. (2016). Radionuclide imaging of liposomal drug delivery. *Expert Opinion on Drug Delivery, 13*(9), 1231–1242. https://doi.org/10.1080/17425247.2016.1205584 (accessed on 4th July 2025).

Gequelin, L. C. F., Riediger, I. N., Nakatani, S. M., Biondo, A. W., & Bonfim, C. M. (2011). Epstein-Barr virus: General factors, virus-related diseases and measurement of viral load after transplant. *Revita Brasileira de Hematologic e Hemoterapia, 33*(5), 383–388. https://doi.org/10.5581/1516-8484.20110103 (accessed on 4th July 2025).

Ghorbani, M., & Hamishehkar, H. (2018). A novel multi stimuli-responsive PEGylated hybrid gold/nanogels for co-delivery of doxorubicin and 6-mercaptopurine. *Materials Science and Engineering: C, 92* (November), 599–611. https://doi.org/10.1016/j.msec.2018.07.019 (accessed on 4th July 2025).

Ghosh, P., Han, G., De, M., Kim, C., & Rotello, V. (2008). Gold nanoparticles in delivery applications☆. *Advanced Drug Delivery Reviews, 60*(11), 1307–1315. https://doi.org/10.1016/j.addr.2008.03.016 (accessed on 4th July 2025).

Gillison, M. L., Koch, W. M., Capone, R. B., Spafford, M., Westra, W. H., Wu, L., Zahurak, M. L., et al. (2000). Evidence for a causal association between human papillomavirus and a subset of head and neck cancers. *Journal of the National Cancer Institute, 92*(9), 709–720. https://doi.org/10.1093/jnci/92.9.709 (accessed on 4th July 2025).

Gogoi, M., Kumar, N., & Patra, S. (2016). Multifunctional magnetic liposomes for cancer imaging and therapeutic applications. In Holban, A. M., & Grumezescu, G. (Eds.), *Nano Architectonics Smart Delivery Drug Targeting* (pp. 743–782).

Gregoriadis, G., & Perrie, Y. (2010). Liposomes. In *ELS*. Wiley. https://doi.org/10.1002/9780470015902.a0002656.pub2 (accessed on 4th July 2025).

Griffin, B. E. (1998). Relation of Burkitt's tumor-associated herpes-type virus to infectious mononucleosis. *Reviews in Medical Virology, 8*(2), 61–66. https://doi.org/10.1002/(sici)1099-1654(199804/06)8:2<61::aid-rmv215>3.0.co;2-h (accessed on 4th July 2025).

Gu, Y. J., Cheng, J., Man, C. W. Y., Wong, W. T., & Cheng, S. H. (2012). Gold-doxorubicin nanoconjugates for overcoming multidrug resistance. *Nanomedicine: Nanotechnology, Biology and Medicine, 8*(2), 204–211. https://doi.org/10.1016/j.nano.2011.06.005 (accessed on 4th July 2025).

Guerrero, C., Jain, T., & Kelemen, K. (2019). HHV-8-associated lymphoproliferative disorders and pathogenesis in an HIV-positive patient. *Case Reports in Hematology, 2019*, 1–4.

Gui, X., Chen, Y., Zhang, Z., Lei, L., Zhu, F., Yang, W., Guo, Y., & Chu, M. (2020). Fluorescent hollow mesoporous carbon spheres for drug loading and tumor treatment through 980-nm laser and microwave co-irradiation. *Biomaterials, 248*, 120009.

Ha, J. H., & Kim, Y. J. (2021). Photodynamic and cold atmospheric plasma combination therapy using polymeric nanoparticles for the synergistic treatment of cervical cancer. *International Journal of Molecular Sciences, 22*(3), 1172. https://doi.org/10.3390/ijms22031172 (accessed on 4th July 2025).

Halata, Z., Grim, M., & Bauman, K. I. (2003). Friedrich Sigmund Merkel and his 'Merkel cell': Morphology, development, and physiology. *The Anatomical Record, 239* (May 2002), 225–239. https://doi.org/10.1002/ar.a.10029 (accessed on 4th July 2025).

Hall, E. J., & Brenner, D. J. (1991). The dose-rate effect revisited: Radiobiological considerations of importance in radiotherapy. *International Journal of Radiation Oncology Biology Physics, 21*(6), 1403–1414.

Han, M., Gao, X., Su, J. Z., & Nie, S. (2001). Quantum-dot-tagged microbeads for multiplexed optical coding of biomolecules. *Nature Biotechnology, 19*(7), 631–635.

Hausen, H. zur. (2009). The search for infectious causes of human cancers: Where and why. *Virology, 392*(1), 1–10. https://doi.org/10.1016/j.virol.2009.06.001 (accessed on 4th July 2025).

Heath, M., Jaimes, N., Lemos, B., Mostaghimi, A., Wang, L. C., Peñas, P., & Nghiem, P. (2008). *NIH Public Access, 58*(3), 375–381.

Hirai, H., Satoh, E., Osawa, M., Inaba, T., Shimazaki, C., Kinoshita, S., Nakagawa, M., Mazda, O., & Imanishi, J. (1997). Use of EBV-based vector/HVJ-liposome complex vector for targeted gene therapy of EBV-associated neoplasms. *Biochemical and*

Biophysical Research Communications, 241(1), 112–118. https://doi.org/10.1006/bbrc.1997.7776 (accessed on 4th July 2025).

Hood, R. R., Vreeland, W. N., & DeVoe, D. L. (2014). Microfluidic remote loading for rapid single-step liposomal drug preparation. *Lab on a Chip, 14*(17), 3359. https://doi.org/10.1039/C4LC00390J (accessed on 4th July 2025).

Hoory, T., Monie, A., Gravitt, P., & Wu, T. C. (2008). Molecular epidemiology of human papillomavirus. *Journal of the Formosan Medical Association, 107*(3), 198–217. https://doi.org/10.1016/S0929-6646(08)60138-2 (accessed on 4th July 2025).

Hoque, J., Sangaj, N., & Varghese, S. (2019). Stimuli-responsive supramolecular hydrogels and their applications in regenerative medicine. *Macromolecular Bioscience, 19*(1), 1800259. https://doi.org/10.1002/mabi.201800259 (accessed on 4th July 2025).

Jackson, S. P., & Bartek, J. (2009). The DNA-damage response in human biology and disease. *Nature, 461*(7267), 1071–1078.

Ji, J., Zuo, P., & Wang, Y. L. (2015). Enhanced antiproliferative effect of carboplatin in cervical cancer cells utilizing folate-grafted polymeric nanoparticles. *Nanoscale Research Letters, 10*(1), 453. https://doi.org/10.1186/s11671-015-1162-2 (accessed on 4th July 2025).

Jones, K. S., Fugo, K., Petrow-Sadowski, C., Huang, Y., Bertolette, D. C., Lisinski, I., Cushman, S. W., Jacobson, S., & Ruscetti, F. W. (2006). Human T-cell leukemia virus type 1 (HTLV-1) and HTLV-2 use different receptor complexes to enter T cells. *Journal of Virology, 80*(17), 8291–8302. https://doi.org/10.1128/jvi.00389-06 (accessed on 4th July 2025).

Kadota, A., Moriguchi, M., Watanabe, T., Sekine, Y., Nakamura, S., Yasuno, T., Ohe, T., Mashino, T., & Fujimuro, M. (2022). A pyridinium-type fullerene derivative suppresses primary effusion lymphoma cell viability via the downregulation of the Wnt signaling pathway through the destabilization of β-catenin. *Oncology Reports, 47*(3), 1–17.

Kayali, Z., Buckwold, V. E., Zimmerman, B., & Schmidt, W. N. (2002). Hepatitis C, cryoglobulinemia, and cirrhosis: A meta-analysis. *Hepatology, 36*(4), 978–985.

Kelkar, S. S., & Reineke, T. M. (2011). Theranostics: Combining imaging and therapy. *Bioconjugate Chemistry, 22*(10), 1879–1903.

Khaled, H., Abu-Taleb, F., & Haggag, R. (2017). Hepatitis C virus and non-Hodgkin's lymphomas: A minireview. *Journal of Advanced Research, 8*(2), 131–137.

Khan, M. A., Zafaryab, M., Mehdi, S. H., Ahmad, I., & Rizvi, M. M. A. (2016). Characterization and anti-proliferative activity of curcumin loaded chitosan nanoparticles in cervical cancer. *International Journal of Biological Macromolecules, 93* (December), 242–253. https://doi.org/10.1016/j.ijbiomac.2016.08.050 (accessed on 4th July 2025).

Kiyosawa, K., Akahane, Y., Nagata, A., & Furuta, S. (1984). Hepatocellular carcinoma after non–A, non-B posttransfusion hepatitis. *American Journal of Gastroenterology, 79*(10).

Krishna, V., Stevens, N., Koopman, B., & Moudgil, B. (2010). Optical heating and rapid transformation of functionalized fullerenes. *Nature Nanotechnology, 5*(5), 330–334.

Lammel, T., Boisseaux, P., Fernández-Cruz, M. L., & Navas, J. M. (2013). Internalization and cytotoxicity of graphene oxide and carboxyl graphene nanoplatelets in the human hepatocellular carcinoma cell line Hep G2. *Particle and Fiber Toxicology, 10*(1), 1–21.

Lammers, T., Aime, S., Hennink, W. E., Storm, G., & Kiessling, F. (2011). Theragnostic nanomedicine. *Accounts of Chemical Research, 44*(10), 1029–1038.

Langereis, S., De Lussanet, Q. G., Van Genderen, M. H. P., Backes, W. H., & Meijer, E. W. (2004). Multivalent contrast agents based on gadolinium- diethylenetriaminepentaacetic acid-terminated poly (propylene imine) dendrimers for magnetic resonance imaging. *Macromolecules, 37*(9), 3084–3091. https://doi.org/10.1021/ma035983+ (accessed on 4th July 2025).

Li, J., Wu, C., Gao, F., Zhang, R., Lv, G., Fu, D., Chen, B., & Wang, X. (2006). *In vitro* study of drug accumulation in cancer cells via specific association with CdS nanoparticles. *Bioorganic & Medicinal Chemistry Letters, 16*(18), 4808–4812.

Li, L., Zhao, J. F., Won, N., Jin, H., Kim, S., & Chen, J. Y. (2012). Quantum dot-aluminum phthalocyanine conjugates perform photodynamic reactions to kill cancer cells via fluorescence resonance energy transfer. *Nanoscale Research Letters, 7*(1), 1–8.

Li, Y., Lu, J., Zhang, J., Zhu, X., Liu, J., & Zhang, Y. (2020). Phase-change nanotherapeutic agents based on mesoporous carbon for multimodal imaging and tumor therapy. *ACS Applied Bio Materials, 3*(12), 8705–8713.

Li, Z., Barnes, J. C., Bosoy, A., Stoddart, J. F., & Zink, J. I. (2012). Mesoporous silica nanoparticles in biomedical applications. *Chemical Society Reviews, 41*(7), 2590. https://doi.org/10.1039/c1cs15246g (accessed on 4th July 2025).

Liang, Y., Xu, Y., Tong, Y., Chen, Y., Chen, X., & Wu, S. (2022). Graphene-based electrochemical sensor for detection of hepatocellular carcinoma markers. *Frontiers in Chemistry, 10*.

Lin, C. Y., Li, W. P., Huang, S. P., Yeh, C. S., & Yang, C. M. (2017). Hollow mesoporous silica nanosphere-supported FePt nanoparticles for potential theragnostic applications. *Journal of Materials Chemistry B, 5*(36), 7598–7607. https://doi.org/10.1039/C7TB01812F (accessed on 4th July 2025).

Liu, C. C., Zhao, J. J., Zhang, R., Li, H., Chen, B., Zhang, L. L., & Yang, H. (2017). Multifunctionalization of graphene and graphene oxide for controlled release and targeted delivery of anticancer drugs. *American Journal of Translational Research, 9*(12), 5197.

Liu, H., Li, C., Qian, Y., Hu, L., Fang, J., Tong, W., Nie, R., Chen, Q., & Wang, H. (2020). Magnetic-induced graphene quantum dots for imaging-guided photothermal therapy in the second near-infrared window. *Biomaterials, 232*, 119700.

Liu, H., Wang, H., Xu, Y., Guo, R., Wen, S., Huang, Y., Liu, W., et al. (2014). Lactobionic acid-modified dendrimer-entrapped gold nanoparticles for targeted computed tomography imaging of human hepatocellular carcinoma. *ACS Applied Materials and Interfaces, 6*(9), 6944–6953. https://doi.org/10.1021/am500761x (accessed on 4th July 2025).

Liu, Y., Li, J., Liu, F., Zhang, L., Feng, L., Yu, D., & Zhang, N. (2015). Theragnostic polymeric micelles for the diagnosis and treatment of hepatocellular carcinoma. *Journal of Biomedical Nanotechnology, 11*(4), 613–622. https://doi.org/10.1166/jbn.2015.1945 (accessed on 4th July 2025).

Llovet, J. M., Kelley, R. K., Villanueva, A., Singal, A. G., Pikarsky, E., Roayaie, S., Lencioni, R., Koike, K., Zucman-Rossi, J., & Finn, R. S. (2021). Hepatocellular carcinoma. *Nature Reviews Disease Primers, 7*(1), 6. https://doi.org/10.1038/s41572-020-00240-3 (accessed on 4th July 2025).

Loutfy, S. A., Salaheldin, T. A., Ramadan, M. A., Farroh, K. Y., Abdallah, Z. F., & Youssef, T. (2017). Synthesis, characterization and cytotoxic evaluation of graphene oxide nanosheets: *In vitro* liver cancer model. *Asian Pacific Journal of Cancer Prevention: APJCP, 18*(4), 955.

Luo, G., Long, J., Zhang, B., Liu, C., Ji, S., Xu, J., Yu, X., & Ni, Q. (2012). Quantum dots in cancer therapy. *Expert Opinion on Drug Delivery, 9*(1), 47–58.

Ma, X., Hui, H., Jin, Y., Dong, D., Liang, X., Yang, X., Tan, K., Dai, Z., Cheng, Z., & Tian, J. (2016). Enhanced immunotherapy of SM5-1 in hepatocellular carcinoma by conjugating with gold nanoparticles and it's *in vivo* bioluminescence tomographic evaluation. *Biomaterials, 87*, 46–56. https://doi.org/10.1016/j.biomaterials.2016.02.007 (accessed on 4th July 2025).

Martín-Saldaña, S., Palao-Suay, R., Aguilar, M. R., Ramírez-Camacho, R., & San Román, J. (2017). Polymeric nanoparticles loaded with dexamethasone or α-tocopheryl succinate to prevent cisplatin-induced ototoxicity. *Acta Biomaterial, 53*, 199–210.

Maruyama, K., Ishida, O., Takizawa, T., & Moribe, K. (1999). Possibility of active targeting to tumor tissues with liposomes. *Advanced Drug Delivery Reviews, 40*(1, 2), 89–102.

Matsuo, K., Kusano, A., Sugumar, A., Nakamura, S., Tajima, K., & Mueller, N. E. (2004). Effect of hepatitis C virus infection on the risk of non-Hodgkin's lymphoma: A meta-analysis of epidemiological studies. *Cancer Science, 95*(9), 745–752.

Meng, H., Yang, S., Li, Z., Xia, T., Chen, J., Ji, Z., Zhang, H., et al. (2011). Aspect ratio determines the quantity of mesoporous silica nanoparticle uptake by a small GTPase-dependent macropinocytosis mechanism. *ACS Nano, 5*(6), 4434–4447. https://doi.org/10.1021/nn103344k (accessed on 4th July 2025).

Mody, V. V., Nounou, M. I., & Bikram, M. (2009). Novel nanomedicine-based MRI contrast agents for gynecological malignancies. *Advanced Drug Delivery Reviews, 61*(10), 795–807.

Moore, P. S., & Chang, Y. (2010). Why do viruses cause cancer? Highlights of the first century of human tumor virology. *Nature Reviews Cancer, 10*(12), 878–889. https://doi.org/10.1038/nrc2961 (accessed on 4th July 2025).

Mousavi, S. M., Behbudi, G., Hashemi, S. A., Babapoor, A., Chiang, W. H., Ramakrishna, S., Rahman, M. M., Lai, C. W., Gholami, A., & Omidifar, N. (2021). Recent progress in electrochemical detection of human papillomavirus (HPV) via graphene-based nano sensors. *Journal of Sensors, 2021*.

Mousseau, F., Berret, J. F., & Oikonomou, E. K. (2019). Design and applications of a fluorescent labeling technique for lipid and surfactant preformed vesicles. *ACS Omega, 4*(6), 10485–10493. https://doi.org/10.1021/acsomega.9b01094 (accessed on 4th July 2025).

Mui, U. N., Haley, C. T., & Tyring, S. K. (2017). Viral oncology: Molecular biology and pathogenesis. *Journal of Clinical Medicine, 6*(12), 1–58. https://doi.org/10.3390/jcm6120111 (accessed on 4th July 2025).

Nindl, I., & Rösl, F. (2008). Molecular concepts of virus infections causing skin cancer in organ transplant recipients. *American Journal of Transplantation, 8*(11), 2199–2204. https://doi.org/10.1111/j.1600-6143.2008.02392.x (accessed on 4th July 2025).

Nygren, P. (2001). What is cancer chemotherapy? *Acta Oncological, 40*(2, 3), 166–174.

Ohtsuki, Y., Akagi, T., Takahashi, K., & Miyoshi, I. (1982). Ultrastructural study on type C virus particles in a human cord T-cell line established by co-cultivation with adult T-cell leukemia cells. *Archives of Virology, 73*(1), 69–73. https://doi.org/10.1007/BF01341729 (accessed on 4th July 2025).

Olusanya, T. O. B., Ahmad, R. R. H., Ibegbu, D. M., Smith, J. R., & Elkordy, A. A. (2018). Liposomal drug delivery systems and anticancer drugs. *Molecules, 23*(4), 907.

Orecchioni, M., Cabizza, R., Bianco, A., & Delogu, L. G. (2015). Graphene as cancer theragnostic tool: Progress and future challenges. *Theragnostic, 5*(7), 710.

Palantavida, S., Guz, N. V., Woodworth, C. D., & Sokolov, I. (2013). Ultrabright fluorescent mesoporous silica nanoparticles for prescreening of cervical cancer. *Nanomedicine: Nanotechnology, Biology and Medicine, 9*(8), 1255–1262. https://doi.org/10.1016/j.nano.2013.04.011 (accessed on 4th July 2025).

Parkin, D. M. (2006). The global health burden of infection-associated cancers in the year 2002. *International Journal of Cancer, 118*(12), 3030–3044. https://doi.org/10.1002/ijc.21731 (accessed on 4th July 2025).

Partridge, J. M., & Koutsky, L. A. (2006). Genital human papillomavirus infection in men. *Lancet Infectious Diseases, 6*(1), 21–31. https://doi.org/10.1016/S1473-3099(05)70323-6 (accessed on 4th July 2025).

Pearson, R. M., Sunoqrot, S., Hsu, H. J., Bae, J. W., & Hong, S. (2012). Dendritic nanoparticles: The next generation of nanocarriers? *Therapeutic Delivery, 3*(8), 941–959.

Petersen, A. L., Hansen, A. E., Gabizon, A., & Andresen, T. L. (2012). Liposome imaging agents in personalized medicine. *Advanced Drug Delivery Reviews, 64*(13), 1417–1435. https://doi.org/10.1016/j.addr.2012.09.003 (accessed on 4th July 2025).

Pollock, S., Nichita, N. B., Böhmer, A., Radulescu, C., Dwek, R. A., & Zitzmann, N. (2010). Polyunsaturated liposomes are antiviral against hepatitis B and C viruses and HIV by decreasing cholesterol levels in infected cells. *Proceedings of the National Academy of Sciences, 107*(40), 17176–17181. https://doi.org/10.1073/pnas.1009445107 (accessed on 4th July 2025).

Pourmadadi, M., Dinani, H. S., Tabar, F. S., Khassi, K., Janfaza, S., Tasnim, N., & Hoorfar, M. (2022). Properties and applications of graphene and its derivatives in biosensors for cancer detection: A comprehensive review. *Biosensors, 12*(5), 269.

Rana, S., Bajaj, A., Mout, R., & Rotello, V. M. (2012). Monolayer coated gold nanoparticles for delivery applications. *Advanced Drug Delivery Reviews, 64*(2), 200–216. https://doi.org/10.1016/j.addr.2011.08.006 (accessed on 4th July 2025).

Ringehan, M., McKeating, J. A., & Protzer, U. (2017). Viral hepatitis and liver cancer. *Philosophical Transactions of the Royal Society B: Biological Sciences, 372*(1732), 20160274.

Rosenholm, J. M., Meinander, A., Peuhu, E., Niemi, R., Eriksson, J. E., Sahlgren, C., & Lindén, M. (2009). Targeting of porous hybrid silica nanoparticles to cancer cells. *ACS Nano, 3*(1), 197–206. https://doi.org/10.1021/nn800781r (accessed on 4th July 2025).

Rowe, M., Young, L. S., Cadwallader, K., Petti, L., Kieff, E., & Rickinson, A. B. (1989). Distinction between Epstein-Barr virus type A (EBNA 2A) and type B (EBNA 2B) isolates extends to the EBNA 3 family of nuclear proteins. *Journal of Virology, 63*(3), 1031–1039. https://doi.org/10.1128/jvi.63.3.1031-1039.1989 (accessed on 4th July 2025).

Saengkrit, N., Saesoo, S., Srinuanchai, W., Phunpee, S., & Rungsardthong Ruktanonchai, U. (2014). Influence of curcumin-loaded cationic liposome on anticancer activity for cervical cancer therapy. *Colloids and Surfaces B: Bio Interfaces, 114*, 349–356.

Saengkrit, N., Sanitrum, P., Woramongkolchai, N., Saesoo, S., Pimpha, N., Chaleawlert-Umpon, S., Tencomnao, T., & Puttipipatkhachorn, S. (2012). The PEI-introduced CS shell/PMMA core nanoparticle for silencing the expression of E6/E7 oncogenes in human cervical cells. *Carbohydrate Polymers, 90*(3), 1323–1329.

Saleem, J., Wang, L., & Chen, C. (2018). Carbon-based nanomaterials for cancer therapy via targeting tumor microenvironment. *Advanced Healthcare Materials, 7*(20), 1800525.

Sample, J., Young, L., Martin, B., Chatman, T., Kieff, E., Rickinson, A., & Kieff, E. (1990). Epstein-Barr virus types 1 and 2 differ in their EBNA-3A, EBNA-3B, and EBNA-3C genes. *Journal of Virology, 64*(9), 4084–4092. https://doi.org/10.1128/jvi.64.9.4084-4092.1990 (accessed on 4th July 2025).

Sawant, R. R., & Torchilin, V. P. (2012). Challenges in development of targeted liposomal therapeutics. *The AAPS Journal, 14*(2), 303–315.

Shastri, V. P. (2003). Non-degradable biocompatible polymers in medicine: Past, present and future. *Current Pharmaceutical Biotechnology, 4*(5), 331–337.

Shen, A. J., Li, D. L., Cai, X. J., Dong, C. Y., Dong, H. Q., Wen, H. Y., Dai, G. H., Wang, P. J., & Li, Y. Y. (2012). Multifunctional nanocomposite based on graphene oxide for *in vitro* hepatocarcinoma diagnosis and treatment. *Journal of Biomedical Materials Research Part A, 100*(9), 2499–2506.

Shi, H., Gu, R., Xu, W., Huang, H., Xue, L., Wang, W., Zhang, Y., Si, W., & Dong, X. (2019). Near-infrared light-harvesting fullerene-based nanoparticles for promoted synergetic tumor photothrombotic. *ACS Applied Materials & Interfaces, 11*(48), 44970–44977.

Simões, S. M. N., Figueiras, A. R., Veiga, F., Concheiro, A., & Alvarez-Lorenzo, C. (2015). Polymeric micelles for oral drug administration enabling locoregional and systemic treatments. *Expert Opinion on Drug Delivery, 12*(2), 297–318. https://doi.org/10.1517/17425247.2015.960841 (accessed on 4th July 2025).

Slowing, I., Vivero-Escoto, J., Wu, C., & Lin, V. (2008). Mesoporous silica nanoparticles as controlled release drug delivery and gene transfection carriers☆. *Advanced Drug Delivery Reviews, 60*(11), 1278–1288. https://doi.org/10.1016/j.addr.2008.03.012 (accessed on 4th July 2025).

Smith, C., & Khanna, R. (2018). Immune-based therapeutic approaches to virus-associated cancers. *Current Opinion in Virology, 32*, 24–29.

Song, S., Qin, Y., He, Y., Huang, Q., Fan, C., & Chen, H. Y. (2010). Functional nanoprobes for ultrasensitive detection of biomolecules. *Chemical Society Reviews, 39*(11), 4234–4243.

Sosnowska, M., Kutwin, M., Jaworski, S., Strojny, B., Wierzbicki, M., Szczepaniak, J., Łojkowski, M., Święszkowski, W., Bałaban, J., & Chwalibog, A. (2019). Mechano-signaling, induced by fullerene C60 nanofilms, arrests the cell cycle in the G2/M phase and decreases proliferation of liver cancer cells. *International Journal of Nanomedicine, 14*, 6197.

Sreekanth, C. N., Bava, S. V., Sreekumar, E., & Anto, R. J. (2011). Molecular evidences for the chemo sensitizing efficacy of liposomal curcumin in paclitaxel chemotherapy in mouse models of cervical cancer. *Oncogene, 30*(28), 3139–3152.

Stanley, M. A., Pett, M. R., & Coleman, N. (2007). *Stanley 2007 Rv, HPV–9*, 35, 1456–1460.

Tai, P. (2013). A practical update of surgical management of Merkel cell carcinoma of the skin. *International Scholarly Research Notices, 2013.*

Talanov, V. S., Regino, C. A. S., Kobayashi, H., Bernardo, M., Choyke, P. L., & Brechbiel, M. W. (2006). Dendrimer-based nanoprobe for dual modality magnetic resonance and fluorescence imaging.

Tang, F., Li, L., & Chen, D. (2012). Mesoporous silica nanoparticles: Synthesis, biocompatibility and drug delivery. *Advanced Materials, 24*(12), 1504–1534. https://doi.org/10.1002/adma.201104763 (accessed on 4th July 2025).

Tang, H., Chen, D., Li, C., Zheng, C., Wu, X., Zhang, Y., Song, Q., & Fei, W. (2019). Dual GSH-exhausting sorafenib loaded manganese-silica nanodrugs for inducing the ferroptosis of hepatocellular carcinoma cells. *International Journal of Pharmaceutics, 572*, 118782. https://doi.org/10.1016/j.ijpharm.2019.118782 (accessed on 4th July 2025).

Tang, J., Kong, B., Wu, H., Xu, M., Wang, Y., Wang, Y., Zhao, D., & Zheng, G. (2013). Carbon nanodots featuring efficient FRET for real-time monitoring of drug delivery and two-photon imaging. *Advanced Materials, 25*(45), 6569–6574.

Tashiro, H., & Brenner, M. K. (2017). Immunotherapy against cancer-related viruses. *Cell Research, 27*(1), 59–73.

Taylor, G. P., & Matsuoka, M. (2005). Natural history of adult T-cell leukemia/lymphoma and approaches to therapy. *Oncogene, 24*(39), 6047–6057. https://doi.org/10.1038/sj.onc.1208979 (accessed on 4th July 2025).

Tohme, S., Simmons, R. L., & Tsung, A. (2017). Surgery for cancer: A trigger for metastases. *Cancer Research, 77*(7), 1548–1552.

Veness, M., & Richards, S. (2003). Role of modern radiotherapy in treating skin cancer. *Australasian Journal of Dermatology, 44*(3), 159–168.

Vijayan, V., Reddy, K. R., Sakthivel, S., & Swetha, C. (2013). Optimization and characterization of repaglinide biodegradable polymeric nanoparticle loaded transdermal patches: *In vitro* and *in vivo* studies. *Colloids and Surfaces B: Bio Interfaces, 111*, 150–155.

Villiers, E. M. de, Fauquet, C., Broker, T. R., Bernard, H. U., & zur Hausen, H. (2004). Classification of papillomaviruses. *Virology, 324*(1), 17–27. https://doi.org/10.1016/j.virol.2004.03.033 (accessed on 4th July 2025).

Vivero-Escoto, J. L., Slowing, I. I., & Lin, V. S. Y. (2010). Tuning the cellular uptake and cytotoxicity properties of oligonucleotide intercalator-functionalized mesoporous silica nanoparticles with human cervical cancer cells HeLa. *Biomaterials, 31*(6), 1325–1333. https://doi.org/10.1016/j.biomaterials.2009.11.009 (accessed on 4th July 2025).

Vousden, K. H., & Farrell, P. J. (1994). Viruses and human cancer. *British Medical Bulletin, 50*(3), 560–581.

Wang, J., Chenivesse, X., Henglein, B., & Bréchot, C. (1990). Hepatitis B virus integration in a cyclin A gene in a hepatocellular carcinoma. *Nature, 343*(6258), 555–557.

Wang, J., Wang, X., Song, Y., Wang, J., Zhang, C., Chang, C., Yan, J., Qiu, L., Wu, M., & Guo, Z. (2013). A platinum anticancer theragnostic agent with magnetic targeting potential derived from maghemite nanoparticles. *Chemical Science, 4*(6), 2605. https://doi.org/10.1039/c3sc50554e (accessed on 4th July 2025).

Wang, Y., Chen, J., Tian, J., Wang, G., Luo, W., Huang, Z., Huang, Y., Li, N., Guo, M., & Fan, X. (2022). Tryptophan-sorbitol based carbon quantum dots for theragnostic against hepatocellular carcinoma. *Journal of Nanobiotechnology, 20*(1), 1–16.

Wang, Z., Shao, D., Chang, Z., Lu, M., Wang, Y., Yue, J., Yang, D., Li, M., Xu, Q., & Dong, W. F. (2017). Janus gold nanoplatform for synergetic chemoradiotherapy and computed tomography imaging of hepatocellular carcinoma. *ACS Nano, 11*(12), 12732–12741. https://doi.org/10.1021/acsnano.7b07486 (accessed on 4th July 2025).

Watanabe, T., Nakamura, S., Ono, T., Ui, S., Yagi, S., Kagawa, H., Watanabe, H., Ohe, T., Mashino, T., & Fujimuro, M. (2014). Pyrrolidinium fullerene induces apoptosis by activation of procaspase-9 via suppression of Akt in primary effusion lymphoma. *Biochemical and Biophysical Research Communications, 451*(1), 93–100.

Watson, A. D., Klaveness, J., Jamieson, G. C., Fellmann, J. D., & Vogt, N. B. (1997). *Use of Fullerenes in Diagnostic and/or Therapeutic Agents*. Google Patents.

Wei, R., Jiang, G., Lv, M., Tan, S., Wang, X., Zhou, Y., Cheng, T., et al. (2019). TMTP1-modified indocyanine green-loaded polymeric micelles for targeted imaging of cervical cancer and metastasis sentinel lymph node *in vivo*. *Theragnostic, 9*(24), 7325–7344. https://doi.org/10.7150/thno.35346 (accessed on 4th July 2025).

Wobser, M., Kürzinger, N., Ugurel, S., Bröcker, E. B., & Becker, J. C. (2009). Therapy of metastasized Merkel cell carcinoma with liposomal doxorubicin in combination with radiotherapy. *Journal der Deutscher Dermatologist Gesellschaft, 7*(6), 521–525. https://doi.org/10.1111/j.1610-0387.2008.06990.x (accessed on 4th July 2025).

Wu, Y., Chakrabortty, S., Gropeanu, R. A., Wilhelmi, J., Xu, Y., Er, K. S., Kuan, S. L., Koynov, K., Chan, Y., & Weil, T. (2010). pH-responsive quantum dots via an albumin polymer surface coating. *Journal of the American Chemical Society, 132*(14), 5012–5014.

Wu, Z., Xu, X. L., Zhang, J. Z., Mao, X. H., Xie, M. W., Cheng, Z. L., Lu, L. J., Duan, X. H., Zhang, L. M., & Shen, J. (2017). Magnetic cationic amylose nanoparticles used to deliver survivin-small interfering RNA for gene therapy of hepatocellular carcinoma *in vitro*. *Nanomaterials, 7*(5), 110. https://doi.org/10.3390/nano7050110 (accessed on 4th July 2025).

Xia, H., Li, F., Hu, X., Park, W., Wang, S., Jang, Y., Du, Y., et al. (2016). pH-sensitive Pt nanocluster assembly overcomes cisplatin resistance and heterogeneous stemness of hepatocellular carcinoma. *ACS Central Science, 2*(11), 802–811. https://doi.org/10.1021/acscentsci.6b00197 (accessed on 4th July 2025).

Xing, E., Du, Y., Yin, J., Chen, M., Zhu, M., Wen, X., Xu, J., Feng, Y., & Meng, S. (2021). Multi-functional nanodrug based on a three-dimensional framework for targeted photo-chemo synergetic cancer therapy. *Advanced Healthcare Materials, 10*(8), 2001874.

Xu, J., Zeng, F., Wu, H., Hu, C., Yu, C., & Wu, S. (2014). Preparation of a mitochondria-targeted and NO-releasing nanoplatform and its enhanced pro-apoptotic effect on cancer cells. *Small, 10*(18), 3750–3760.

Yamakoshi, Y., Umezawa, N., Ryu, A., Arakane, K., Miyata, N., Goda, Y., Masumizu, T., & Nagano, T. (2003). Active oxygen species generated from photoexcited fullerene (C60) as potential medicines: $O2^{-}$• versus $^{1}O_2$. *Journal of the American Chemical Society, 125*(42), 12803–12809.

Yang, J., Li, S., Guo, F., Zhang, W., Wang, Y., & Pan, Y. (2013). Induction of apoptosis by chitosan/HPV16 E7 siRNA complexes in cervical cancer cells. *Molecular Medicine Reports, 7*(3), 998–1002.

Yang, Z., Lin, H., Huang, J., Li, A., Sun, C., Richmond, J., & Gao, J. (2019). A gadolinium-complex-based theragnostic prodrug for *in vivo* tumor-targeted magnetic resonance imaging and therapy. *Chemical Communications, 55*(31), 4546–4549. https://doi.org/10.1039/C9CC01816F (accessed on 4th July 2025).

Yokoyama, M. (2014). Polymeric micelles as drug carriers: Their lights and shadows. *Journal of Drug Targeting, 22*(7), 576–583. https://doi.org/10.3109/1061186X.2014.934688 (accessed on 4th July 2025).

Yu, M. W., & Chen, C. J. (1994). Hepatitis B and C viruses in the development of hepatocellular carcinoma. *Critical Reviews in Oncology/Hematology, 17*(2), 71–91.

Zamboni, C. G., Kozielski, K. L., Vaughan, H. J., Nakata, M. M., Kim, J., Higgins, L. J., Pomper, M. G., & Green, J. J. (2017). Polymeric nanoparticles as cancer-specific DNA delivery vectors to human hepatocellular carcinoma. *Journal of Controlled Release, 263*, 18–28. https://doi.org/10.1016/j.jconrel.2017.03.384 (accessed on 4th July 2025).

Zeng, Y., Zhang, D., Wu, M., Liu, Y., Zhang, X., Li, L., Li, Z., Han, X., Wei, X., & Liu, X. (2014). Lipid-AuNPs@PDA nanohybrid for MRI/CT imaging and photothermal therapy of hepatocellular carcinoma. *ACS Applied Materials & Interfaces, 6*(16), 14266–14277. https://doi.org/10.1021/am503583s (accessed on 4th July 2025).

Zhang, X., Gao, Q., Zhuang, Q., Zhang, L., Wang, S., Du, L., Yuan, W., et al. (2021). A dual-functional nano vehicle with fluorescent tracking and its targeted killing effects on hepatocellular carcinoma cells. *RSC Advances, 11*(18), 10986–10995. https://doi.org/10.1039/D0RA10486H (accessed on 4th July 2025).

Zhang, Y., Li, M., Gao, X., Chen, Y., & Liu, T. (2019). Nanotechnology in cancer diagnosis: Progress, challenges and opportunities. *Journal of Hematology and Oncology, 12*(1), 1–13. https://doi.org/10.1186/s13045-019-0833-3 (accessed on 4th July 2025).

Zhao, Q., Sun, X., Wu, B., Shang, Y., Huang, X., Dong, H., Liu, H., Chen, W., Gui, R., & Li, J. (2021). Construction of homologous cancer cell membrane camouflage in a nano-drug delivery system for the treatment of lymphoma. *Journal of Nanobiotechnology, 19*(1), 8. https://doi.org/10.1186/s12951-020-00738-8 (accessed on 4th July 2025).

Zhou, B., Song, J., Wang, M., Wang, X., Wang, J., Howard, E. W., Zhou, F., Qu, J., & Chen, W. R. (2018). BSA-bioinspired gold nanorods loaded with immunoadjuvant for the treatment of melanoma by combined photothermal therapy and immunotherapy. *Nanoscale, 10*(46), 21640–21647. https://doi.org/10.1039/C8NR05323E (accessed on 4th July 2025).

CHAPTER 7

Nanotechnological Approaches for the Treatment of Influenza Viruses

U. P. S. HASARA, H. T. D. R. KARUNADASA, H. H. LOKUGE, N. N. WEERAPERUMA, and GOBIKA THIRIPURANATHAR*

College of Chemical Sciences, Institute of Chemistry Ceylon, Welikada, Rajagiriya, Sri Lanka

*Corresponding author

ABSTRACT

With the advent of nanotechnology, the prevention, diagnosis, and treatment of diseases caused by countless viruses have become viable. The main categories of treatments used for influenza viruses include the usage of surface protein inhibitors, RNA polymerase blockers, and vaccines. Various nanomaterials could be employed in the aforementioned approaches. This chapter discusses the use of lipid-based nanoformulations such as liposomes, nanoemulsions, and dendrimers; polymer-based nanoformulations including chitosan, polymeric micelles, and poly (lactic-co-glycolic acid); inorganic-based nanoparticles (NPs) such as quantum dots, gold NPs, silver NPs, iron oxide NPs, selenium NPs, and zinc oxide NPs; and carbon-based nanoformulations like carbon nanotubes, fullerenes, and graphene, and their potential applications in the treatment of influenza viruses. Furthermore, it explores the use of nanogels, nanotraps, and nano-vaccines, as well as the application of nanotechnology in gene silencing for treating influenza virus diseases using antisense oligonucleotides, RNA interference, and DNAzymes.

Nanotechnological Management of Viral Infections.
Radhakrishnan EK, Shiji Mathew, and Riya Alex (Eds.)

DOI: 10.1201/9781779640895-7

7.1 INTRODUCTION

Viral infections caused by influenza viruses pose significant health challenges globally due to their rapidly evolving nature. As a respiratory pathogen, influenza viruses contribute significantly to both seasonal, endemic infections and periodic, pandemic infections. These viruses belong to the relatively small family of Orthomyxoviridae viruses, enveloping a negative single-stranded genomic RNA (Hayden and Palese, 2018; Ison, 2011; Szewczyk et al., 2014). The Orthomyxoviridae family comprises seven genera: *Influenza A virus* (Figure 7.1), *Influenza B virus*, *Influenza C virus*, *Influenza D virus*, *Quaranjavirus*, *Thogovirus*, and *Isavirus* (Hayden and Palese, 2018; Szewczyk et al., 2014; Tamura and Kurata, 2004; Zhumatov et al., 2020).

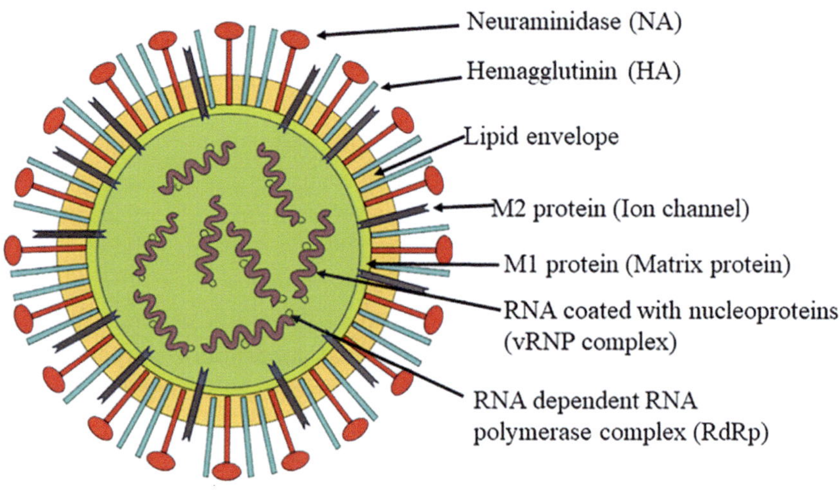

FIGURE 7.1 Structure of the *Influenza A virus*.
Source: Adapted from Hayden and Palese (2018).

Human influenza A virus (IAV) was initially isolated in 1933, followed by the identification of the influenza B virus (IBV) and the influenza C virus (ICV) in 1940 and 1947, respectively (Theodoridis et al., 2000). These viral agents, namely IAV and IBV, cause annual epidemics resulting in 3–5 million cases of severe morbidity and approximately 300,000 deaths, with mortality rates of 16% and 10%, respectively (Zhumatov et al., 2020). IAV, IBV, and ICV can infect humans and certain other mammals, while

Quaranjavirus and *Thogovirus* are found among invertebrates such as ticks and are not recognized as human pathogens. Isavirus, on the other hand, affects fish (Hayden and Palese, 2018; Szewczyk et al., 2014; Tamura and Kurata, 2004; Zhumatov et al., 2020).

Influenza viruses are roughly spherical with a diameter of approximately 120 nm, featuring an outer lipid layer originating from the host's plasma membranes (Hayden and Palese, 2018; Szewczyk et al., 2014). About 500 projections/virions exist outside the lipid envelope, with approximately 80% of these projections appearing as rods composed of hemagglutinin (HA), while the remaining projections take the shape of mushrooms and are constructed from neuraminidase (NA) molecules (Hayden and Palese, 2018; Szewczyk et al., 2014; Yoon et al., 2014). The M2 protein, unique to IAV, is also incorporated into virions as a third integral membrane protein, playing a pivotal role in the uncoating of viruses in the endosomes and in the regulation of virus assembly through its ion channel activity (Hayden and Palese, 2018). The matrix protein M1, the most abundant protein in virions, underlies the lipid layer and is crucial for the attachment of the ribonucleoprotein (RNP) (Szewczyk et al., 2014).

IAV and IBV consist of eight different RNA gene segments, each coding for at least one protein, whereas the ICV genome has only seven segments, with only one surface glycoprotein (Hayden and Palese, 2018; Taubenberger and Morens, 2008; Zhumatov et al., 2020). For a single virus particle to be infectious, it must contain all eight unique RNA segments, and the eight IAV RNA segments encode 11 recognized gene products (Yoon et al., 2014). The IAV genome consists of eight single-stranded negative-sense RNAs ((-) RNA), which bind with viral proteins to form viral ribonucleoprotein complexes (vRNP). Each RNA segment is coated with nucleoproteins and bound to RNA-dependent RNA polymerase (RdRp) (Wieczorek et al., 2020). ICVs lack the NA gene (Hayden and Palese, 2018). Additionally, each HA subtype can combine with the subtypes of the NA, resulting in a substantial and highly flexible pool of genetic variations (Khanna et al., 2008). However, subtypes only occur in IAV, with 16 distinct HA and nine distinct NA subtypes recognized in animal influenza viruses, of which only 3 HA subtypes (H1, H2, and H3) and 2 NA subtypes (N1 and N2) are known to have caused widespread outbreaks in humans (Hayden and Palese, 2018; Ison, 2011; Resa-Infante et al., 2011). While the H2N2 subtype of IAV has persisted for an extended period, only subtypes H1N1 and

H3N2 follow an epidemiological pattern in humans and are considered endemic (Wahlgren, 2011).

7.1.1 INFLUENZA VIRUS LIFE CYCLE

To design anti-influenza molecules and drugs, it is vital to understand the replication life cycle of the influenza virus. This description focuses on the IAV. The first stage of the influenza virus life cycle is to identify the host cell in the respiratory tract by its receptor molecule, α-sialic acid. The binding site to the sialic acid of the IAV is located at each subunit of trimeric HA (Luo, 2012). Binding of the virus particle to the host cell occurs as a multivalent binding event due to the presence of multiple HA copies on each virus particle. After successful binding of the host cell and the virus particle, the virus particle can enter the host cell through different routes such as clathrin-mediated endocytosis or CME, caveolae-dependent endocytosis or CDE, clathrin-caveolae-independent endocytosis, or micropinocytosis. In the CME pathway, the cell entry mostly occurs by internalizing the virus particle into an endosomal compartment called the endosome (Zheng and Tao, 2013). The RNPs of the virus particle is released into the cytosol when the viral membrane fusion occurs in the envelope. To translate, transcribe, and replicate the viral genome, RNPs should reach the host nucleus. RNPs serve as active templates for viral mRNA synthesis and the synthesis of anti-genomic complementary RNA, cRNA. These cRNAs direct the synthesis of virus RNAs (vRNAs), acting as replication intermediates. The nucleoproteins and other proteins such as M1, PA, PB1, and PB2, which are synthesized in the cytoplasm, need to be imported back to the nucleus and reconstituted into RNPs. Viral mRNAs are not encapsidated into RNP structures, but nascent cRNAs and vRNA are. These influenza virus RNPs are then transported to the cytoplasmic membrane (Gasparini et al., 2014; Watanabe et al., 2010).

The final step of the viral life cycle is budding/capsid assembly and release. Budding can be simply explained as the formation of viral particles by the abundant accumulation of viral proteins (Ryu, 2017). Mainly initiated by HA protein, the process of budding takes place at the apical membrane, around the RNP complex, where HA, NA, M1, and M2 proteins are abundant (Gasparini et al., 2014). M1 and M2 proteins have been proven important in closing off the budding process. The formed buds are then covered in a viral envelope and released from the host cell.

Envelopment of the buds can be performed through two mechanisms (Ryu, 2017): a random packaging model (Samji, 2009) and a specific packaging model. These two models differ in whether there is a signal that leads the genomic segments into virions or not. In the last part of budding, the release of the capsids, the M2 protein plays a crucial role. The M2 protein makes the positive curvature of the cell membrane allowing the removal of capsids from the host cell. Finally, the capsid completely breaks free from the host cell by removing sialic acid units, which bond the capsids to HA proteins (Gasparini et al., 2014; Samji, 2009).

The respiratory tract is affected due to direct viral infection of the influenza virus or due to a failure of the immune system. The HA molecule of the influenza virus is successfully cleaved only at the respiratory epithelium in humans and produces infectious viral particles. The influenza virus can affect other cell types, such as multiple immune cells, and initiate protein production even though the effective generation of the infectious virus particles takes place in the human respiratory epithelium. When a susceptible person comes in contact with aerosols or respiratory particles from an infected person, the virus is transmitted (Braciale, 2013; Mehle and McCullers, 2013). Additionally, the influenza virus directly infects the respiratory epithelium, resulting in lung inflammation and damage. The effects of lung inflammation brought on by immune responses increase when there is an urge to stop the spread of the virus (Kalil and Thomas, 2019).

Furthermore, the influenza viruses cause acute inflammation in the respiratory tract, along with symptoms such as fever, cough, fatigue, and body aches (Fukuyama and Kawaoka, 2011), due to the immune response to viral infection and interferon reaction. These symptoms are often coupled with respiratory tract sickness symptoms such as a runny nose, sore throat, and nonproductive cough, which lead to uncomplicated influenza. In addition, influenza can more severely harm other organs such as the heart, brain, and lungs than the respiratory system and result in hospitalization (Moghadami, 2017). Severe complications occur in individuals who belong to the higher risk group, such as pregnant women, elderly adults, and patients who suffer from underlying diseases such as cardiac diseases, chronic lung diseases, and other chronic diseases. Viral pneumonia is the primary complication of the influenza virus that results from damage to the alveolar epithelium, unlike the damage to the tracheobronchial epithelium in uncomplicated influenza (Kuiken and Taubenberger, 2008).

7.2 CURRENT APPROACHES FOR TREATING INFLUENZA VIRUSES AND THEIR LIMITATIONS

Three major categories of treatments have been identified for influenza viruses, which include the use of surface protein (M2, NA) inhibitors, RNA polymerase blockers (PB2, PB1, PA), and vaccines (Gansukh et al., 2018). According to the different drug target locations on the surface, two main classes of commonly used drugs have been identified to treat influenza virus diseases. One class targets the Matrix 2 (M2) ion channels, and the other group targets the NA proteins expressed and located in the viral envelope (Gansukh et al., 2017). The M2 protein is a transmembrane protein located in the virus envelope, forming ion channels to equilibrate pH across the viral membrane when entering cells and across the trans-Golgi membrane during viral maturation (Manzoor et al., 2017). Amantadine and rimantadine are protein channel inhibitor drugs effective against the IAV. These inhibitors can block the release and migration of vRNP into the host cell nucleus. However, the use of these drugs, known as adamantanes, has been discontinued and replaced by neuraminidase inhibitors (NAI) as these drugs are only effective after diagnosis and have the potential to inhibit only IAV as IBV proteins lack M2 ion channels (Barik 2012; Sheu et al., 2011). Oseltamivir and zanamivir are used as NAI drugs to treat and prevent uncomplicated flu caused by IAV and IBV. Peramivir is the only available intravenous drug formulation among anti-influenza NAIs (Spanakis et al., 2014). Recently, Japan approved the NAI laninamivir for treating influenza viral infections, and found that this drug is long-acting and acts against viruses that are even resistant to oseltamivir (Ikematsu and Kawai, 2011).

Blocking the RNA polymerase is a new approach for treating influenza viruses (Enkhtaivan et al., 2017; Gansukh et al., 2016) as the natural and synthesized compounds used have the ability to inhibit influenza viruses by blocking RNA polymerases (Gansukh et al., 2016). Vaccines support the immune system to start immune mechanisms before the virulent species enter the body. Various types of vaccines have been used to treat influenza viral diseases that consist of live, attenuated virus particles (Kandel and Hartshorn, 2001). According to the World Health Organization, the two main types of influenza vaccines available are the inactivated influenza vaccine (IIV) and the live attenuated influenza vaccine (LAIV). They protect against either 3 influenza virus variants, influenza A(H3N2), pandemic A (H1N1), and one of two influenza B lineage viruses, or four influenza virus variants, which are the previously mentioned influenza A(H3N2), pandemic A (H1N1), and both influenza B lineage viruses.

Due to various factors, treating and preventing influenza is challenging, and it greatly contributes to the threat caused by this disease. The influenza virus possesses an RNA genome that lacks proofreading ability. Additionally, it undergoes rapid mutations and increases resistance to existing vaccines and antiviral drugs (Beigel and Bray, 2008). Antigenic drift, or the small changes in viral HA and NA antigen sequences, is a reason for such mutations occurring in the genome, which may allow the virus to escape from the host's adaptive immunity. Furthermore, increased infection ability and virulence cause horizontal and vertical spread of the disease (Wolf et al., 2006). Moreover, if coinfection occurs, genetic reassortment takes place, leading to an antigenic shift. The segmented genome of the influenza virus eases the genetic reassortment during this situation. New hybrid viral strains result due to genetic reassortment, causing global pandemics due to a lack of immunity (Dunham et al., 2009). Certain populations, such as the elderly, pregnant women, and people with diabetes or immune deficiencies (such as those with AIDS), are especially vulnerable to influenza. In fact, despite constituting only about 15% of the population, people aged 65 and older account for 90% of seasonal influenza-related deaths. Drug tolerance decreases with genetic mutations, and genetic reassortment occurs in influenza viruses (Metersky et al., 2012).

In addition to all the above reasons, the rise of drug-resistance of influenza virus strains has increased significantly in recent years and is now a significant global public health concern (Yang et al., 2017). Strengthening the host's defenses and stopping diseases brought on by influenza virus infections is considered essential. Therefore, novel approaches for treating influenza viruses are vital to meet the challenges head-on. Recent developments in nanotechnology have opened numerous possibilities for drug development. Nanomaterials, the outcomes of nanotechnology, have piqued the interest of researchers due to their unique and distinguishable characteristics compared to bulk materials. Therefore, nanotechnological approaches could serve as promising candidates for treating these diseases.

7.3 NANOTECHNOLOGY-BASED METHODS FOR THE TREATMENT OF INFLUENZA

Conventional medications have significant limitations due to undesirable outcomes resulting from non-specificity and lack of effectiveness due to improper or inadequate dosages (Aminu et al., 2020). However, minimizing these adverse effects and increasing the effectiveness of drugs could be achieved by designing drugs with higher cell specificity (Navya et al., 2019). Various types of nanostructures with distinctive physicochemical and biological features have been synthesized using size reduction techniques, turning them into materials suitable for biomedical applications, which has increased the significance of pharmaceutical sciences. Thus, this technology could be employed to treat influenza viral diseases (Surendiran et al., 2009), as summarized in Figure 7.2 and the following sections.

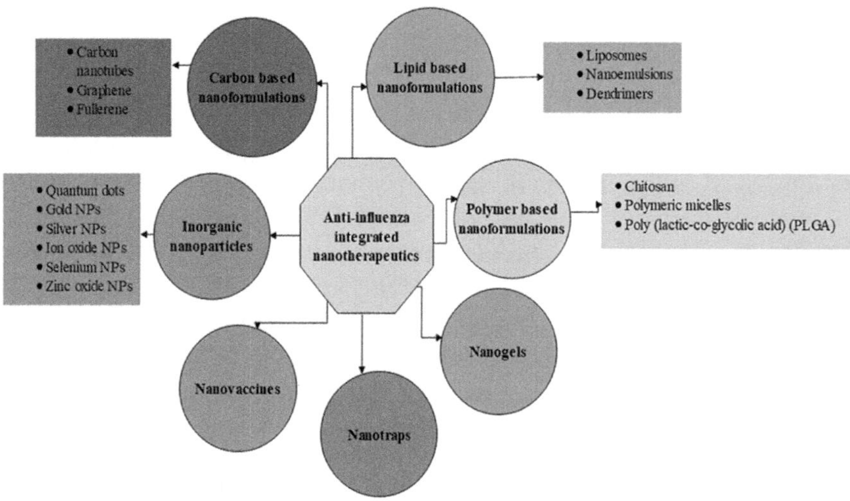

FIGURE 7.2 Summary of anti-influenza integrated nanotherapeutics.

Nanomaterials belong to various categories, such as lipid-based nanoformulations, polymer-based nanoformulations, or polymeric nanoparticles (PNP), inorganic-based nanoformulations, and carbon-based nanoformulations. They have the potential to treat diseases caused by influenza virus infections. Additionally, the application of nanotubes, nanotraps, nanovaccines, nanogels, and gene silencing techniques based on nanotechnological approaches are also considered ideal candidates for treating influenza virus diseases (Chakravarty and Vora, 2021).

7.3.1 LIPID-BASED NANOFORMULATIONS TO TREAT INFLUENZA VIRUSES

Lipids possess unique characteristics, such as small size, large surface area, improved interface interactions, high drug-loading capacity, controlled release, and improved overall performance of the drug delivery process. Some lipid-based nanoformulations used to treat influenza viruses include liposomes and nanoemulsions (Chakravarty and Vora, 2021).

7.3.1.1 LIPOSOMES

Liposomes have been studied for more than six decades due to their potential as a drug delivery system. They vary in size, ranging from 30–1000 nm, a significant parameter that influences the circulation half-life of the liposomes. They consist of hollow spheres or vesicles bordered by a lipid bilayer composed of phospholipids, which can be naturally occurring or synthetic (Figure 7.3). The lipid bilayers, a distinctive feature of liposomes, enclose a hydrophilic interior, enabling the storage of aqueous drugs within the vesicle. The number of bilayers surrounding the liposome is another principal parameter governing the bundling and encapsulation of the drug (Akbarzadeh et al., 2013; Ftouh et al., 2021).

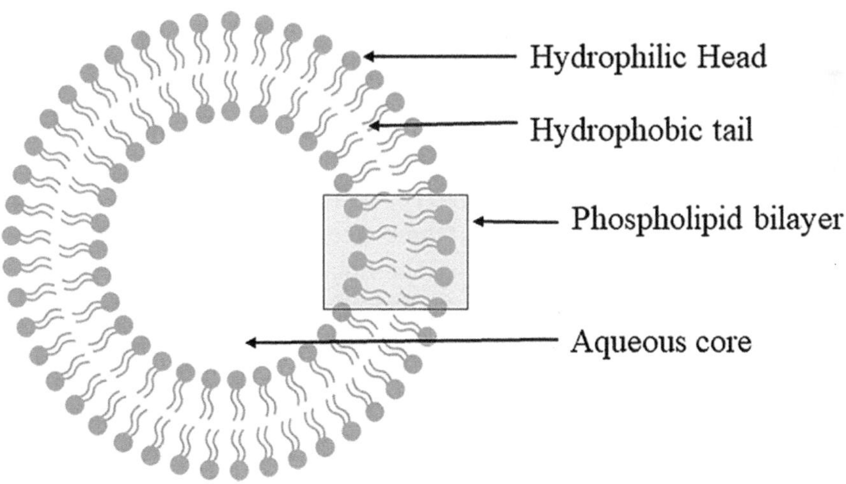

FIGURE 7.3 Structure of the liposome.

Source: Adapted from Hendricks et al. (2013).

Liposomes with ligands embedded in the surface can ensure targeted delivery and consequently reduce the required drug dosage compared to conventional ingestion or inhalation. Ionization of liposomes surviving in different media with varying pH values, aqueous and organic environments, has been proposed to ensure targeted delivery. This feature offers an advantage, as the drug inside the vesicle can traverse adverse environments, thereby preventing the possibility of drug degradation along the way. Thus, uninterrupted drug circulation is also guaranteed. Given that liposomes are naturally occurring organic lipid-based nanoparticles (NPs), their reduced toxicity (Ftouh et al., 2021) is an additional advantage of liposome-based nanomedicine for influenza viruses.

Furthermore, influenza viruses can attach to sialic acid-bearing cells through various weak ligand-binding interactions. Although polymerized sialic acid analogs can form multivalent interactions with influenza viruses, their toxicity and solubility render them unsuitable for therapeutic use. Liposomal decoys (LSTc) were employed as a novel approach for delivering the glycan sialylneolacto-N-tetraose c (Hendricks et al., 2013). Inhibition of IAV was examined by assessing the capacity of LSTc-carrying decoy liposomes to capture IAV. The influenza virus engages with decoy liposomes containing LSTc to establish multivalent polymer-like connections. Hemagglutination inhibition assays revealed that decoy liposomes competitively bind influenza viruses, leading to the dose-dependent inhibition of infection in target cells (Hendricks et al., 2013).

A liposome NP-based subunit vaccine was formulated, containing 10 encapsulated highly conserved B and T cell epitope peptides, aiming to enhance protective immune activity against a zoonotic swine influenza A virus (SwIAV) H1N1 challenge infection in a pig model (Dhakal et al., 2018). Piglets in a flu-free nursery received two doses of the vaccine formulation as an intranasal mist at three-week intervals, along with monosodium urate crystals as adjuvants. The liposome peptide flu vaccination administered with MSU adjuvant improved the hemagglutination inhibition antibody titer and mucosal IgA response against the SwIAV challenge, as well as against two other highly genetically variant IAVs. An increase in the frequency of peptides and virus-specific T-helper/memory cells and IFN responses was observed with the use of liposomal vaccines. The MSU adjuvant-based liposomal peptide flu vaccine enhanced the cellular and mucosal humoral immune responses of partially shielded pigs against flu-induced fever and pneumonic lesions, reduced nasal virus shedding, and decreased viral load in the lungs. This study demonstrates the potential of liposome and MSU adjuvant-based subunit flu vaccines for development as intranasal subunit flu vaccines, with preclinical investigations in a pig model (Dhakal et al., 2018).

7.3.1.2 NANOEMULSIONS (NE)

NE are single-phase, thermodynamically stable systems composed of oil, water, surfactants, and co-surfactants, with sizes ranging from 20–500 nm. They offer significant advantages, including increased aqueous solubility, improved loading capacity, superior absorption and bioavailability, and lymphatic uptake (Chakravarty and Vora, 2021). In an *in-vivo* study conducted by Donovan et al., two nanoemulsion formulations, 8N8 and 20N10, made from soybean oil, tributyl phosphate, and Triton X-100, significantly improved the survival rate of mice exposed to IAV when used as a prophylaxis (Mehendale et al., 2013; Zhou et al., 2021). A subsequent study demonstrated that polyphenol nanoemulsions made from *Ginkgo biloba* leaves acted as a nanocarrier, providing a virucidal and protective effect when tested against the influenza H3N2 virus (Aguilera-Correa et al., 2021).

7.3.1.3 DENDRIMERS

Dendrimers are nanoscale polymeric molecules characterized by a highly branched and globular structure. This unique structural feature contributes to the distinctive physical properties of dendrimers, which include a uniform structure with terminal groups that facilitate interactions and targeted delivery (Ftouh et al., 2021; Gurunathan et al., 2020; Maus et al., 2021). The globular portion of a dendrimer consists of three layers: a central core, dendrons as branches, and terminal functional groups. The hydrophobic central core of a dendrimer enables the loading of hydrophobic drugs, and modifications in the core structure can alter certain properties of the adsorbed drug (Figure 7.4). The functional groups on the outer shell can be easily modified to deliver the drug to the desired location through chemical bonds or electrostatic interactions (Ftouh et al., 2021).

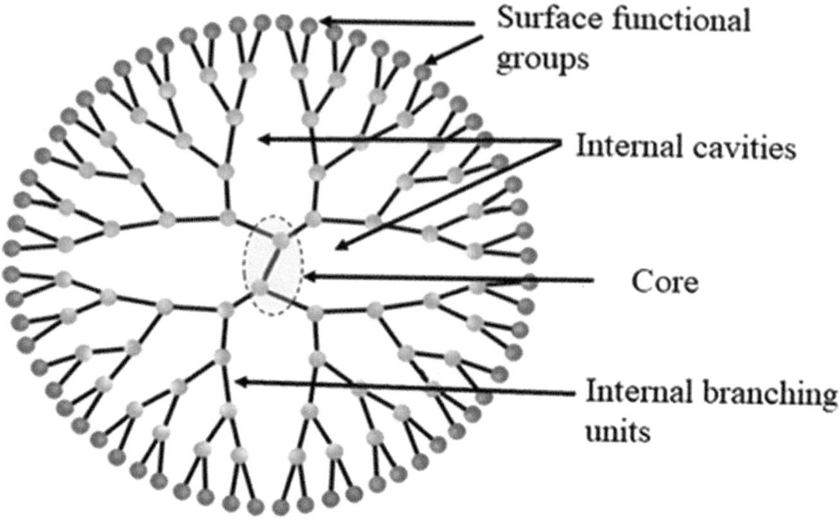

FIGURE 7.4 Structure of the dendrimer.
Source: Adapted from Rabiee et al. (2020).

Dendrimers have already been utilized in the treatment of influenza and human respiratory syncytial viruses, demonstrating their ability to prevent host cell penetration. Therefore, the use of dendrimers is recommended for the early-stage detection of virus attacks, and positive results have been reported against the H5N1 virus (Ftouh et al., 2021; Maus et al., 2021). Due to their lower molecular weight and suitability for delivery through vaccination, dendrimers can be modified by conjugating with proteins to develop other delivery methods (Ftouh et al., 2021).

A series of systematically synthesized carbosilane dendrimers were functionalized with an HA-binding peptide, consisting of an Ala-Arg-Leu-Pro-Arg amino acid sequence, to examine their ability to inhibit influenza viruses. While sialylated dendrimers were digested by viral neuraminidase, carbosilane dendrimers were not. Peptide dendrimers of various shapes exhibited significant biological activities, with a dumbbell-shaped peptide dendrimer showing potent inhibitory effects against two human influenza viruses, A/PR/8/34 (H1N1) and A/Aichi/2/68 (H3N2). This dumbbell-shaped carbosilane dendrimer, serving as the ideal core scaffold for HA-binding peptide dendrimers, exhibited the highest IC50 value among all HA-binding peptide derivatives, which was 0.60 μM (Hatano et al., 2014).

7.3.2 POLYMER-BASED NANOFORMULATIONS TO TREAT INFLUENZA VIRUSES

Various types of polymers are employed in the preparation of nanoformulations, including natural hydrophilic polymers such as proteins (gelatin, albumin, lectin), and polysaccharides (alginate, dextran, chitosan, and agarose), as well as synthetic hydrophobic polymers such as polylactic acid (PLA), polylactide-co-glycolic acid (PLGA), polystyrene, poly(epsilon-caprolactone) (PECL), and polymerized in process, poly(isobutylcyanoacrylate) (PICA), polybutylcyanoacrylate, polyhexylcyanoacrylate, and polymethacrylate (PMMA) (Chakravarty and Vora, 2021). The following are leading polymer-based nanoformulations that have been studied for their effectiveness against influenza viruses.

7.3.2.1 CHITOSAN

Chitosan is a biopolymeric nanoparticle and biodegradable polymer derived from a natural polysaccharide, chitin. It is commonly used in nasal vaccination due to its ability to bind to the negatively charged cell membranes of mucus (mucoadhesive property), owing to its cationic/positively charged surface. These particles have demonstrated effective results in opening tight junctions, thereby enhancing antigen transportation (Dehghan et al., 2013; Ftouh et al., 2021).

Chitosan nanoparticles possess a hydrophilic nature, allowing for the loading of hydrophilic drugs such as proteins and antivirals. To address its low stability, derivatized chitosan nanoparticles have been developed. Despite their limited stability hindering mass production, they are suitable for the transportation of certain hydrophilic drugs and encapsulation with antigens and immunological adjuvants, significantly enhancing immunity (Dehghan et al., 2013; Ftouh et al., 2021).

Intranasal administration of chitosan nanoparticles alone resulted in the complete protection of BALB/C mice against lethal dosages of H7N9 virus (Zheng et al., 2016). The same study was conducted to assess the suppression of A/California/7/2009 (H1N1) and A/Chicken/Jiangsu/7/2002 (H9N2) virus strains to determine whether the protective effects of chitosan are universal. Chitosan was administered in two 100 μg doses, and the mice were challenged with 10 times the lethal dose of A/California/7/2009 (H1N1) and A/Chicken/Jiangsu/7/2002 (H9N2).

The complete protection of mice against these two virus strains confirmed that chitosan is an ideal candidate for development as a universal anti-influenza agent (Zheng et al., 2016).

To overcome the lack of effective delivery methods for antigenic molecules to the cytosol of antigen-presenting cells, a biodegradable delivery system was developed using influenza whole inactivated viruses and CpG oligodeoxynucleotides formulated with chitosan nanoparticles and a Th1-specific adjuvant. BALB/c mice used in this study were challenged with the mouse-adapted influenza virus A/PR8/34 (H1N1). Significant stimulation of both humoral and cellular immunity was observed when this formulation was administered at both low and high doses (Sadati et al., 2018).

7.3.2.2 POLYMERIC MICELLES

Micelles are spherical particles ranging in size from 5–100 nm, with a hydrophilic outer layer and a hydrophobic core. The hydrophobic core can encapsulate hydrophobic drugs, and several micelles' hydrophilic surfaces can be aggregated together, allowing a greater amount of the drug to be loaded and preventing the premature release of drugs (Ftouh et al., 2021; Maus et al., 2021). Micelles are commonly used for accurate and targeted drug delivery, and the development of micelles with amphiphilic polymers has been undertaken to maximize this purpose. These polymeric micelles are highly efficient in drug delivery as they can boost the bioavailability of the encapsulated drug (Ftouh et al., 2021). Complexing the surface of the micelle with specific ligands or monoclonal antibodies provides the advantages of targeted drug delivery using polymeric micelles (Chakravarty and Vora, 2021). A study that employed a multifunctional PLA-b-PEG copolymer modified with a sialic acid derivative, methyl-b-neuraminic acid (MNA), as a drug delivery system to treat the influenza virus reported that amantadine loaded in the micelles inhibits hemagglutination by binding to the hemagglutinin of influenza viruses and efficiently alleviates viral infection (Rana, 2021).

7.3.2.3 POLY(LACTIC-CO-GLYCOLIC ACID) (PLGA)

Poly(lactic-co-glycolic acid) (PLGA) is the most widely used nanoparticle in the treatment of viruses, such as influenza and respiratory syncytial viruses. PLGAs are synthetic polymeric particles made from lactic acid and glycolic acid monomers. These starting materials play a vital role in reducing the toxicity of these particles as they are naturally occurring in the body following the Krebs cycle by polymeric hydrolyzation (Ftouh et al., 2021; Mirakabad et al., 2014). The polymers that form PLGA particles can be branched, linear, or spherical and can encapsulate a desired drug inside the polymer or adsorb onto the surface branches. Further encapsulation of drugs in PLGAs has proven to increase the solubility and stability of the drug (Mirakabad et al., 2014).

As these particles are naturally occurring compounds in the body, they tend to interact with other compounds in the bloodstream and direct to the liver or spleen instead of the intended destination. However, this issue can be overcome by modifying the particle, such as PEGylation. Further developments, such as ligand-embedded surfaces, can be used to ensure targeted drug delivery and increase the antigen and antiviral half-life (Ftouh et al., 2021). In a study using Diphyllin-loaded polyethylene glycol (PEG)-functionalized PLGA diblock copolymeric nanoparticles, a broad range of antiviral activity was demonstrated against two strains of influenza virus, H1N1 and H3N2 (Hu et al., 2018). In another study, it was shown that hollow PLGA nanoparticles induced dendritic cell maturation, leading to the expression of IL-1β, IL-6, IL-12, and IFN-γ, demonstrating potent immunostimulation when used with cytosine-guanine repetition antiviral agents for the Avian influenza virus H6N1 strain (Lin et al., 2020; Shah et al., 2021).

7.3.3 INORGANIC-BASED NANOPARTICLES USED TO TREAT INFLUENZA VIRUSES

7.3.3.1 QUANTUM DOTS (QD)

Although there are relatively fewer studies on QDs, the experimental results suggest a promising future in the treatment of influenza virus infections associated with QDs due to their unique antiviral properties. While the exact structure of these QDs is not finalized yet, they have been considered as graphene fragments with a size below 10 nm. With their numerous functional groups, they can bind to the surface and exhibit outstanding optical properties and strong luminescence, making them suitable for biosensing and biological labeling (Lim et al., 2021; Maus et al., 2021; Wu et al., 2020). Consequently, QD-based biological labeling has proven to be highly sensitive and reproducible in various studies, leading to their development as viral pathogen detectors (Wu et al., 2020). Various types of QDs are available, such as amorphous QDs, partially graphitized core-shell QDs, amorphous fluorescent polymeric QDs, and graphene quantum dots (GQDs) (Innocenzi and Stagi, 2020), with core-shell QDs being the most commonly used type.

In a study aiming to create a QD-based detection system for H5 and H9 subtypes, researchers developed a QD-based lateral flow immunoassay system (QD-LFIAS). QD-LFIAS enabled the analysis of the assay in less than 15 minutes, successfully detecting both H5 and H9 subtypes simultaneously. The system demonstrated competent accuracy and reproducibility, suggesting that QD-LFIAS could be a reliable method to detect H5 and H9 subtypes (Wu et al., 2020). Another promising candidate, CdSe/CdS/ZnS-linked QDs, has also been the subject of research as a rapid fluorescent immunochromatographic test. By incorporating anti-influenza antibodies with CdSe/CdS/ZnS QD compounds, the test was able to detect H1N1 and H3N2 viruses, demonstrating 93.75% sensitivity in clinical samples. Therefore, the CdSe/CdS/ZnS QD complex is an effective component in fluorescent-based influenza detection tests (Lim et al., 2021).

7.3.3.2 GOLD NANOPARTICLES (AuNPs)

Gold nanoparticles (AuNPs) have recently been extensively tested and developed as drug carrier systems due to their adjustable surface-to-volume ratio, charge, and other chemical and physical properties (Farooq et al., 2018). The outer layer of AuNPs typically consists of organic compounds, while the core remains inorganic. The physical properties are dependent on the inorganic core, while the other properties can be modified to desired levels. Typically, the antiviral drug is also linked to the functional groups on the surface (Ftouh et al., 2021). Furthermore, AuNPs can infiltrate the virus-host cell and/or target specific viral genes to prevent the virus from reproducing (Ftouh et al., 2021; Maus et al., 2021). In the case of influenza treatments, AuNPs have demonstrated increased mucosal immunity against the influenza virus. Conjugating the AuNP with the M2 protein of the influenza virus has been shown to increase immunity against H1N1, H3N2, and H5N1 IAVs in mice. Additionally, the toxicity of the particles can be reduced by coating them with biocompatible compounds (Ftouh et al., 2021).

Anionic AuNPs were tested for their potential to inhibit various influenza virus strains, including A/Israel/119/2009 (H1N1), A/Brisbane/10/2007 (H3N2), A/Puerto Rico/8/1934 (H1N1), B/Brisbane/60/2008, and B/Shandong/7/1997 (referred to as H1N1, H3N2, PR8, B-Bris, and B-Shan, respectively) in Madin-Darby canine kidney cells (MDCK) (Sametband et al., 2011). In this case, the NPs were prepared with an Au core and mercaptoethanesulfonate (MES) molecules where the MES bonded to the AuNP surface through the thiol group (AuNP-MES). The AuNP-MES exhibited potential in reducing virus activity when a hemagglutination inhibition assay was conducted (Sametband et al., 2011). Another study used multivalent sialic-acid-functionalized AuNPs to inhibit influenza virus activity. These sialic-acid-functionalized AuNPs were prepared in 2 nm and 14 nm sizes (Papp et al., 2010). The study demonstrated the inhibition of the A/X-31 (H3N2) virus by sialic-acid-functionalized AuNPs of 14 nm, suggesting that multivalent interactions depend on the size of the interacting particle surfaces (Papp et al., 2010).

7.3.3.3 SILVER NANOPARTICLES (AgNPs)

Silver nanoparticles (AgNP) have been one of the most appealing types of metallic nanoparticles in biomedicine due to their distinctive physicochemical characteristics. Silver has been used to treat illnesses in various forms and compositions since ancient times. As nanotechnology research has advanced, it has become evident that AgNPs can be utilized to treat several diseases, including those caused by viral infections (Xu et al., 2020). Studies have been conducted to determine the antiviral activity against the influenza A/New Caledonia/20/99 (H1N1) strain in MDCK cells. AgNPs were found to be non-toxic to MDCK cells up to a concentration of 1 μg/mL, showing a destructive effect on the virus membrane glycoprotein knobs and the cells (Mehrbod et al., 2009). Similar studies were conducted to identify the antiviral activity of AgNPs against A/Puerto Rico/8/1934 (H1N1) (Dongxi Xiang et al., 2011) and A/Human/Hubei/3/2005 (H3N2) (Dongxi Xiang et al., 2013) virus strains, further emphasizing the potential of AgNPs to inhibit the IAV strains.

AgNPs prepared using green synthesis, *Cinnamomum cassia*, have been used to evaluate their activity against the H7N3 strain and showed antiviral activity. A concentration of 200 μg/mL caused an inhibition level of 76% when AgNPs were incubated with the virus before infection (Fatima et al., 2015). A similar study using the ultrasonication method to synthesize AgNPs with a Panax ginseng aqueous extract observed low inhibition levels, 7.10% inhibition at 0.02 M and 15.12% inhibition at 0.25 M (Sreekanth et al., 2018). These results suggest that green-synthesized AgNPs are also promising candidates for combating influenza viruses, warranting further research.

7.3.3.4 IRON OXIDE NANOPARTICLES (IONPs)

Ferrimagnetic iron oxide nanoparticles (IONPs) have found numerous biomedical and bioengineering applications. Maghemite (γFe_2O_3), mixed ferrites (MFe_2O_4), and magnetite (Fe_3O_4) are three different forms of iron oxide-based nanoparticles (Figuerola et al., 2010). These nanoparticles have been thoroughly researched for targeted drug delivery, magnetic resonance imaging (MRI), magnetic hyperthermia, thermoablation, bioseparation, and biosensing during the past 10 years (Wu et al., 2015).

A study analyzing the inhibition of the influenza H1N1 (2009) virus using polymer-coated superparamagnetic Fe_3O_4 nanoparticles confirmed their potential to inhibit influenza viral RNA synthesis in MDCK cells. The non-toxic nature of the samples was confirmed by cell viability studies using a standard MTT assay. Additionally, RT-PCR analysis confirmed the potential of Fe_3O_4 nanoparticles to inhibit influenza viral RNA synthesis in MDCK cells (Kumar et al., 2014). A similar investigation using monkey African green kidney (MA104) cells revealed that IONPs in the size range of 10–15 nm have the potential to inhibit the pandemic influenza strain A/H1N1/Eastern India/66/PR8-H1N1 (Kumar et al., 2019). The study assessed cell viability and anti-influenza activity in a dose- and time-dependent manner using the MTT assay, plaque inhibition, and quantitative real-time PCR with IONPs. The results indicated a significant decrease in virus measured by RT-PCR within 24 hours of virus infection, suggesting a new opportunity for using IONPs against influenza viral infections.

7.3.3.5 SELENIUM NANOPARTICLES (SENPS)

Selenium (Se) is an essential nutrient in human metabolism and has a higher bioavailability compared to other nanomaterials, resulting in lower toxicity in the nano form. SeNPs in the range of 5–15 nm have shown an increased ability to remove free radicals, making them suitable for medicinal purposes (He et al., 2021). Among nanomaterials, SeNPs have been shown to play a significant role in medication for the prevention of influenza virus infections. Various studies have revealed that adequate supplements of Se can boost the immune system's response to the H1N1 influenza virus and reduce the risk of infection (Lin et al., 2018; Liu et al., 2022). SeNPs are also effective against HSV-1 by promoting cell apoptosis (He et al., 2021). Furthermore, they are currently being used as drug carriers, with studies demonstrating the effective inhibition of the influenza virus when Oseltamivir is loaded onto SeNPs (Lin et al., 2018; Liu et al., 2022).

7.3.3.6 ZINC OXIDE NANOPARTICLES (ZnONPs)

Zinc oxide Nanoparticles (ZnONPs) have demonstrated antimicrobial properties, similar to previously discussed metallic nanoparticles (Siddiqi et al., 2018). Limited studies have been conducted to observe the anti-influenza potential of ZnO-NPs. However, further investigations hold promise for the development of ZnO-NPs to treat diseases caused by influenza viruses.

A study evaluating the inhibition of the virus strain A/Puerto Rico/8/34 (H1N1) utilized ZnO-NP and PEG-coated ZnO-NP (PEG-ZnO-NP) (Ghaffari et al., 2019). The research found that PEGylated ZnO-NP exhibited better activity and displayed lower toxicity in treating the influenza H1N1 virus, suggesting that the PEGylated coating significantly lowered the toxicity of the NPs by reducing the release of $Zn2^{+}$ ions. *In vitro* studies demonstrated that both ZnO-NPs and PEGylated ZnO-NPs have inhibitory properties against the influenza virus after the virus enters the host cell (Ghaffari et al., 2019).

7.3.4 CARBON-BASED NANO FORMULATIONS

Various nanoformulations based on carbon include carbon nanotubes, fullerenes, graphene, and carbon dots. Research is being conducted to explore the ability of derivatives of these nano formulations to resist influenza viruses.

7.3.4.1 CARBON NANOTUBES (CNTs)

Carbon nanotubes (CNTs) are nano-scaled cylindrical structures made with sp2 hybridization of carbon atoms, giving them a honeycomb shape. The structure of a carbon nanotube can be simply explained as a rolled graphene sheet with single or multiple layers. Depending on the number of layers, CNT is categorized into two main groups: single-wall carbon nanotubes (SWCNT) and multiwall carbon nanotubes (MWCNT). Regardless of the characterization, CNT generally possesses several properties that lead to various applications (Lim et al., 2021). Recent studies have successfully used CNT in developing DNA sensors, as interest has been raised in the quick identification and inhibition of viral and genetic diseases due to the economic feasibility of the process. With CNT-based immunosensors, it is possible to detect and remove the viral DNA of IAV in a short period. This study confirmed that as a result of the outstanding electrical conductivity properties of CNT, even 1 pM of the sample could be detected eminently, proving the efficiency of CNT-based immunosensors (Zhu, 2017).

Polydiallyldimethylammonium chloride (PDDA) based CNT is another efficient candidate for CNT-based biosensors. PDDA can be strongly adsorbed onto CNT through π-π interactions, leading to engagement with various types of functional groups while preserving the unique structure of the CNT. These properties of PDDA-adsorbed CNT can significantly increase the surface area and electrical activity that can lead to efficient targeting of viruses (Tao et al., 2017). In other studies applying CNT-based techniques for inhibiting and preventing influenza viruses, scientists have experimented with CNT size-tunable enrichment microdevice (CNT-STEM) technology. These studies have revealed that CNT-STEM can identify viral pathogens without the aid of antibodies or devices customized for the said pathogen by adjusting the inner diameter of CNT to the size of the virus. It is also reported that when the low pathogenic avian influenza virus H5N2 (H5N2 LP AIV) was used, CNT-STEMs indicated a very high density of captured viruses. The efficiency of the process, measured with real-time reverse transcription PCR (RRT-PCR), revealed that the CNT-STEM with a 25 nm diameter resulted in 96.5±0.5% efficiency. This technique eliminates the need to boost the number of pathogens to identify and remove (Lim et al., 2021; Yeh et al., 2016).

7.3.4.2 FULLERENES

Fullerenes are nanosized caged hollow spheres made entirely of carbon atoms. The most prevalent type of fullerenes is buckyball, also known as buckminsterfullerene (C60), which has 60 carbon atoms organized in a spherical configuration with excellent symmetry (Goodarzi et al., 2017). Limited research has been conducted to determine the anti-influenza activity of fullerenes, with one of the most promising investigations focusing on 12 different water-soluble fullerene derivatives (Shoji et al., 2013). In this study, IAV strains A/Puerto Rico (PR)/8/34 (H1N1) or A/Aichi/2/68 (H3N2) were utilized. The study targeted the PA subunit of RNA polymerase in the influenza virus among the three subunits PA, PB1, and PB2. An assay was conducted to inhibit the PA endonuclease activity, and eight fullerene derivatives among the 12 inhibited the endonuclease activity of the PA N-terminal domain *in vitro* by suppressing the nucleoprotein synthesis, suggesting that fullerene derivatives could be developed for anti-influenza treatments (Shoji et al., 2013).

In a subsequent study, α-N-acetylneuraminyl-(2-6)-D-galactopyranose was synthesized and bonded to a water-soluble fullerene derivative using a 1,3-dipolar cycloaddition click reaction to observe the inhibition of various virus strains, including A/H1N1, A/H3N2, and influenza B, by binding to hemagglutinin in the influenza virus. Although this compound did not show inhibition of virus hemagglutinin, it moderately inhibited the neuraminidase with an IC50 of 81 μM (Tollas et al., 2014). Another study conducted using C70 fullerene derivatives determined the suppression of virus activity against H1N1 and three different strains of subtype H3N2. The fullerene derivatives were prepared from two different chlorofullerenes, $C_{70}Cl_{10}$ and $C_{70}Cl_8$, and then with the derivatives $C_{70}[p\text{-}C_6H_4(CH_2)nCOOH]_8$ ($n = 2, 3$) to assess the anti-influenza inhibition (Kornev et al., 2011).

7.3.4.3 GRAPHENE

Graphene is one of the most promising carbon-based nanomaterials with great potential for antiviral applications. It is a two-dimensional (2-D) planar sheet of hexagonally arranged sp2-hybridized carbon atoms and is chemically oxidized to graphene oxide (GO), acquiring functional groups containing oxygen such as hydroxyl, epoxide, and carboxylic acids (Singh et al., 2017). Another study demonstrated that GO nanomaterial could disinfect IAV H9N2 in aqueous solutions in a temperature-dependent manner (Chen and Liang, 2020). GO and reduced GO (rGO) have been utilized to identify the anti-influenza activity of H9N2 (endemic gastrointestinal avian influenza A virus). At a temperature of 56°C, the inactivation of the virus was observed when the virus was in direct contact with GO (Song et al., 2015).

7.3.5 NANOGELS (NGs)

Nanogels (NGs) are unique three-dimensional structures consisting of a cross-linked polymer complex. NGs contain up to 95% water and are often referred to as hydrogels. Cross-linked polymers enable the swelling of the NG structure, allowing it to retain this high percentage of water. The solid part or shell of the NG can be made with both natural and synthetic polymers, preventing the NG from dissolving in water and facilitating its retention in an aqueous medium (Aderibigbe and Naki, 2018; Maus et al., 2021).

Nanogels are often categorized in nanomedicine as drug delivery vessels. They possess unique properties that enhance the efficiency of drug delivery. Their hydrophilicity allows them to coexist in biological media without causing harm and prevents the degradation of encapsulated drugs in biological systems. NGs also exhibit very high encapsulation efficiency, making them an excellent option for drug delivery (Maus et al., 2021). Another critical property of NGs is their ability to respond to internal and external changes in their environment, such as fluctuations in pH, ion/charge imbalances, temperature, and protein concentrations. These changes can cause structural adjustments in NGs that lead to the release of the drugs encapsulated in the gel. As a biological system becomes infected with a viral pathogen, it often experiences changes and fluctuations in its environment. Thus, the NG can precisely target the infected site and release the drug (Maus et al., 2021; Wu et al., 2020). Furthermore, when NGs are coated with a PEG layer, they are shielded from unnecessary interactions with proteins and other biological systems, providing additional protection (Chakravarty and Vora, 2021).

Recent experiments have utilized nanogel-based vaccines as potential drug carriers to inhibit and decrease the spread of viral pathogens.

In vivo studies were conducted to determine the effectiveness of nanogels in preventing viral infection, and for this study, poly-γ-glutamic acid/chitosan (PC) NG was used. The combination of oppositely charged poly-γ-glutamic acid and chitosan was specifically chosen because the compound had demonstrated increased cellular immunity against Ovalbumin, a general antigen. In the study conducted on mice infected with the H1N1 influenza virus, the PC NG vaccine recorded better immunity against the virus, and no mouse had died or lost body weight. Additionally, the study documented an *in vivo* experiment on H1N1 infected ferrets using the same PC NG vaccines intranasally. Lung sections were analyzed for five days and showed no influenza virus traits in the samples. Therefore, PC NG vaccines can achieve protective immunity against the H1N1 influenza virus (Yang et al., 2017).

Another study focused on nanogel-induced immunization against the influenza virus tested an NG drug delivery system consisting of pullulan, which has a cholesteryl group, along with a non-toxic Clostridium botulinum fragment. After intranasal injection, the NG did not accumulate in the olfactory bulbs or the brain, indicating its safety, and the injected mice survived without any severe side effects. Hence, the delivery of drugs through NG systems induces a respiratory immune response (Aderibigbe and Naki, 2018). In a subsequent study, mice were intranasally vaccinated with an NG made with N-[(2-hydroxy-3-trimethylammonium) propyl] chitosan chloride (HTCC) and a, b-glycerophosphate as a drug delivery method to inhibit the H5N1 influenza virus. Since this thermal-sensitive fluorescent NG tends to gelatinize at body temperature, the residence time of the virus in the nasal route could be observed accurately. Strong fluorescence indicated that 54% of the NG-delivered antigen was retained in the nasal cavity even after 2 hours of injection. Therefore, NG-based drug delivery could be considered an outstanding method for better vaccines that do not require adjuvants (Singh et al., 2014).

7.3.6 NANOTRAPS

Nanotraps are thermoresponsive hydrogels that can attach to various proteins and antigens via coupling affinity baits to the particles (Shafagati et al., 2016). They efficiently capture various proteins, including viral proteins, live infectious viruses, and viral RNA, even from complex mixtures such as serum. Nanotraps concentrate analytes and ensure their protection, making them an excellent tool for sample preparation in the identification of biomarkers and the development of diagnostic assays (Shafagati et al., 2014).

Studies on this technology demonstrated the ability of nanotraps to capture various viral particles, including respiratory pathogens. To assess the capturing ability of IAVs and IBVs, five different types of nanotraps were used, labeled as NT45, NT46, NT53, NT69, and NT120. Quantitative reverse transcription polymerase chain reaction (qRT-PCR) was employed to determine the quantity of viruses captured. NT46 particles outperformed other nanotrap particles by tenfold, with NT46 prepared with immobilized reactive red dye as the bait. In plaque assays conducted to ensure the capturing of the entire infectious virus, the NT46 particles showed an eightfold increase in detection compared to the control, which had no nanotraps. Even when the influenza variant and subtype were changed, NT46 provided the best results for detecting the influenza viruses with qRT-PCR and plaque assays, emphasizing the enriched performance of NT46 (Shafagati et al., 2014).

7.3.7 NANO-VACCINES

The global prevalence of the influenza virus has long been a significant health concern. Vaccination using weakened virus DNA to generate antibodies within the human body has been the most effective method to mitigate the spread of these influenza-type viruses, including the SARS-CoV, which resulted in over 6 million deaths worldwide (worldometer). This method serves as a precaution taken before viral infection, while post-infection measures involve administering drugs that inhibit the breach of cell membranes by the virus and its reproduction.

To enhance the efficacy of influenza-type virus vaccines, novel nanotechnology-based vaccine methods have been introduced. These methods are based on three primary mechanisms of inhibiting the virus, namely delivering deactivated viral antigens by NPs, delivering mRNA fragments through NPs to produce viral antigens, and delivering the deactivated virus encapsulated in NPs. Various antigens are utilized to inhibit or decrease the spread of influenza viruses. These antigens can be classified into those against internal viral proteins, including anti-nucleoprotein, anti-Matrix protein 1 (M1), and anti-nonstructural proteins (PB1-F2), and those against external viral proteins, including anti-Hemagglutinin, anti-Neuraminidase, and anti-Matrix protein 2 (M2). The role of these nano-based antigens is to transport these antibodies into the cells, allowing for the production and release of the aforementioned antibodies, thereby disrupting the viral spread (Lin et al., 2020).

Furthermore, *in vitro* studies have demonstrated the effective influence of AuNP combined with trimetric HA from the H3N2 virus and flagellin, a bacterial flagella protein, on T cell-mediated immunity (Wang et al., 2017). Additionally, the delivery of HA encapsulated in sodium tripolyphosphate cross-linked chitosan NP was reported to provide 100% protection against a lethal dose of influenza in infected mice (Sawaengsak et al., 2014). Subsequent studies revealed the effectiveness of HA combined with ferritin NP against H1N1 IAV (Kanekiyo et al., 2013), and HA encapsulated in polyanhydride NPs was shown to enhance the immune response against H5N1 and H5N2 viruses (Kingstad-Bakke et al., 2019).

Alongside the accumulation of mutations in the virus genes (antigenic drift), the immune response to the antibodies against HA and NA may be reduced. To counteract this, recent research has focused on antigens against matrix proteins, as M2 proteins play a role in virus entry into the host cell and its growth (Manzoor et al., 2017). Although immunity against M2 protein is weak, subdomains of the M2 protein, such as the extracellular N-terminal, incorporated into protein carriers, have proven effective (Schepens et al., 2018). Nanovaccines generated from AuNP and Virus-Like-Particles (VLP) incorporating M2 proteins have shown positive results against H1N1 and H5N1 viruses in studies conducted on infected mice (Tao et al., 2017). Moreover, PLGA NPs entrapping IAV H1N1 peptides resulted in vaccinated pigs showing no flu symptoms and a reduced virus load in the pig airways (Hiremath et al., 2016).

Another key area of interest in nano-vaccination is the delivery of inactivated influenza viruses encapsulated in vaccines incorporated with nanomaterials. Studies have shown that polyanhydride NP incorporated inactivated IAV virus reduced the number of viral antigens in the airways of infected pigs (Hiremath et al., 2016). Furthermore, calcium phosphate NPs incorporated with inactivated IAV were found to increase the inhibition of HA in virus-infected mice (Lin et al., 2020). The strategy of treating influenza viruses by transporting mRNA fragments to infected host cells through nano-based materials has shown great promise. These mRNA strands mimic defective interfering particles (DIP), which can increase the immune response through the activation of pathogen recognition receptors, and DIP-like NPs can act similarly (Vasou et al., 2017) as well as stabilize RNA (Tang et al., 2021).

For mRNA vaccination, dendrimers have been effectively used, demonstrating action against the influenza A/NWS/33 H1N1 virus strain (Chahal et al., 2016). Immunizing mice with vaccines prepared using liposome NPs containing mRNA has shown enhanced immunity in mice against the influenza A/Northern Territory/60/1968 (H3N2) strain. The mRNA encoding influenza virus nucleoprotein was encapsulated into cholesterol/phosphatidylcholine/phosphatidylserine liposomes through the detergent removal technique. This study revealed that induced cytotoxic T cells were similar to those produced by a real viral infection (Martinon et al., 1993). Moreover, a similar study conducted using lipid NPs containing mRNA encoding HA protein of A/Jiangxi-Donghu/346/2013 ($H_{10}N_8$) or A/Anhui/1/2013 (H7N9) IAV strains demonstrated enhanced immune responses in mice, ferrets, and nonhuman primates, as measured by hemagglutination inhibition and microneutralization assays (Bahl et al., 2017).

7.3.8 APPLICATION OF NANOTECHNOLOGY IN GENE SILENCING STRATEGIES TO TREAT INFLUENZA VIRUS DISEASES

Gene silencing is a natural mechanism for inactivating genes, often achieved by using silencers that target various fragments of the genome or transcriptome. Synthetic nucleic acids, including antisense oligonucleotides (ASO), ribozymes, DNAzymes, short interfering RNA (siRNA), microRNA (miRNA), short hairpin RNA (shRNA), and peptide nucleic acids (PNAs), are utilized as silencers (Kesy et al., 2019; Piasecka et al., 2020; Weng et al., 2019). However, introducing synthetic nucleic acids into cells is often limited by inefficient systems. Current biochemical and physical transfection methods may influence the cellular condition, necessitating the development of new transfection methods with improved efficiency and reduced cytotoxicity (Kim and Eberwine, 2010). NPs show promise as tools for developing new delivery systems for silencers.

7.3.8.1 ANTISENSE OLIGONUCLEOTIDES (ASOs)

Antisense oligonucleotides (ASOs), also known as RNA-modified oligonucleotides, are typically 12–30 nucleotides long and interact with specific RNAs. The enzyme ribonuclease H (RNase H) cleaves the RNA of RNA/DNA hybrids, a process critical for DNA stability during replication and repair. ASO action involves various mechanisms, including RNase H cleavage of mRNA in RNA-DNA duplex, steric hindrance of the ribosome by binding ASO near the translation initiation site, destabilization and degradation of the transcript by ASO near the poly (A) or cap of the mRNA, and blocking or destabilization of the functional RNA structure (Frazier, 2015). Additional techniques such as mRNA maturation inhibition and mRNA precursor alternative splicing induction are employed for gene silencing using ASOs (Mescalchin and Restle, 2011).

An intriguing approach involved targeting the noncoding 3′-terminal region of segment 5 (-) RNA using ASO DNAs. These ASOs were noncovalently attached to titanium dioxide NPs (TiO_2 NPs) through a polylysine linker (PL), creating the NP delivery system for cell penetration without the use of any transfection agent. Nanocomposites (NCs) inhibiting H3N2 IAV replication in MDCK cells showed high antiviral activity with low cytotoxicity. At a concentration of 30 nM for DNA (1.5 g/mL TiO_2), nearly half of the virus inhibition concentration (IC50) was achieved, while the toxic concentration (TC50) was calculated to be 1800 g/mL (Levina et al., 2015). A subsequent study demonstrated that covalently binding the same ASO sequence to PL resulted in higher antiviral activity than association with electrostatic interactions (Levina et al., 2014). Targeting the conserved region of segment 5 IAV, higher antiviral activity was obtained when inhibiting H1N1 and H5N1 strains using the same NCs. Another study designed ASOs targeting both the negative (-) RNA and positive (+) RNA sense strands of IAV, with the NCs containing DNA targeting (-) RNA displaying higher antiviral activity compared to those targeting (+) RNA (Levina et al., 2015). In a new NC, ASO targeted the 3′-noncoding regions of IAV segment 5 viral (-) RNA, bound to silicon-organic ($Si\text{-}NH_2$) NPs via electrostatic interactions, demonstrating selective and effective inhibition of IAV replication in cell culture (Levina et al., 2015). These findings and subsequent investigations suggest the potential development of efficient antiviral drugs using ASOs to combat emerging IAV strains that could lead to pandemics.

7.3.8.2 RNA INTERFERENCE (RNAi)

RNA interference (RNAi) is a post-transcriptional gene regulation process where siRNA or miRNA, incorporated into the RNA-induced silencing complex (RISC), targets mRNA in a sequence-specific manner. This strategy has been employed against various viruses, including influenza. Advances in siRNA design, synthesis, and the use of nanotechnology-based delivery methods have further improved the effectiveness of this approach. A multi-shell NP composed of a CaP core covered with siRNAs encapsulated in PLGA, forming siRNA-loaded CaP/PLGA NPs, coated with polyethylenimine (PEI), was utilized to decrease gene expression of CCL-2, IP-10, and IFN-γ in inflamed lung tissue. Mice treated with siRNA-loaded CaP/PLGA NPs exhibited reduced lung inflammation and lower expression of the targeted genes (Frede et al., 2017). Chitosan NPs encapsulating siRNA targeting viral nucleoprotein inhibited IAV growth in cells and provided protection to mice against a lethal viral dose (Jamali et al., 2018).

7.3.8.3 DNAzymes

DNAzymes are DNA fragments with the ability to cleave complementary RNA. While natural DNAzymes have yet to be detected, artificial DNAzymes are employed to determine gene silencing activity. DNAzymes immobilized on TiO_2 NPs pre-covered with PL, targeting (+) RNA of IAV segment 5, demonstrated a significant reduction in IAV replication by 2700-fold in MDCK cells (Repkova et al., 2017).

7.4 CONCLUSIONS

The distinctive characteristics of nanomaterials have enabled creative solutions to numerous issues in the field of medicine. Nanotechnology has facilitated novel approaches to the prevention, diagnosis, and treatment of various viral diseases, particularly those associated with influenza viruses. The unique properties of nanomaterials, such as their small particle size, high surface area to volume ratio, the ability to achieve desired selectivity and biocompatibility by altering the surface, their suitability as targets for various ligands and nucleic acids, and their utility as imaging agents, have provided added potential in the fight against influenza viruses. In the medical industry, nanotechnology has overcome several challenges in drug delivery to the target site, serving as exceptional drug delivery systems and nanodrugs.

Given the genetic characteristics that allow influenza viruses to rapidly evolve, the emergence of drug resistance poses a significant threat. Because NPs and virus particles share similar dimensions, they preferentially interact with each other, enhancing the speed and efficiency of treatment. Virus-like particles and other NPs carrying proteins or segments of influenza viruses trigger immune responses in the body, resembling the activity of vaccines. Combining anti-influenza medications with nanosystems holds considerable potential for treating influenza viral diseases. The results of numerous studies demonstrate that materials based on nanotechnology have the capability to prevent the transmission of the influenza virus and related diseases. Inhibiting disease transmission can be achieved through various nanotechnological approaches, including the use of self-sterilizing surfaces. Although the results of this innovative technology are promising, it is important to explore methods to enhance the development of less toxic nanodrugs, reduce drug-drug interactions, and address the complexities of large-scale nanomedicine production. Several antiviral NP-based medications have already received approval, exhibiting minimal to no toxicity and showing promise for therapeutic application in the near future. By overcoming these minor obstacles and focusing on clinical trials, nanotechnology can play a promising role in effectively eradicating the influenza virus and preventing the emergence of global pandemics.

KEYWORDS

- **lipid-based nanoformulations**
- **nanogels**
- **nanomaterials**
- **nanotechnology**
- **nanotraps**
- **RNA polymerase**
- **vaccines**

REFERENCES

Aderibigbe, B. A., & Naki, T. (2018). Design and efficacy of nanogels formulations for intranasal administration. *Molecules, 23*(6). https://doi.org/10.3390/molecules23061241 (accessed on 4th July 2025).

Aguilera-Correa, J. J., Esteban, J., & Vallet-Regí, M. (2021). Inorganic and polymeric nanoparticles for human viral and bacterial infections prevention and treatment. *Nanomaterials, 11*(1), 1–26. https://doi.org/10.3390/nano11010137 (accessed on 4th July 2025).

Akbarzadeh, A., Rezaei-Sadabady, R., Davaran, S., Joo, S. W., & Zarghami, N. (2013). Liposome: Classification, preparation, and applications. *Nanoscale Research Letters, 8*, 102. http://www.nanoscalereslett.com/content/8/1/102 (accessed on 4th July 2025).

Aminu, N., Bello, I., Umar, N. M., Tanko, N., Aminu, A., & Audu, M. M. (2020). The influence of nanoparticulate drug delivery systems in drug therapy. *Journal of Drug Delivery Science and Technology, 60*, 101961. https://doi.org/10.1016/j.jddst.2020.101961 (accessed on 4th July 2025).

Bahl, K., Senn, J. J., Yuzhakov, O., Bulychev, A., Brito, L. A., Hassett, K. J., Laska, M. E., et al. (2017). Preclinical and clinical demonstration of immunogenicity by mRNA vaccines against H10N8 and H7N9 influenza viruses. *Molecular Therapy, 25*(6), 1316–1327. https://doi.org/10.1016/j.ymthe.2017.03.035 (accessed on 4th July 2025).

Beigel, J., & Bray, M. (2008). Current and future antiviral therapy of severe seasonal and avian influenza. *Antiviral Research, 78*(1), 91–102. https://doi.org/10.1016/j.antiviral.2008.01.003 (accessed on 4th July 2025).

Chahal, J. S., Khan, O. F., Cooper, C. L., McPartlan, J. S., Tsosie, J. K., Tilley, L. D., Sidik, S. M., et al. (2016). Dendrimer-RNA nanoparticles generate protective immunity against lethal Ebola, H1N1 influenza, and *Toxoplasma gondii* challenges with a single dose. *Proceedings of the National Academy of Sciences of the United States of America, 113*(29), E4133–E4142. https://doi.org/10.1073/pnas.1600299113 (accessed on 4th July 2025).

Chakravarty, M., & Vora, A. (2021). Nanotechnology-based antiviral therapeutics. *Drug Delivery and Translational Research, 11*(3), 748–787. https://doi.org/10.1007/s13346-020-00818-0 (accessed on 4th July 2025).

Chen, L., & Liang, J. (2020). An overview of functional nanoparticles as novel emerging antiviral therapeutic agents. *Materials Science and Engineering C, 112*, 110924. https://doi.org/10.1016/j.msec.2020.110924 (accessed on 4th July 2025).

Dehghan, S., Tavassoti Kheiri, M., Tabatabaiean, M., Darzi, S., & Tafaghodi, M. (2013). Dry-powder form of chitosan nanospheres containing influenza virus and adjuvants for nasal immunization. *Archives of Pharmacal Research, 36*(8), 981–992. https://doi.org/10.1007/s12272-013-0043-4 (accessed on 4th July 2025).

Dhakal, S., Cheng, X., Salcido, J., Renu, S., Bondra, K., Lakshmanappa, Y. S., Misch, C., et al. (2018). Liposomal nanoparticle-based conserved peptide influenza vaccine and monosodium urate crystal adjuvant elicit protective immune response in pigs. *International Journal of Nanomedicine, 13*, 6699–6715. https://doi.org/10.2147/IJN.S178809 (accessed on 4th July 2025).

Dunham, E. J., Dugan, V. G., Kaser, E. K., Perkins, S. E., Brown, I. H., Holmes, E. C., & Taubenberger, J. K. (2009). Different evolutionary trajectories of European avian-like and classical swine H1N1 influenza A viruses. *Journal of Virology, 83*(11), 5485–5494. https://doi.org/10.1128/jvi.02565-08 (accessed on 4th July 2025).

Enkhtaivan, G., Muthuraman, P., & Kim, D. H. (2017). Inhibitory effect of 2,4-dichlorophenoxyacetic acid on ROS, autophagy formation, and mRNA replication for influenza virus infection. *Journal of Molecular Recognition, 30*(8), 1–10. https://doi.org/10.1002/jmr.2616 (accessed on 4th July 2025).

Farooq, M. U., Novosad, V., Rozhkova, E. A., Wali, H., Ali, A., Fateh, A. A., Neogi, P. B., Neogi, A., & Wang, Z. (2018). Gold nanoparticles-enabled efficient dual delivery of anticancer therapeutics to HeLa cells. *Scientific Reports, 8*(1), 1–12. https://doi.org/10.1038/s41598-018-21331-y (accessed on 4th July 2025).

Ftouh, M., Kalboussi, N., Abid, N., Sfar, S., Mignet, N., & Bahloul, B. (2021). Contribution of nanotechnologies to vaccine development and drug delivery against respiratory viruses. *PPAR Research, 2021*. https://doi.org/10.1155/2021/6741290 (accessed on 4th July 2025).

Fukuyama, S., & Kawaoka, Y. (2011). The pathogenesis of influenza virus infections: The contributions of virus and host factors. *Current Opinion in Immunology, 23*(4), 481–486. https://doi.org/10.1016/j.coi.2011.07.016 (accessed on 4th July 2025).

Gansukh, E., Anthonydhason, V., Jung, S., Kim, D. H., Muthu, M., Gopal, J., & Chun, S. (2018). Nanotherapeutic anti-influenza solutions: Current knowledge and future challenges. *Journal of Cluster Science, 29*(6), 933–941. https://doi.org/10.1007/s10876-018-1417-z (accessed on 4th July 2025).

Gansukh, E., Kazibwe, Z., Pandurangan, M., Gopal, J., & Kim, D. H. (2016). Probing the impact of quercetin-7-O-glucoside on influenza virus replication influence. *Phytomedicine, 23*(9), 958–967. https://doi.org/10.1016/j.phymed.2016.06.001 (accessed on 4th July 2025).

Gansukh, E., Muthu, M., Paul, D., Ethiraj, G., Chun, S., & Gopal, J. (2017). Nature nominee quercetin's anti-influenza combat strategy—Demonstrations and remonstrations. *Reviews in Medical Virology, 27*(3), 1–14. https://doi.org/10.1002/rmv.1930 (accessed on 4th July 2025).

Gasparini, R., Amicizia, D., Lai, P. L., Bragazzi, N. L., & Panatto, D. (2014). Compounds with anti-influenza activity: Present and future of strategies for the optimal treatment and management of influenza. Part I: Influenza life-cycle and currently available drugs. *Journal of Preventive Medicine and Hygiene, 55*(3), 69–85.

Hatano, K., Matsubara, T., Muramatsu, Y., Ezure, M., Koyama, T., Matsuoka, K., Kuriyama, R., Kori, H., & Sato, T. (2014). Synthesis and influenza virus inhibitory activities of carbosilane dendrimers peripherally functionalized with hemagglutinin-binding peptide. *Journal of Medicinal Chemistry, 57*(20), 8332–8339. https://doi.org/10.1021/jm5007676 (accessed on 4th July 2025).

Hayden, F. G., & Palese, P. (2018). Influenza virus. *Trends in Microbiology, 26*(9), 809–810. https://doi.org/10.1016/j.tim.2018.05.013 (accessed on 4th July 2025).

Hendricks, G. L., Weirich, K. L., Viswanathan, K., Li, J., Shriver, Z. H., Ashour, J., Ploegh, H. L., et al. (2013). Sialylneolacto-N-tetraose c (LSTc)-bearing liposomal decoys capture influenza A virus. *Journal of Biological Chemistry, 288*(12), 8061–8073. https://doi.org/10.1074/jbc.M112.437202 (accessed on 4th July 2025).

Hu, C. M. J., Chen, Y. T., Fang, Z. S., Chang, W. S., & Chen, H. W. (2018). Antiviral efficacy of nanoparticulate vacuolar ATPase inhibitors against influenza virus infection.

International Journal of Nanomedicine, 13, 8579–8593. https://doi.org/10.2147/IJN.S185806 (accessed on 4th July 2025).

Ikematsu, H., & Kawai, N. (2011). Laninamivir octanoate: A new long-acting neuraminidase inhibitor for the treatment of influenza. *Expert Review of Anti-Infective Therapy, 9*(10), 851–857. https://doi.org/10.1586/eri.11.112 (accessed on 4th July 2025).

Ison, M. G. (2011). Antivirals and resistance: Influenza virus. *Current Opinion in Virology, 1*(6), 563–573. https://doi.org/10.1016/j.coviro.2011.09.002 (accessed on 4th July 2025).

Kalil, A. C., & Thomas, P. G. (2019). Influenza fisiopatología. *Critical Care, 23*, 258. https://doi.org/10.1186/s13054-019-2539-x (accessed on 4th July 2025).

Kandel, R., & Hartshorn, K. L. (2001). Prophylaxis and treatment of influenza virus infection. *BioDrugs, 15*(5), 303–323. https://doi.org/10.2165/00063030-200115050-00003 (accessed on 4th July 2025).

Khanna, M., Choudhary, K., Kumar, P., & Vijayan, V. K. (2008). Emerging influenza virus: A global threat. *Indian Journal of Medical Research, 33*(November), 475–482.

Kornev, A. B., Peregudov, A. S., Martynenko, V. M., Balzarini, J., Hoorelbeke, B., & Troshin, P. A. (2011). Synthesis and antiviral activity of highly water-soluble polycarboxylic derivatives of [70] fullerene. *Chemical Communications, 47*(29), 8298–8300. https://doi.org/10.1039/c1cc12209f (accessed on 4th July 2025).

Kuiken, T., & Taubenberger, J. K. (2008). Pathology of human influenza revisited. *Vaccine, 26*(Suppl. 4). https://doi.org/10.1016/j.vaccine.2008.07.025 (accessed on 4th July 2025).

Lim, J. W., Ahn, Y. R., Park, G., Kim, H. O., & Haam, S. (2021). Application of nanomaterials as an advanced strategy for the diagnosis, prevention, and treatment of viral diseases. *Pharmaceutics, 13*(10). https://doi.org/10.3390/pharmaceutics13101570 (accessed on 4th July 2025).

Lin, S. Y., Yao, B. Y., Hu, C. M. J., & Chen, H. W. (2020). Induction of robust immune responses by CpG-ODN-loaded hollow polymeric nanoparticles for antiviral and vaccine applications in chickens. *International Journal of Nanomedicine, 15*, 3303–3318. https://doi.org/10.2147/IJN.S241492 (accessed on 4th July 2025).

Luo, M. (2012). Influenza virus entry. In *Advances in Experimental Medicine and Biology* (Vol. 726, pp. 201–221). https://doi.org/10.1007/978-1-4614-0980-9_9 (accessed on 4th July 2025).

Manzoor, R., Igarashi, M., & Takada, A. (2017). Influenza A virus M2 protein: Roles from ingress to egress. *International Journal of Molecular Sciences, 18*(12), 1–16. https://doi.org/10.3390/ijms18122649 (accessed on 4th July 2025).

Martinon, F., Krishnan, S., Lenzen, G., Magné, R., Gomard, E., Guillet, J. G., Lévy, J. P., & Meulien, P. (1993). Induction of virus-specific cytotoxic T lymphocytes *in vivo* by liposome-entrapped mRNA. *European Journal of Immunology, 23*(7), 1719–1722. https://doi.org/10.1002/eji.1830230749 (accessed on 4th July 2025).

Maus, A., Strait, L., & Zhu, D. (2021). Nanoparticles as delivery vehicles for antiviral therapeutic drugs. *Engineered Regeneration, 2*, 31–46. https://doi.org/10.1016/j.engreg.2021.03.001 (accessed on 4th July 2025).

Mehendale, R., Joshi, M., & Patravale, V. (2013). Nanomedicines for treatment of viral diseases. *Critical Reviews in Therapeutic Drug Carrier Systems, 30*(1), 1–49. https://doi.org/10.1615/CritRevTherDrugCarrierSyst.2013005469 (accessed on 4th July 2025).

Mehle, A., & McCullers, J. A. (2013). Structure and function of the influenza virus replication machinery and PB1-F2. In *Textbook of Influenza* (pp. 133–145). https://doi.org/10.1002/9781118636817.ch8 (accessed on 4th July 2025).

Metersky, M. L., Masterton, R. G., Lode, H., File, T. M., & Babinchak, T. (2012). Epidemiology, microbiology, and treatment considerations for bacterial pneumonia complicating influenza. *International Journal of Infectious Diseases, 16*(5), e321–e331. https://doi.org/10.1016/j.ijid.2012.01.003 (accessed on 4th July 2025).

Moghadami, M. (2017). A narrative review of influenza: A seasonal and pandemic disease. *Iranian Journal of Medical Sciences, 42*(1), 2–13.

Navya, P. N., Kaphle, A., Srinivas, S. P., Bhargava, S. K., Rotello, V. M., & Daima, H. K. (2019). Current trends and challenges in cancer management and therapy using designer nanomaterials. *Nano Convergence, 6*(1). https://doi.org/10.1186/s40580-019-0193-2 (accessed on 4th July 2025).

Resa-Infante, P., Jorba, N., Coloma, R., & Ortin, J. (2011). The influenza virus RNA synthesis machine. *RNA Biology, 8*(2), 207–215. https://doi.org/10.4161/rna.8.2.14513 (accessed on 4th July 2025).

Ryu, W. S. (2017). Virus life cycle. In *Molecular Virology of Human Pathogenic Viruses* (No. 1, pp. 31–45). https://doi.org/10.1016/b978-0-12-800838-6.00003-5 (accessed on 4th July 2025).

Samji, T. (2009). Influenza A: Understanding the viral life cycle. *Yale Journal of Biology and Medicine, 82*(4), 153–159.

Shafagati, N., Fite, K., Patanarut, A., Baer, A., Pinkham, C., An, S., Foote, B., Lepene, B., & Kehn-Hall, K. (2016). Enhanced detection of respiratory pathogens with Nanotrap particles. *Virulence, 7*(7), 756–769. https://doi.org/10.1080/21505594.2016.1185585 (accessed on 4th July 2025).

Shafagati, N., Patanarut, A., Luchini, A., Lundberg, L., Bailey, C., Petricoin, E., Liotta, L., Narayanan, A., Lepene, B., & Kehn-Hall, K. (2014). The use of Nanotrap particles for biodefense and emerging infectious disease diagnostics. *Pathogens and Disease, 71*(2), 164–176. https://doi.org/10.1111/2049-632X.12136 (accessed on 4th July 2025).

Shah, S., Chougule, M. B., Kotha, A. K., Kashikar, R., Godugu, C., Raghuvanshi, R. S., Singh, S. B., & Srivastava, S. (2021). Nanomedicine based approaches for combating viral infections. *Journal of Controlled Release, 338*, 80–104. https://doi.org/10.1016/j.jconrel.2021.08.011 (accessed on 4th July 2025).

Singh, L., Kruger, H. G., Maguire, G. E. M., Govender, T., & Parboosing, R. (2017). The role of nanotechnology in the treatment of viral infections. *Therapeutic Advances in Infectious Disease, 4*(4), 105–131. https://doi.org/10.1177/2049936117713593 (accessed on 4th July 2025).

Song, Z., Wang, X., Zhu, G., Nian, Q., Zhou, H., Yang, D., Qin, C., & Tang, R. (2015). Virus capture and destruction by label-free graphene oxide for detection and disinfection applications. *Small, 11*(9, 10), 1771–1776. https://doi.org/10.1002/smll.201401706 (accessed on 4th July 2025).

Surendiran, A., Sandhiya, S., Pradhan, S. C., & Adithan, C. (2009). Novel applications of nanotechnology in medicine. *Indian Journal of Medical Research, 130*(6), 689–701.

Szewczyk, B., Bieńkowska-Szewczyk, K., & Król, E. (2014). Introduction to molecular biology of influenza A viruses. *Acta Biochimica Polonica, 61*(3), 397–401. https://doi.org/10.18388/abp.2014_1857 (accessed on 4th July 2025).

Tamura, S. I., & Kurata, T. (2004). *Flu–8.pdf* (pp. 236–247).

Taubenberger, J. K., & Morens, D. M. (2008). The pathology of influenza infections. *Annual Review of Pathology: Mechanisms of Disease, 3*, 499–522. https://www.ncbi.nlm.nih.gov/pmc/articles/PMC3624763/pdf/nihms412728.pdf (accessed on 4th July 2025).

Theodoridis, G., Bahr, J. T., Hotzman, F. W., Sehgel, S., & Suarez, D. P. (2000). New generation of protox-inhibiting herbicides. *Crop Protection, 19*(8), 533–535. https://doi.org/10.1016/S0261-2194(00)00069-7 (accessed on 4th July 2025).

Tollas, S., Bereczki, I., Borbás, A., Batta, G., Vanderlinden, E., Naesens, L., & Herczegh, P. (2014). Synthesis of a cluster-forming sialylthio-D-galactose fullerene conjugate and evaluation of its interaction with influenza virus hemagglutinin and neuraminidase. *Bioorganic and Medicinal Chemistry Letters, 24*(11), 2420–2423. https://doi.org/10.1016/j.bmcl.2014.04.032 (accessed on 4th July 2025).

Wahlgren, J. (2011). Influenza A viruses: An ecology review. *Infection Ecology & Epidemiology, 1*(1), 6004. https://doi.org/10.3402/iee.v1i0.6004 (accessed on 4th July 2025).

Watanabe, T., Watanabe, S., & Kawaoka, Y. (2010). Cellular networks involved in the influenza virus life cycle. *Cell Host and Microbe, 7*(6), 427–439. https://doi.org/10.1016/j.chom.2010.05.008 (accessed on 4th July 2025).

Wieczorek, K., Szutkowska, B., & Kierzek, E. (2020). Anti-influenza strategies based on[Title incomplete]. pp. 1–24.

Wolf, Y. I., Viboud, C., Holmes, E. C., Koonin, E. V., & Lipman, D. J. (2006). Long intervals of stasis punctuated by bursts of positive selection in the seasonal evolution of influenza A virus. *Biology Direct, 1*, 1–19. https://doi.org/10.1186/1745-6150-1-34 (accessed on 4th July 2025).

Yang, J., Shim, S. M., Nguyen, T. Q., Kim, E. H., Kim, K., Lim, Y. T., Sung, M. H., Webby, R., & Poo, H. (2017). Poly-γ-glutamic acid/chitosan nanogel greatly enhances the efficacy and heterosubtypic cross-reactivity of H1N1 pandemic influenza vaccine. *Scientific Reports, 7*, 44839. https://doi.org/10.1038/srep44839 (accessed on 4th July 2025).

Yeh, Y. T., Tang, Y., Sebastian, A., Dasgupta, A., Perea-Lopez, N., Albert, I., Lu, H., Terrones, M., & Zheng, S. Y. (2016). Tunable and label-free virus enrichment for ultrasensitive virus detection using carbon nanotube arrays. *Science Advances, 2*(10). https://doi.org/10.1126/sciadv.1601026 (accessed on 4th July 2025).

Yoon, S. W., Webby, R. J., & Webster, R. G. (2014). Evolution and ecology of influenza A viruses. *Current Topics in Microbiology and Immunology, 385*(1), 359–375. https://doi.org/10.1007/82_2014_396 (accessed on 4th July 2025).

Zheng, W., & Tao, Y. J. (2013). Structure and assembly of the influenza A virus ribonucleoprotein complex. *FEBS Letters, 587*(8), 1206–1214. https://doi.org/10.1016/j.febslet.2013.02.048 (accessed on 4th July 2025).

Zhou, J., Krishnan, N., Jiang, Y., Fang, R. H., & Zhang, L. (2021). Nanotechnology for virus treatment. *Nano Today, 36*, 101031. https://doi.org/10.1016/j.nantod.2020.101031 (accessed on 4th July 2025).

Zhumatov, K. K., Kydyrmanov, A. I., & Sayatov, M. (2020). Influenza D viruses–pathogens forming. pp. 12–19.

CHAPTER 8

Nanotechnological Approaches for Management of Coronaviruses

SHIJI MATHEW[1] and RADHAKRISHNAN EK[2,*]

[1]*Department of Biology, College of Science and Technology, Temple University, Philadelphia, Pennsylvania, United States*

[2]*School of Biosciences, Mahatma Gandhi University, Kottayam, Kerala, India*

*Corresponding author

ABSTRACT

The ongoing pandemic outbreak of the SARS-CoV-2 virus, which began in late 2019, continues to impact the world. Despite the development of new antivirals and widespread administration of effective vaccines, we are still struggling to overcome this virus. The most effective approach to combat this virus is to minimize its contact with our bodily surfaces. Nanotechnology offers various effective strategies for managing coronaviruses both before and after they enter the human body. These strategies include detection methods, as well as preventive, therapeutic, and curative approaches. This chapter primarily reviews the conventional preventive, diagnostic, and treatment strategies implemented against SARS-CoV-2, and focuses on the potential for improving the limitations of these strategies using nanotechnology. Nanotechnology has the potential to provide significant advancements in the prevention, diagnosis, and detection, as well as in the therapy and vaccinology, of COVID-19, offering benefits such as improved speed, efficiency, accuracy, and convenience.

Nanotechnological Management of Viral Infections.
Radhakrishnan EK, Shiji Mathew, and Riya Alex (Eds.)

DOI: 10.1201/9781779640895-8

8.1 INTRODUCTION

Coronaviruses belong to the family Coronaviridae, subfamily Coronavirinae, and order Nidovirales. Based on their phylogenetic relationships and genomic structures, coronaviruses are divided into four genera: Alphacoronavirus, Betacoronavirus, Gammacoronavirus, and Deltacoronavirus. Both Alphacoronaviruses and Betacoronaviruses infect mammals, causing respiratory illnesses in humans and gastroenteritis in animals. While gammacoronaviruses and deltacoronaviruses primarily infect birds, some strains may also affect mammals (Woo et al., 2012). The betacoronaviruses are also known as severe acute respiratory syndrome coronavirus 2 (SARS-CoV-2). These enveloped positive-sense RNA viruses are the causative agent of the novel COVID-19 pandemic outbreak. SARS-CoV-2 infection exhibits certain salient features, such as nonspecific symptoms, high infectivity without any signs of illness, a long incubation period (7–30 days), transmission from asymptomatic patients, tropism for mucosal surfaces like the conjunctiva, prolonged duration of illness (10–45 days), transmission even after clinical recovery, and recurrence of infection even in a cured patient (Singhal, 2020). These features, combined with the lack of proper treatment, make its management a difficult task.

COVID-19 is an acute viral infection, and its clinical severity may range from mild symptoms to a terminal illness. Primarily affecting the respiratory system, COVID-19 targets the lung parenchyma and typically presents with symptoms such as fever, shortness of breath, and cough. Recent studies have also indicated that COVID-19 can lead to extrapulmonary symptoms and affect multiple organs (Mehta et al., 2021). Although individuals of all age groups can be infected with COVID-19, elderly people and individuals with pre-existing medical conditions are more vulnerable to developing severe symptoms (Cascella et al., 2020).

Individuals with compromised immune responses and various underlying health conditions such as cardiovascular diseases (hypertension, heart diseases, heart failure), cerebrovascular diseases (Parkinson's disease, multiple sclerosis, cerebral palsy), diabetes, asthma, severe obesity, chronic lung, kidney and liver disease, cancer, pregnancy, and tobacco smoking habits are at greater risk of experiencing serious implications from COVID-19 infection (CDC, 2020; Li et al., 2020). Additionally, older males are found to be highly susceptible to COVID-19, with an increased fatality rate compared to older females. Evidence suggests that the incidence of COVID-19 in children below 15 years of age is significantly lower, and even when infected, they typically present milder symptoms compared to adults (Harapan et al., 2020; Lee et al., 2020; Wang et al., 2020). While many pediatric cases of COVID-19 have been reported worldwide with mild symptoms and a good prognosis, the possibility of children acting as potential carriers and contributing to the spread of the virus across the population is a cause for concern (Kelvin and Halperin, 2020; Michelle Fernandes, 2020). More information on the sources of infection, pathogenesis, modes of transmission, and clinical symptoms of COVID-19 is explained in Chapter 1 of this book. This chapter mainly summarizes the latest nanotechnology-based developments in managing the prevention, cure, and treatment of coronavirus infections, with special emphasis on SARS-CoV-2 infection.

8.2 COVID-19 TREATMENTS AVAILABLE

Understanding the pathogenesis of COVID-19 is crucial for the development of efficient treatment options. Clinical research has demonstrated the effectiveness of various antiviral drugs such as ribavirin, nelfinavir, niclosamide, ciclesonide, pitavastatin, oseltamivir, tocilizumab, perampanel, favipiravir, abidol, and praziquantel against the direct cytopathic effects of SARS-CoV-2. Additionally, treatments involving corticosteroids and immunosuppressive/immunomodulatory agents targeting immune responses have been considered theoretically appropriate (Agostini et al., 2018; Bartoli et al., 2021; Singh et al., 2020). Below are detailed descriptions of some important antiviral therapies that can serve as promising treatment options for COVID-19.

8.2.1 REMDESIVIR

Remdesivir, a 1′-cyano-substituted adenosine nucleotide analogue prodrug developed by Gilead for treating Ebola virus infection, has shown successful inhibition of SARS-CoV and MERS-CoV *in vitro*. Its mechanism of action involves the inhibition of viral replication by mediating the inhibition of RNA-dependent RNA polymerase (RdRp). Notably, it has also demonstrated inhibitory effects against SARS-CoV-2 *in vitro*. The first case of COVID-19 in the U.S. was successfully treated with a one-day intravenous administration of remdesivir (Amirian and Levy, 2020; Holshue et al., 2020). On May 2, 2020, the U.S. Food and Drug Administration granted emergency use authorization for remdesivir in the treatment of severely ill COVID-19 patients (Erika Edwards, 2020).

8.2.2 LOPINAVIR/RITONAVIR (KALETRA)

Lopinavir/Ritonavir, manufactured by Abbott and sold under the brand names Kaletra or Aluvia, has been an effective protease-inhibiting drug used against human immunodeficiency syndrome (HIV). Studies have reported the ability of Kaletra to inhibit the endopeptidase C30 of the SARS-CoV-2 protease, thereby inhibiting protein synthesis. This drug alone or in combination with other antiviral drugs has shown improved outcomes in severe cases. A combination therapy involving Kaletra with arbidol and a traditional Chinese medicine called *Shufeng Jiedu* capsule has been found to be effective in treating the novel coronavirus in China (Wang et al., 2020). Arbidol or umifenovir, a small indole derivative molecule, has also been effective against Influenza and Hepatitis viruses, and it has shown activity against SARS-CoV *in vitro* (Khamitov et al., 2008).

8.2.3 INTERFERON-ALPHA (INF-A)

Interferons, broad-spectrum antiviral agents that are glycoproteins, can trigger antiviral immune responses in virus-infected patients. They can enhance both innate and adaptive immune responses in the host and suppress viral replication. *In vitro* studies have demonstrated the efficacy of INF-α in inhibiting the replication of SARS-CoV (Ströher et al., 2004; Zorzitto et al., 2006).

8.2.4 CHLOROQUINE AND HYDROXYCHLOROQUINE

Chloroquine, used for over 70 years to treat malaria and autoimmune diseases, has recently shown activity against certain viral infections due to its unknown mechanisms. Potential mechanisms of chloroquine include its ability to inhibit viral replication by altering the pH-dependent steps of viral replication, its immunomodulatory effects by inhibiting the release of TNF-α and IL-6, its interference with viral infection and replication by acting as an autophagy inhibitor, and its interference with the glycosylation of cellular receptors in SARS-CoV. Recent *in vitro* studies conducted by Wang et al. have demonstrated the efficiency of chloroquine in suppressing SARS-CoV-2 (Wang et al., 2020). Additionally, hydroxychloroquine (HCQ), an anti-rheumatic drug, has been reviewed for its potential to decrease the host response in COVID-19 patients (Baghchechi et al., 2020; Schrezenmeier and Dörner, 2020). Gauret et al. reported that the combination of azithromycin and hydroxychloroquine had beneficial effects in the treatment of COVID-19 (Gautret et al., 2020).

8.2.5 CONVALESCENT PLASMA THERAPY

Patients who have recovered from COVID-19 are likely to produce specific anti-COVID-19 antibodies. Thus, the plasma collected from recovered patients can be used to prepare plasma globulin specific to SARS-CoV-2. Convalescent plasma therapy is another promising method for treating severe and critically ill patients (Zhang et al., 2020).

The efficiency of existing antiviral agents against SARS-CoV-2 is still under investigation. The use of combination therapy has been shown to reduce viral replication, subsequently lowering inflammation and leading to the production of virus-specific antibodies, resulting in the cure of the disease. *In vitro* studies have demonstrated the efficacy of a combinatorial therapy of remdesivir with chloroquine in fighting against COVID-19 (Wang et al., 2020). However, certain factors need to be considered before widespread use, such as evaluating the interaction of antiviral agents with other therapeutics and avoiding the use of more than three antiviral agents simultaneously (Zhai et al., 2020).

8.3 NANOTECHNOLOGY FOR MANAGING COVID-19

Nanotechnology is defined as the design and application of particles with dimensions ranging from 1–100 nm. Over the decades, nanoparticles have been extensively utilized in medicine for various purposes, including the detection, prevention, and treatment of numerous diseases, including viral infections. In the future, nanotechnological approaches could be the primary choice for viral theragnostics. Nanoparticles offer a broad range of opportunities in combating COVID-19, as they are primarily deposited in the respiratory tract through a diffusion process (Singh et al., 2017).

Nanotechnology has already proven its preclinical efficacy in combating several viruses such as HIV, HPV, HSV, and respiratory viruses (Laudon et al., 2011; Singh et al., 2017). In the case of COVID-19, the unique functionalities of nanoparticles can be advantageous, especially in drug delivery. These functionalities can be summarized as follows: (i) some nanoparticles (such as gold and silver) possess intrinsic antiviral activity (McNeil, 2011); (ii) the large surface area to volume ratio of nanoparticles enables high drug loading (Petros and DeSimone, 2010); (iii) the small size and surface area of nanoparticles enable the delivery of drugs into normally inaccessible sites (Yadavalli and Shukla, 2017); and (iv) surface charge modification of nanoparticles enables them to cross negatively charged membranes. Nanotechnology offers diverse strategies for managing viruses before and after they enter the human body. These strategies include detection methods, preventive, therapeutic, and curative approaches. Figure 8.1 summarizes the major nanotechnological contributions to the management of COVID-19 such as:

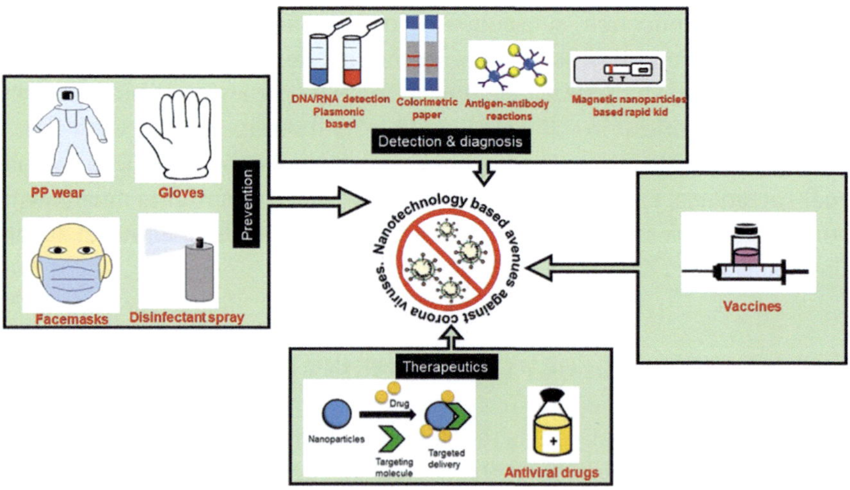

FIGURE 8.1 Nanotechnological avenues in management of COVID-19.

1. **Preventive Measures:** The use of nanomaterials in air filters and Personal Protective Equipment (PPE), such as masks, can aid in filtering and inactivating viruses, thereby providing maximum

safety for healthcare professionals. The use of nano-based disinfection sprays and the fabrication of nanomodified surfaces to inactivate and prevent viral adhesion and spread are other preventive measures of nanotechnology.

2. **Detection Methods:** Using nanotechnology, rapid, highly sensitive, and specific tests can be designed to detect both viral infections (antigen tests) and immunological responses (antibody tests). Sophisticated tools for tracing contacts can also be manufactured.
3. **Therapeutic Measures:** Development of nano antiviral agents for treatment with less toxicity, greater sustainability, and targeted delivery.
4. **Vaccines:** Nanomaterial-based vaccines offer targeted delivery, increased antigenic stability, and controlled release.
5. **Nanomarkers:** Help elucidate the mechanism by which the virus infects the host.

8.3.1 NANOTECHNOLOGY IN THE PREVENTION OF COVID-19

SARS-CoV-2 can remain viable on various surfaces, such as plastics and stainless steel, for up to 3 days, on copper for four hours, and on cardboard for 1 day. Therefore, proper sanitization and the application of disinfectants, such as 62%–71% ethanol, 0.1% sodium hypochlorite, or 0.5% hydrogen peroxide, surfactants, or soaps on infected or exposed surfaces, have been found effective in inactivating SARS-CoV-2 (Kampf et al., 2020; Wang et al., 2020). Despite their effectiveness, these chemical disinfection processes are associated with certain drawbacks, including the requirement of high concentrations for 100% viral inhibition, short duration of effect, and potential risks to the environment and health. Additionally, according to a recent study, water- or alcohol-based disinfectants may not necessarily work successfully on all surfaces (Huang et al., 2020). In this context, nanotechnology offers alternative options for the inactivation of viruses through long-lasting, non-toxic disinfection processes, based on chemical, biological, and physical methods. Nanotechnology-based chemical disinfection can be achieved using metal ion-coated surfaces or hydrogen peroxide steam, while biological methods include the use of biosurfactants or probiotics. Physical methods include UV irradiation.

8.3.1.1 NANOTECHNOLOGY-BASED SURFACE DISINFECTANTS

Nanotechnology, due to its intrinsic antiviral activity, which involves the release of reactive oxygen species (ROS), has enabled the development of new materials that release antimicrobial agents in a controlled manner in response to various stimuli, such as electrothermal, photothermal, and photocatalytic responses for disinfecting surfaces. In India, the Defense Institute of Advanced Technology (DIAT), Pune, has developed a nanotechnology-based water disinfectant spray named "Ananya" to combat COVID-19. This spray is claimed to be effective in sanitizing various surfaces, including PPE kits, masks, and contaminated fomites (Disinfectant Spray of DIAT, 2020).

According to reports, a special nanotechnology-based disinfectant spray made of titanium dioxide and silver ions, developed by Nanotech Surface company, was used as a key measure to disinfect buildings and stop the spread of coronavirus in Milan, Italy (NBIC+, 2020). This nanospray is expected to leave the surface self-sterilized for up to two years. The Prelynx Portal, a first-response nano-polymer-based scanning/sanitizing portal developed by Design.123, is used to disinfect environments contaminated with COVID-19. This product is designed to scan the body temperature as soon as an individual passes beneath it. If the individual's temperature is within the expected range, the light bar changes from blue to green. This portal can be used in laboratories and hospital wards, where a high-powered blast of disinfectant vapor sanitizes the person as soon as they enter the room (Hannah Davis, 2020). A list of nanotechnology-based disinfectant sprays and surface coatings developed against COVID-19 is summarized in Table 8.1.

8.3.1.2 NANOTECHNOLOGY-BASED PERSONAL PROTECTIVE EQUIPMENT (PPE) AND FACEMASKS

As the SARS-CoV-2 virus is primarily transmitted through close contact and respiratory secretions of infected individuals, the use of appropriate PPE, such as masks and gloves, is crucial to control the spread of the virus. However, ordinary masks have several limitations, including reduced performance during extended use due to the high moisture absorption of exhaled breath, development of breathing problems during prolonged use,

TABLE 8.1 Nanotechnology Based Disinfectant Sprays and Surface Coatings For Combating COVID-19

Developers	Product Name	Product Type	Properties	References
University of Guleph and EnvisionSQ company	NanoCleanSQ solution	Photocatalytic Nanocoating	Uses photocatalytic technology to protect high touch surfaces	NBIC+ (2020)
NanoTouch Materials, LLC	Nanotouch self-cleaning surface	Photocatalytic self-cleaning Nanocoating films	Composed of mineral nanocrystal that are charged by any kind of visible light (LED, incandescent, fluorescent and sunlight)	https://nanotouch.com (2020)
Nano4life Europe L.P. Greece	Nano4-hygienelife	Surface sanitizer	On the applied surface, the positive charge of the sanitizer attracts negatively charged microbes and kills physically	https://www.nano4life.co/nano4-hygienelife (2020)
Shepros SDN BHD, Malaysia	Nanosilver multipurpose sanitiser (NSMS)	Multipurpose Sanitizer	Non skin irritating, non-foaming, environment friendly and non-toxic nanocolloid agent	www.NEWPAGES.com.my (2020)
FN Nano Inc., USA	Functional coatings FN Nano	Photocatalytic Nanocoating	Titanium dioxide based nanocoating for surface sterilization	FN NANO (2020)
MVX Prime Ltd, UK	MVX Protex	Antimicrobial coat nanospray	Antimicrobial coat spray composed of nanoparticles of titanium dioxide and silver zeolite based which provides effect for five years	Nanotechnology Products Database (2020a)
Nanoveu Inc, Australia	Nanoshield screen protector	Antiviral screen protector nanocoating	Copper oxide nanoparticles-based nanoshield screen coating for phone front glass and cover	Nanotechnology Products Database (2020b)
Ben-Gurian University of the Negev	-	Surface coating	Copper and polymer-based nanoparticle spray coatings which can be used in hospital and healthcare facilities and public places such as schools, airports, buses etc.	Statnano (2020)

incomplete prevention of virus spread if not properly fitted to the face, and environmental concerns associated with the disposal of single-use masks.

In this context, nanotechnology offers promising improvements in PPE, such as facemasks, aprons, and gloves. One such approach involves introducing hydrophobicity in PPE, which provides an intrinsic barrier against airborne droplets released during sneezing or coughing. This can be achieved through: (i) nanoengineering of materials (e.g., development of nanowhiskers, nanocomposites, and nanofibers); (ii) inclusion of nanoscale 3D surfaces; and (iii) coating with hydrophobic nanoparticles (Mansi et al., 2019; Srinivas et al., 2014). Another approach is the modification of textile surfaces by including antiviral polymeric or peptidyl nanoparticles, metallic nanoparticles such as silver and copper, and quaternary ammonium or quaternary phosphonium salts (Yetisen et al., 2016). Figure 8.2 highlights the different nanoparticle-based technologies used in face masks and their various functionalities.

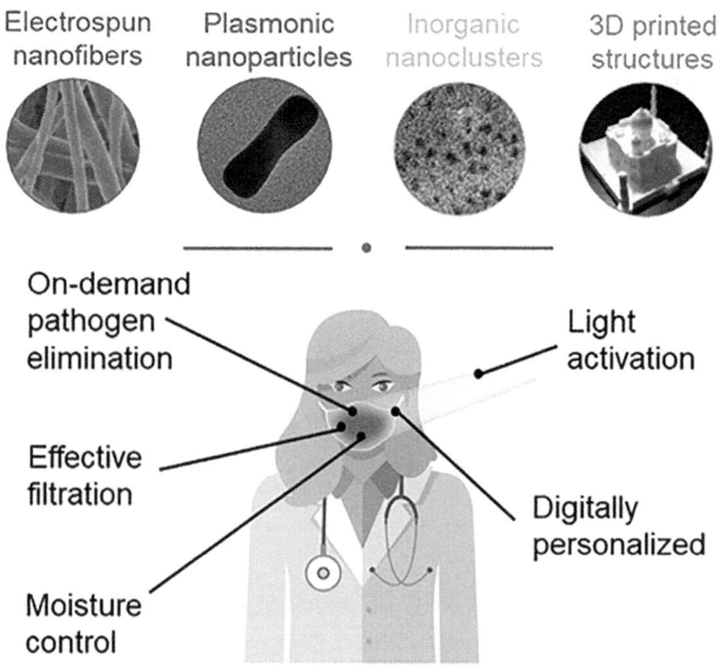

FIGURE 8.2 Multifunctional nano-based face masks against COVID-19.

Source: Reprinted with permission from De Sio et al. (2021), Copyright © 2020 Wiley-VCH GmbH

Nanoengineering of face masks can be achieved through the use of nanofiber membrane technology, where dense networks of nanofibers resembling spiderwebs are formed, providing a larger surface area, a high number of pores, and a small pore size. Such nanofibers or nanowhiskers can be included in face masks, resulting in excellent filterability and improved breathability. These masks are particularly beneficial for individuals with pre-existing respiratory symptoms and for those who need to wear masks for extended periods.

For instance, researchers at the Queensland University of Technology (QUT) developed a highly breathable, disposable, and biodegradable cellulose nanofiber-based material designed to block out coronaviruses (Statnano, 2020a). Additionally, Zen Graphene Solutions Ltd. (ZEN) in collaboration with the UK-based Graphene Composites Ltd. (GC) created a graphene-based virucidal nanocomposite ink that can be applied to PPE and facemasks, including N95 masks, to enhance their protective properties by potentially neutralizing trapped viruses (www.mining.com, 2020). In another case, the USA-based company Intetgricote Inc., in collaboration with the University of Houston, developed a hydrophobic nanotech coating that could effectively shield against coronaviruses (Statnano, 2020b). Other examples of nanotechnology-based protection systems applied to PPE and masks are summarized in Table 8.2.

8.4 NANO-BASED VIRAL DETECTION AND DIAGNOSIS TOOLS

Coronaviruses, like other viruses, are intracellular pathogens that cannot be observed using an ordinary microscope, making their detection and isolation particularly challenging (Udugama et al., 2020). Therefore, early detection and diagnosis are crucial measures for the isolation, control, and tracking of COVID-19. Standard COVID-19 testing kits typically function by detecting either nucleic acids, such as viral RNA using reverse transcriptase-polymerase chain reaction (RT-PCR), or antibodies through methods like enzyme-linked immunosorbent assay (ELISA). The most widely accepted method is protein-based or serological tests, which detect specific antigen-antibody reactions in the body. However, these kits suffer from certain drawbacks, including the occurrence of false negative reactions due to cross-reactivity between antibodies, prolonged reactivity time, and ineffectiveness in detecting mutated strains. These limitations can be addressed with the implementation of nanotechnology for early viral detection using highly sensitive and accurate nano-based sensors (Rocchitta et al., 2016).

TABLE 8.2 Some Examples of Nanotechnological Applications in Personal Protective Equipment (PPE)

Nanotechnology Used	Manufacturers	Product Type	Specifications	References
Nanofiber membrane technology	Yamashin Filter Corporation, Japan	Nanofiber mask inner sheet	3D surface mask made of synthetic polymers with high trapping properties.	http://www.yamashin-filter.co.jp/eng/ (2020)
	Avalon nanofiber, Taiwan	Nanopoly Nanofiber mask	4 layered masks made of water repellent non-woven first layer, followed by two layers of nanofiber, and the innermost silky skin friendly layer	https://www.avalon-nanofiber.com (2020)
	Nanovia, Czech Republic	Nano-based Respiratory mask	Forms barrier for microbes by principle of mechanical detection	https://www.nanovia.org (2020)
	Nano Fanavaran Khavar, Iran	NFK nano mask	Polyacrylonitrile nanofibers with high porosity and high surface to volume ratio	https://en.nanoproduct.ir (2020)
	Metamask Ltd., New Zealand	Nano-coco-carbon filter	Unique combination of natural coconut shell carbon and nanofiber allows an extremely thin membrane with 99.99% filterability	https://www.metamasks.com (2020)
Nanocomposite membrane technology	Copper3D, Chile	NanoHack	Three layers of non-woven polypropylene infused with 5% copper oxide nanoparticles	https://3dprintingcenter.net (2020)
	Verdex technologies, Inc., USA	Face mask	Nanofibers functionalized with miniscule particulates of 30–60 microns	https://verdextech.com (2020)
Nanoparticles technology	Respilon Group s.r.p, Czech Republic	Respimask ® VK	Contains copper dioxide nanoparticles incorporated which not only traps virus, but also kills it. Accelerated copper oxide gives the mask a natural skin like colour	https://www.respilon.com (2020)
	Hong Kong Polytechnic University	Graphene coated photolytic reusable mask	Nanocarbon coatings deposited on masks makes it superhydrophobic, and self-sterilizing on exposure to light	Zhong et al. (2020)
	X.TiO_2 Inc. (XTI), USA	XTITM Active Nano Facemask	Self-regenerating germicidal Titanium dioxide and silver nanoparticle incorporated facemask	https://product.statnano.com (2020)

Nanomaterials such as metallic nanoparticles, polymeric nanoparticles, carbon nanotubes, graphene nanoparticles, quantum dots, silica nanoparticles, and photonic crystals are already being utilized in viral detection tools. The main nanotechnological approaches for virus detection include the development of biosensors and the magnetic extraction of viral particles from body fluids (blood/nasal swabs) using magnetic nanoparticles, a technology known as nanotrap technology.

Another highly efficient technology involves the application of nanotechnology to improve the efficacy of PCR tests through nano-PCR methods, enabling the simultaneous detection of both DNA and RNA viruses (Talebian et al., 2020). A team of researchers led by Prof. Cheong developed a one-pot PCR tool with magneto-plasmonic nanoparticles (MPNs) at its core and a gold shell with plasmonic properties. These MPNs were applied to PCR to develop a nano-PCR tool, which significantly improved the detection time of RT-PCR while maintaining the test's full accuracy (*see* Figure 8.3). By utilizing the plasmonic property of the nanoparticle, light energy was converted to thermal energy, resulting in the shortening of the thermocycling step of RT-PCR from 1–2 hours to 11 minutes. Furthermore, the magnetic properties of the nanoparticles allowed for an additional magnetic field for enhanced fluorescent detection of amplified genes (Cheong et al., 2020).

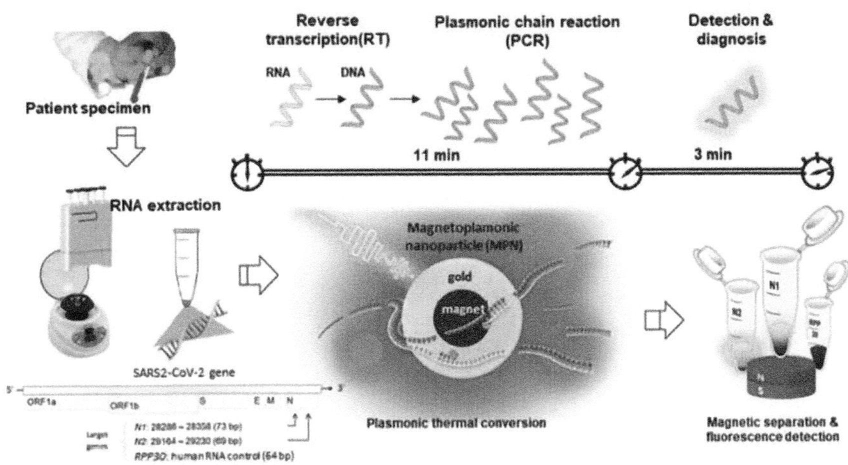

FIGURE 8.3 High-speed nano-polymerase chain reaction (PCR) technology for point-of-care diagnosis of COVID-19.

Source: Reprinted with permission from Cheong et al. (2020).

A nanobiosensor is an essential tool that utilizes nano-based probes to facilitate the high-intensity detection of analytes present in body fluids or other solutions. The large surface area-to-volume ratio of the nanoprobe efficiently enhances the interaction between the sensor and the analyte, ultimately transforming it into easily measurable and quantifiable signals (Rocchitta et al., 2016). To achieve this, nanomaterials must be functionalized with viral biomolecules such as viral enzymes, nucleic acids, antibodies, microorganisms, cells, tissues, organic receptors, or even biomimicking substances. Assays can be performed based on various methods including colorimetry, antigen-antibody reactions, photothermal and light reactions (Talebian et al., 2020).

In a recent study, a dual-functional plasmonic biosensor was developed that combined the plasmonic photothermal effect and localized surface plasmon resonance (LSPR) sensing transduction, showing promising applications in COVID-19 diagnosis (Qiu et al., 2020). In this work, two-dimensional gold nanoislands (AuNIs) were functionalized with complementary DNA receptors for the detection of specific sequences of the SARS-CoV-2 virus via a nucleic acid hybridization process. For accurate performance, thermoplasmonic heat was generated on the same AuNIs chips when illuminated at their plasmonic resonance frequency. Additionally, for the rapid and sensitive detection of the SARS-CoV-2 virus from a nasopharyngeal swab, a field-effect transistor (FET)-based biosensor device was prepared, where a graphene sheet was chosen as the sensing material and was conjugated with SARS-CoV-2 virus spike antibody via 1-pyrenebutyric acid N-succinimide ester (Seo et al., 2020). Moitra et al. reported the development of a rapid colorimetric assay (providing naked-eye detection of results within 10 minutes) using gold nanoparticles capped with thiol-modified antisense oligonucleotides specific to the N gene of SARS-CoV-2 (Moitra et al., 2020).

8.5 NANOTHERAPEUTICS AGAINST SARS-COV-2

As mentioned in the treatment section of this chapter, no specific therapy is presently available for COVID-19. Unfortunately, the currently prescribed medications raise certain problems of side effects, ineffectiveness in the case of viral mutations, and, in some cases, the requirement of higher doses of drugs posing toxicity to host cells (Sanders et al., 2020).

Researchers have already explored the attractive benefits that nanotechnology offers to treat viral infections.

8.5.1 NANOPARTICLES FOR ANTIVIRAL THERAPY

Nano-based antiviral agents can inhibit viral infection through various mechanisms: (i) by blocking cell attachment and viral entry; (ii) blocking viral replication and proliferation; (iii) inactivating the virus; and (iv) by combining these multiple approaches. Nanoparticles that block viral attachment and entry can be used as both drug-delivering agents and direct antiviral agents. The standard drug that acts through this mechanism is chloroquine. Encapsulation of chloroquine into polymeric nanoparticles acts as an efficient drug carrier system that can mediate the targeted delivery of chloroquine. Polylactic acid (PLA) is the most commonly used polymeric nanoparticle to facilitate the delivery of chloroquine (Lima et al., 2018). Nanoparticles that block viral replication and proliferation: Various nanoparticles have been investigated for inhibiting viral replication. Silver nanoparticles (AgNPs) are one such candidate that offers promise as a therapeutic agent. Functionalized nanoparticles can also interfere directly with viral aggregation. Carbon dots (Ting et al., 2018), silver nanoparticles (Yang et al., 2016), selenium nanoparticles (Li et al., 2018), graphene quantum dots (Iannazzo et al., 2018), gold nanoparticles (Huang et al., 2019), mesoporous silicon dioxide (de Souza e Silva et al., 2016), and chitosan nanoparticles (Raghuwanshi et al., 2012) have already been used and proven to be efficient in viral inhibition.

8.5.2 NANOCARRIERS FOR DRUG DELIVERY

COVID-19 being a respiratory illness, one of the main reasons for treatment failure is the obstacles faced in the direct delivery of drugs to the respiratory tract. The upper respiratory tract has a smaller surface area, decreased blood flow, and mechanisms of infiltration of foreign bodies and mucous layers that block foreign substances (Clarke and McMillan, 2015). Additionally, in some cases, drugs must be administered in high amounts, which may result in toxic effects on the host body. Another problem associated with antiviral agents is their side effects on off-targeted organs. Other challenges such as short half-life, decreased bioavailability, limited aqueous solubility, and toxicity of conventional therapeutics against COVID-19 urge the immediate need for an alternative remedy. In this milieu, nano-based carriers can gain success in the targeted and controlled delivery of antiviral agents, thereby facilitating the therapy. The use of nanoparticles as drug carriers or encapsulating agents for the preparation of nanoformulations can be a boon in the treatment of COVID-19 as it can selectively enhance the delivery of repurposed drugs to targeted sites in a controlled release manner, thereby eliminating the chances of side effects. In nanomedicine, for drug delivery purposes, soft nanoparticles of polymers, polymeric micelles, protein nanoparticles, surfactants and lipids (liposomes, nanostructured lipid carriers, lipid-solid nanoparticles), as well as metal nanoparticles, have been extensively applied. Nanoformulation-based drug delivery systems can increase the drug efficiency by improving pharmacokinetic, pharmodynamic, and biopharmaceutical aspects of drug loading, facilitating local and specific sustained release (Ansari et al., 2020).

8.5.3 NANOVACCINES AGAINST SARS-COV-2

Vaccines play an essential role in the termination of highly infectious and dreadful pandemics by providing an adaptive immune response against the pathogens once they enter our body. As of now, researchers have proposed and validated several conventional coronavirus vaccine candidates, which include live-attenuated, inactivated, viral-vector, nucleic acids, and subunit vaccines. For detailed information on each type of vaccine, readers are suggested to go through the review by Huang et al. 2020. Despite the significant success of these vaccines, they all exhibit moderate side effects and fail to generate long-term antiviral responses. Moreover, these conventional vaccines are ineffective against high antigenic diversity and mutation rates. Taking this into account, researchers have tried to focus on nanotechnology-based vaccine strategies. Currently, several nano-based vaccines have been developed, and out of them, 26 nanoparticle-based vaccines have been recommended for human clinical trials, and more than 60 vaccine candidates are in different preclinical stages (Vu et al., 2021). A nanovaccine comprises nanoparticles that can act as antigen delivery agents to elicit protective immunity or the use of nanoparticles that possess intrinsic immunostimulatory function. Examples of nanoparticles used in the field of vaccinology include virus-like particles (VLPs), lipid nanoparticles (LPNs), nanoparticles of gold, protein assemblies, liposomes, polymers such as chitosan, PLGA, and PEI (Mortola and Roy, 2004). For vaccine nanoformulations, these nanoparticles are associated with SARS-CoV-2 antigens, inactivated viruses, spike proteins, and so forth. The diverse nanoparticle-based vaccine technology approaches are discussed briefly.

8.5.3.1 ANTIGEN PRESENTING/BIOMIMETIC NANO-BASED VACCINES

Biomimetic nanotechnology is one of the promising vaccinology approaches that can be exploited for the development of COVID-19 vaccine formulations, as it offers increased circulation duration, accumulated delivery in targeted sites, good biocompatibility, and unique antigenic and immunostimulatory characteristics (Yang et al., 2019). Biomimetic nano-based vaccines are found to be more effective and safer than conventional vaccines, as they provide sufficient stimulatory signals to elicit humoral and cell-mediated immune responses. Biomimetic nanoparticle vaccines retain the surface properties of nanoparticles and mimic the physiochemical structure of viral pathogens without being antigenic (Meyer et al., 2015). A biomimetic nanoparticle vaccine basically comprises a protein scaffold, an adjuvant, and viral antigen molecules. The adjuvants are intended to elicit innate immunity, whereas the viral antigens can confer acquired immunity. The biomimetic nanoparticles currently used for this purpose include VLPs, virosomes, self-assembling nanoparticles, and synthetic nanoparticles (Yang et al., 2019).

VLPs: Among these, VLPs are highly immunogenic macromolecular complexes that carry both adjuvants and antigens, making them a promising candidate for the development of biomimetic nanoparticle vaccines (Meyer et al., 2015). Virus-like particles, as the name suggests, share a structure similar to viruses but lack the viral genome. They are composed of non-infectious protein capsids conjugated with virus-derived structural proteins. Vaccine formulations made of VLPs have proved to provide protective immunity against many viral diseases such as HBV, HPV, hand-foot-and-mouth disease, and influenza (Bryan, 2007; Low et al., 2014). Several VLP vaccines against SARS-CoV-2 are in the clinical and pre-clinical development process. Studies have reported the development of VLPs similar to SARS-CoV-2 in the baculovirus/insect cell system by the individual or simultaneous expression of S, M, E, and N proteins (Mi et al., 2021). Huang et al. 2020 have proposed the development of a novel biosynthetic SARS-CoV-2 VLPs combined with CpG, named the CpG-VLP SARS-CoV-2 vaccine.

Self-assembling nanoparticles: An adjuvanted, recombinant spike protein-based nanoparticle vaccine NVX-CoV2373, targeting SARS-CoV-2, developed by Novavax, is currently authorized for use in several countries (Dunkle et al., 2022). Another example of a self-assembling protein nanoparticle-based vaccine is the SARS-CoV-2 spike protein ferritin nanoparticle (SpFN), which is currently in phase 1 clinical trial (Joyce et al., 2022).

8.5.3.2 ANTIGEN-ENCAPSULATED NANOPARTICLES

8.5.3.2.1 Lipid nanoparticles (LPN)

The first two COVID-19 vaccines approved for clinical trials and mass administered in humans were mRNA-1273 SARS-CoV-2 and BNT162b2 mRNA vaccine by Moderna and Pfizer/BioNTech, respectively. Both of these vaccines were non-viral complexes based on LPN delivering encapsulated mRNA encoding the SARS-CoV-2 spike protein or receptor-binding domain (Baden et al., 2021; Polack et al., 2020).

8.6 CONCLUSION AND FUTURE OUTLOOK

In recent years, we have been warned many times by Coronaviruses. The lessons we learned from previous CoV outbreaks (SARS-CoV and MERS-CoV) have provided us valuable experiences and insights about the common nature of these viruses. However, compared to SARS-CoV and MERS-CoV, the ongoing SARS-CoV-2 pandemic is a serious public health threat as it has spread around the globe very rapidly, causing millions of deaths. As of now, no specific therapy is available for COVID-19, and hence prevention is the mainstay to fight the infection. This chapter mainly reviews the main preventive, diagnostic, and treatment strategies implemented against SARS-CoV-2 and focuses on the various promising avenues of improving the limitations of these strategies using nanotechnology. Nanotechnology can offer promising innovations in the prevention, diagnosis, detection, therapy, and vaccinology of COVID-19 with better speed, efficiency, accuracy, and convenience.

We also hope that with close collaboration with various societal investors, the development of an effective vaccine or antiviral drug will be made soon, which could be useful during any possible additional waves of the infection that may occur later. We also emphasize that in the future, plans and measures needed to handle and control a pandemic should be the major issue to be addressed and researched worldwide. Advanced preparations and investments should be undertaken to manage a pandemic, as viruses are always present in nature and can attack humans at any time. A step ahead alert on pandemics may bring us many benefits such as support for healthcare, sufficient surveillance, encouragement for vaccine research and development, biosafety management, and the promotion of a balanced development of health and security worldwide.

KEYWORDS

- **antiviral agents**
- **coronaviruses**
- **COVID-19**
- **nano-diagnostics**
- **nanotechnology**
- **nano-vaccines**
- **pandemic**
- **SARS-CoV-2 virus**

REFERENCES

3D Printing Center. (2020). NANOHACK 2.0 face mask. *3DPC | We Speak 3D Printing.* https://3dprintingcenter.net/nanohack-2-0-face-mask/ (accessed on 4th July 2025).

Agostini, M. L., Andres, E. L., Sims, A. C., Graham, R. L., Sheahan, T. P., Lu, X., Smith, E. C., et al. (2018). Coronavirus susceptibility to the antiviral remdesivir (GS-5734) is mediated by the viral polymerase and the proofreading exoribonuclease. *mBio, 9*(2). https://doi.org/10.1128/mBio.00221-18 (accessed on 4th July 2025).

Amirian, E. S., & Levy, J. K. (2020). Current knowledge about the antivirals remdesivir (GS-5734) and GS-441524 as therapeutic options for coronaviruses. *One Health, 9*, 100128. https://doi.org/10.1016/j.onehlt.2020.100128 (accessed on 4th July 2025).

Ansari, M. A., Almatroudi, A., Alzohairy, M. A., AlYahya, S., Alomary, M. N., Al-Dossary, H. A., & Alghamdi, S. (2020). Lipid-based nano delivery of Tat-peptide conjugated drug or vaccine–promising therapeutic strategy for SARS-CoV-2 treatment. *Expert Opinion on Drug Delivery*, 1–4. https://doi.org/10.1080/17425247.2020.1813712 (accessed on 4th July 2025).

Arabi, Y. M., Shalhoub, S., Mandourah, Y., Al-Hameed, F., Al-Omari, A., Al Qasim, E., Jose, J., et al. (2020). Ribavirin and interferon therapy for critically ill patients with Middle East respiratory syndrome: A multicenter observational study. *Clinical Infectious Diseases, 70*(9), 1837–1844. https://doi.org/10.1093/cid/ciz544 (accessed on 4th July 2025).

Avalon Nanofiber. (2020). NanoPoly nanofiber mask–Avalon Nanofiber. https://www.avalon-nanofiber.com/product/nanopoly-nanofiber-mask/ (accessed on 4th July 2025).

Baden, L. R., El Sahly, H. M., Essink, B., Kotloff, K., Frey, S., Novak, R., Diemert, D., et al. (2021). Efficacy and safety of the mRNA-1273 SARS-CoV-2 vaccine. *New England Journal of Medicine, 384*(5), 403–416. https://doi.org/10.1056/NEJMoa2035389 (accessed on 4th July 2025).

Baghchechi, M., Dunn, J., Jaipaul, N., & Jacob, S. E. (2020). Art of prevention: Life in the time of coronavirus. *International Journal of Women's Dermatology*. https://doi.org/10.1016/j.ijwd.2020.03.046 (accessed on 4th July 2025).

Bartoli, A., Gabrielli, F., Alicandro, T., Nascimbeni, F., & Andreone, P. (2021). COVID-19 treatment options: A difficult journey between failed attempts and experimental drugs. *Internal and Emergency Medicine, 16*(2), 281–308. https://doi.org/10.1007/s11739-020-02569-9 (accessed on 4th July 2025).

Bryan, J. T. (2007). Developing an HPV vaccine to prevent cervical cancer and genital warts. *Vaccine, 25*(16), 3001–3006. https://doi.org/10.1016/j.vaccine.2007.01.013 (accessed on 4th July 2025).

Cao, B., Wang, Y., Wen, D., Liu, W., Wang, J., Fan, G., Ruan, L., et al. (2020). A trial of lopinavir–ritonavir in adults hospitalized with severe COVID-19. *New England Journal of Medicine, 382*(19), 1787–1799. https://doi.org/10.1056/NEJMoa2001282 (accessed on 4th July 2025).

Cascella, M., Rajnik, M., Cuomo, A., Dulebohn, S. C., & Di Napoli, R. (2020). Features, evaluation, and treatment of coronavirus (COVID-19). In *StatPearls*. Treasure Island (FL): StatPearls Publishing. http://www.ncbi.nlm.nih.gov/books/NBK554776/ (accessed on 4th July 2025).

CDC. (2020). Coronavirus disease 2019 (COVID-19) | People who are at higher risk for severe illness. *www.cdc.gov*. https://www.cdc.gov/coronavirus/2019-ncov/index.html (accessed on 4th July 2025).

Cheong, J., Yu, H., Lee, C. Y., Lee, J. U., Choi, H. J., Lee, J. H., Lee, H., & Cheon, J. (2020). Fast detection of SARS-CoV-2 RNA via the integration of plasmonic thermocycling and fluorescence detection in a portable device. *Nature Biomedical Engineering, 4*(12), 1159–1167. https://doi.org/10.1038/s41551-020-00654-0 (accessed on 4th July 2025).

Clarke, D., & McMillan, N. (2015). Targeted drug delivery to the virus-infected airway; complications and remedies. *Current Drug Delivery, 12*(1), 86–97. https://doi.org/10.2174/1567201811666140918114528 (accessed on 4th July 2025).

Davis, H. (2020). PRELYNX PORTAL, coronavirus (COVID-19) first response scanner + sanitizer. *123 Design Blog*. https://blog.123.design/health-2/prelynx-portal-covid-19-corona-virus-covid-19-first-response-scanner-sanitizer/ (accessed on 4th July 2025).

De Sio, L., Ding, B., Focsan, M., Kogermann, K., Pascoal-Faria, P., Petronela, F., Mitchell, G., Zussman, E., & Pierini, F. (2021). Personalized reusable face masks with smart nano-assisted destruction of pathogens for COVID-19: A visionary road. *Chemistry–A European Journal, 27*(20), 6112–6130. https://doi.org/10.1002/chem.202004875 (accessed on 4th July 2025).

Disinfectant Spray of DIAT. (2020). Disinfectant spray of DIAT | Pune news–Times of India. https://timesofindia.indiatimes.com/city/pune/disinfectant-spray-of-diat/articleshow/76311161.cms (accessed on 4th July 2025).

Dunkle, L. M., Kotloff, K. L., Gay, C. L., Áñez, G., Adelglass, J. M., Barrat Hernández, A. Q., Harper, W. L., et al. (2022). Efficacy and safety of NVX-CoV2373 in adults in the United States and Mexico. *New England Journal of Medicine, 386*(6), 531–543. https://doi.org/10.1056/NEJMoa2116185 (accessed on 4th July 2025).

Edwards, E. (2020). FDA grants remdesivir emergency use authorization for COVID-19. *NBC News*. https://www.nbcnews.com/health/health-news/fda-grants-remdesivir-emergency-use-authorization-covid-19-n1197576 (accessed on 4th July 2025).

Fernandes, M. (2020). Why children are not immune to Covid-19–BBC Future. https://www.bbc.com/future/article/20200330-coronavirus-are-children-immune-to-covid-19 (accessed on 4th July 2025).

FN NANO. (2020). FN-NANO| Against COVID-19 and for a healthy and clean environment | FN NANO. https://fn-nano.com/?lang=en (accessed on 4th July 2025).

Gautret, P., Lagier, J. C., Parola, P., Hoang, V. T., Meddeb, L., Mailhe, M., Doudier, B., et al. (2020). Hydroxychloroquine and azithromycin as a treatment of COVID-19: Results of an open-label non-randomized clinical trial. *International Journal of Antimicrobial Agents*, 105949. https://doi.org/10.1016/j.ijantimicag.2020.105949 (accessed on 4th July 2025).

Harapan, H., Itoh, N., Yufika, A., Winardi, W., Keam, S., Te, H., Megawati, D., Hayati, Z., Wagner, A. L., & Mudatsir, M. (2020). Coronavirus disease 2019 (COVID-19): A literature review. *Journal of Infection and Public Health*. https://doi.org/10.1016/j.jiph.2020.03.019 (accessed on 4th July 2025).

Holshue, M. L., DeBolt, C., Lindquist, S., Lofy, K. H., Wiesman, J., Bruce, H., Spitters, C., et al. (2020). First case of 2019 novel coronavirus in the United States. *New England Journal of Medicine, 382*(10), 929–936. https://doi.org/10.1056/NEJMoa2001191 (accessed on 4th July 2025).

Huang, H., Fan, C., Li, M., Nie, H. L., Wang, F. B., Wang, H., Wang, R., et al. (2020). COVID-19: A call for physical scientists and engineers. *ACS Nano, 14*(4), 3747–3754. https://doi.org/10.1021/acsnano.0c02618 (accessed on 4th July 2025).

Huang, L., Rong, Y., Pan, Q., Yi, K., Tang, X., Zhang, Q., Wang, W., Wu, J., & Wang, F. (2020). SARS-CoV-2 vaccine research and development: Conventional vaccines and biomimetic nanotechnology strategies. *Asian Journal of Pharmaceutical Sciences*. https://doi.org/10.1016/j.ajps.2020.08.001 (accessed on 4th July 2025).

Huang, X., Li, M., Xu, Y., Zhang, J., Meng, X., An, X., Sun, L., et al. (2019). Novel gold nanorod-based HR1 peptide inhibitor for Middle East respiratory syndrome coronavirus. *ACS Applied Materials & Interfaces, 11*(22), 19799–19807. https://doi.org/10.1021/acsami.9b04240 (accessed on 4th July 2025).

Iannazzo, D., Pistone, A., Ferro, S., De Luca, L., Monforte, A. M., Romeo, R., Buemi, M. R., & Pannecouque, C. (2018). Graphene quantum dots-based systems as HIV inhibitors. *Bioconjugate Chemistry, 29*(9), 3084–3093. https://doi.org/10.1021/acs.bioconjchem.8b00448 (accessed on 4th July 2025).

Iran Nano Product. (2020). Iran Nano Product | Products | Mask containing polymeric nanofiber for dust absorption. https://en.nanoproduct.ir/product/2894/nfk%20nano%20mask (accessed on 4th July 2025).

Joyce, M. G., King, H. A. D., Elakhal-Naouar, I., Ahmed, A., Peachman, K. K., Cincotta, C. M., Subra, C., et al. (2022). A SARS-CoV-2 ferritin nanoparticle vaccine elicits protective immune responses in nonhuman primates. *Science Translational Medicine, 14*(632), eabi5735. https://doi.org/10.1126/scitranslmed.abi5735 (accessed on 4th July 2025).

Kampf, G., Todt, D., Pfaender, S., & Steinmann, E. (2020). Persistence of coronaviruses on inanimate surfaces and their inactivation with biocidal agents. *Journal of Hospital Infection, 104*(3), 246–251. https://doi.org/10.1016/j.jhin.2020.01.022 (accessed on 4th July 2025).

Kang, S., Peng, W., Zhu, Y., Lu, S., Zhou, M., Lin, W., Wu, W., et al. (2020). Recent progress in understanding 2019 novel coronavirus (SARS-CoV-2) associated with human respiratory disease: Detection, mechanisms and treatment. *International Journal of Antimicrobial Agents*, 105950. https://doi.org/10.1016/j.ijantimicag.2020.105950 (accessed on 4th July 2025).

Kelvin, A. A., & Halperin, S. (2020). COVID-19 in children: The link in the transmission chain. *The Lancet Infectious Diseases*. https://doi.org/10.1016/S1473-3099(20)30236-X (accessed on 4th July 2025).

Keyaerts, E., Li, S., Vijgen, L., Rysman, E., Verbeeck, J., Van Ranst, M., & Maes, P. (2009). Antiviral activity of chloroquine against human coronavirus OC43 infection in newborn mice. *Antimicrobial Agents and Chemotherapy, 53*(8), 3416–3421. https://doi.org/10.1128/AAC.01509-08 (accessed on 4th July 2025).

Khamitov, R. A., Loginova, S. I., Shchukina, V. N., Borisevich, S. V., Maksimov, V. A., & Shuster, A. M. (2008). [Antiviral activity of arbidol and its derivatives against the pathogen of severe acute respiratory syndrome in the cell cultures]. *Voprosy Virusologii, 53*(4), 9–13.

Laudon, M., Romanowicz, B., & Nano-Science and Technology Institute. (2011). Nanotechnology 2011: Advanced materials, CNTs, particles, films and composites. In *Technical Proceedings of the 2011 NSTI Nanotechnology Conference and Expo, NSTI-Nanotech 2011*, Vol. 1. Boca Raton, FL: CRC Press.

Lee, P. I., Hu, Y. L., Chen, P. Y., Huang, Y. C., & Hsueh, P. R. (2020). Are children less susceptible to COVID-19? *Journal of Microbiology, Immunology and Infection*. https://doi.org/10.1016/j.jmii.2020.02.011 (accessed on 4th July 2025).

Li, H., Liu, S. M., Yu, X. H., Tang, S. L., & Tang, C. K. (2020). Coronavirus disease 2019 (COVID-19): Current status and future perspectives. *International Journal of*

Antimicrobial Agents, March, 105951. https://doi.org/10.1016/j.ijantimicag.2020.105951 (accessed on 4th July 2025).

Li, Y., Lin, Z., Guo, M., Zhao, M., Xia, Y., Wang, C., Xu, T., & Zhu, B. (2018). Inhibition of H1N1 influenza virus-induced apoptosis by functionalized selenium nanoparticles with amantadine through ROS-mediated AKT signaling pathways. *International Journal of Nanomedicine, 13*, 2005–2016. https://doi.org/10.2147/IJN.S155994 (accessed on 4th July 2025).

Lima, T., Feitosa, R., dos Santos-Silva, E., dos Santos-Silva, A., Siqueira, E., Machado, P., Cornélio, A., et al. (2018). Improving encapsulation of hydrophilic chloroquine diphosphate into biodegradable nanoparticles: A promising approach against herpes virus simplex-1 infection. *Pharmaceutics, 10*(4), 255. https://doi.org/10.3390/pharmaceutics10040255 (accessed on 4th July 2025).

Low, J. G. H., Lee, L. S., Ooi, E. E., Ethirajulu, K., Yeo, P., Matter, A., Connolly, J. E., et al. (2014). Safety and immunogenicity of a virus-like particle pandemic influenza A (H1N1) 2009 vaccine: Results from a double-blinded, randomized phase I clinical trial in healthy Asian volunteers. *Vaccine, 32*(39), 5041–5048. https://doi.org/10.1016/j.vaccine.2014.07.011 (accessed on 4th July 2025).

Mansi, A., Boccuni, F., & Iavicoli, S. (2019). Nanomaterials as a new opportunity for protecting workers from biological risk. *Industrial Health, 57*(6), 668–675. https://doi.org/10.2486/indhealth.2018-0197 (accessed on 4th July 2025).

McNeil, S. E. (2011). Unique benefits of nanotechnology to drug delivery and diagnostics. In S. E. McNeil (Ed.), *Characterization of nanoparticles intended for drug delivery* (Vol. 697, pp. 3–8). Totowa, NJ: Humana Press. https://doi.org/10.1007/978-1-60327-198-1_1 (accessed on 4th July 2025).

Mehta, O. P., Bhandari, P., Raut, A., Kacimi, S. E. O., & Huy, N. T. (2021). Coronavirus disease (COVID-19): Comprehensive review of clinical presentation. *Frontiers in Public Health, 8*, 582932. https://doi.org/10.3389/fpubh.2020.582932 (accessed on 4th July 2025).

MetaMasks. (2020). Nano filter | MetaMasks | Coconut shell activated carbon. https://www.metamasks.com/nanotech (accessed on 4th July 2025).

Meyer, R. A., Sunshine, J. C., & Green, J. J. (2015). Biomimetic particles as therapeutics. *Trends in Biotechnology, 33*(9), 514–524. https://doi.org/10.1016/j.tibtech.2015.07.001 (accessed on 4th July 2025).

Mi, Y., Xie, T., Zhu, B., Tan, J., Li, X., Luo, Y., Li, F., et al. (2021). Production of SARS-CoV-2 virus-like particles in insect cells. *Vaccines, 9*(6), 554. https://doi.org/10.3390/vaccines9060554 (accessed on 4th July 2025).

Moitra, P., Alafeef, M., Dighe, K., Frieman, M. B., & Pan, D. (2020). Selective naked-eye detection of SARS-CoV-2 mediated by N gene targeted antisense oligonucleotide capped plasmonic nanoparticles. *ACS Nano, 14*(6), 7617–7627. https://doi.org/10.1021/acsnano.0c03822 (accessed on 4th July 2025).

Mortola, E., & Roy, P. (2004). Efficient assembly and release of SARS coronavirus-like particles by a heterologous expression system. *FEBS Letters, 576*(1, 2), 174–178. https://doi.org/10.1016/j.febslet.2004.09.009 (accessed on 4th July 2025).

Nano4Life. (2020). COVID-19? 3 years permanent antivirus-antibacterial protection. https://www.nano4life.co/nano4-hygienelife (accessed on 4th July 2025).

Nanotechnology Products Database. (2020a). MVX Protex antimicrobial coat spray. https://product.statnano.com/product/11638/mvx-protex-antimicrobial-coat-spray (accessed on 4th July 2025).

Nanotechnology Products Database. (2020b). Nano shield. https://product.statnano.com/product/11713/nanoshield (accessed on 4th July 2025).

Nanotouch. (2020). *Nano Touch*. https://nanotouch.com/ (accessed on 4th July 2025).

Nanovia. (2020). Nanovia face mask. https://www.nanovia.org/en/portfolio-item/nanovia-face-mask/ (accessed on 4th July 2025).

NBIC+. (2020). Coronavirus: Nanotech surface sanitizes Milan with nanomaterials remaining self-sterilized for years | STATNANO. https://statnano.com/news/67531/Coronavirus-Nanotech-Surface-Sanitizes-Milan-with-Nanomaterials-Remaining-Self-sterilized-for-Years (accessed on 4th July 2025).

Petros, R. A., & DeSimone, J. M. (2010). Strategies in the design of nanoparticles for therapeutic applications. *Nature Reviews Drug Discovery, 9*(8), 615–627. https://doi.org/10.1038/nrd2591 (accessed on 4th July 2025).

Polack, F. P., Thomas, S. J., Kitchin, N., Absalon, J., Gurtman, A., Lockhart, S., Perez, J. L., et al. (2020). Safety and efficacy of the BNT162b2 mRNA Covid-19 vaccine. *New England Journal of Medicine, 383*(27), 2603–2615. https://doi.org/10.1056/NEJMoa2034577 (accessed on 4th July 2025).

Qiu, G., Gai, Z., Tao, Y., Schmitt, J., Kullak-Ublick, G. A., & Wang, J. (2020). Dual-functional plasmonic photothermal biosensors for highly accurate severe acute respiratory syndrome coronavirus 2 detection. *ACS Nano, 14*(5), 5268–5277. https://doi.org/10.1021/acsnano.0c02439 (accessed on 4th July 2025).

Raghuwanshi, D., Mishra, V., Das, D., Kaur, K., & Suresh, M. R. (2012). Dendritic cell targeted chitosan nanoparticles for nasal DNA immunization against SARS CoV nucleocapsid protein. *Molecular Pharmaceutics, 9*(4), 946–956. https://doi.org/10.1021/mp200553x (accessed on 4th July 2025).

Respilon. (2020). Home | Protective facemask ReSpimask. https://www.respilon.com/products/protective-facemask/home/ (accessed on 4th July 2025).

Rocchitta, G., Spanu, A., Babudieri, S., Latte, G., Madeddu, G., Galleri, G., Nuvoli, S., et al. (2016). Enzyme biosensors for biomedical applications: Strategies for safeguarding analytical performances in biological fluids. *Sensors, 16*(6), 780. https://doi.org/10.3390/s16060780 (accessed on 4th July 2025).

Sanders, J. M., Monogue, M. L., Jodlowski, T. Z., & Cutrell, J. B. (2020). Pharmacologic treatments for coronavirus disease 2019 (COVID-19): A review. *JAMA*, April. https://doi.org/10.1001/jama.2020.6019 (accessed on 4th July 2025).

Schrezenmeier, E., & Dörner, T. (2020). Mechanisms of action of hydroxychloroquine and chloroquine: Implications for rheumatology. *Nature Reviews Rheumatology, 16*(3), 155–166. https://doi.org/10.1038/s41584-020-0372-x (accessed on 4th July 2025).

Seo, G., Lee, G., Kim, M. J., Baek, S. H., Choi, M., Ku, K. B., Lee, C. S., et al. (2020). Rapid detection of COVID-19 causative virus (SARS-CoV-2) in human nasopharyngeal swab specimens using field-effect transistor-based biosensor. *ACS Nano, 14*(4), 5135–5142. https://doi.org/10.1021/acsnano.0c02823 (accessed on 4th July 2025).

Singh, A. K., Singh, A., Shaikh, A., Singh, R., & Misra, A. (2020). Chloroquine and hydroxychloroquine in the treatment of COVID-19 with or without diabetes: A systematic search and a narrative review with a special reference to India and other developing countries. *Diabetes & Metabolic Syndrome: Clinical Research & Reviews, 14*(3), 241–246. https://doi.org/10.1016/j.dsx.2020.03.011 (accessed on 4th July 2025).

Singh, L., Kruger, H. G., Maguire, G. E. M., Govender, T., & Parboosing, R. (2017). The role of nanotechnology in the treatment of viral infections. *Therapeutic Advances in Infectious Disease, 4*(4), 105–131. https://doi.org/10.1177/2049936117713593 (accessed on 4th July 2025).

Singhal, T. (2020). A review of coronavirus disease-2019 (COVID-19). *The Indian Journal of Pediatrics, 87*(4), 281–286. https://doi.org/10.1007/s12098-020-03263-6 (accessed on 4th July 2025).

Souza e Silva, J. M. de, Hanchuk, T. D. M., Santos, M. I., Kobarg, J., Bajgelman, M. C., & Cardoso, M. B. (2016). Viral inhibition mechanism mediated by surface-modified silica nanoparticles. *ACS Applied Materials & Interfaces, 8*(26), 16564–16572. https://doi.org/10.1021/acsami.6b03342 (accessed on 4th July 2025).

Srinivas, A. D., Peng, C., Chow Mittal, A., & Agarwal, P. (2014). Surfaces having particles and related methods. United States US20140041905A1, filed October 18, 2013, and issued February 13, 2014. https://patents.google.com/patent/US20140041905A1/en (accessed on 4th July 2025).

StatNano. (2020). ACTIVE-NANO facemask. https://product.statnano.com/product/542/active-nano-facemask (accessed on 4th July 2025).

Statnano. (2020a). Looking for a highly breathable mask that can block out coronavirus? Here it is! *STATNANO*. https://statnano.com/news/67589/Looking-for-a-Highly-Breathable-Mask-That-Can-Block-out-Coronavirus-Here-It-Is (accessed on 4th July 2025).

Statnano. (2020b). This nanotech-based coating can make regular masks resistant to coronavirus. *STATNANO*. https://statnano.com/news/67599/This-Nanotech-based-Coating-Can-Make-Regular-Masks-Resistant-to-Coronavirus (accessed on 4th July 2025).

Statnano. (2020c). Anti-coronavirus nanoparticle-based coatings for healthcare and public settings. *STATNANO*. https://statnano.com/news/67676/Anti-coronavirus-Nanoparticle-based-Coatings-for-Healthcare-and-Public-Settings (accessed on 4th July 2025).

Statnano. (2020d). Guelph researchers: Self-sterilizing nano-coating and no more coronavirus-infected surfaces. *STATNANO*. https://statnano.com/news/67675/Guelph-Researchers-Self-sterilizing-Nano-coating-and-No-More-Coronavirus-infected-Surfaces (accessed on 4th July 2025).

Ströher, U., DiCaro, A., Li, Y., Strong, J. E., Aoki, F., Plummer, F., Jones, S. M., & Feldmann, H. (2004). Severe acute respiratory syndrome–related coronavirus is inhibited by interferon-α. *The Journal of Infectious Diseases, 189*(7), 1164–1167. https://doi.org/10.1086/382597 (accessed on 4th July 2025).

Talebian, S., Wallace, G. G., Schroeder, A., Stellacci, F., & Conde, J. (2020). Nanotechnology-based disinfectants and sensors for SARS-CoV-2. *Nature Nanotechnology, 15*(8), 618–621. https://doi.org/10.1038/s41565-020-0751-0 (accessed on 4th July 2025).

Ting, D., Dong, N., Fang, L., Lu, J., Bi, J., Xiao, S., & Han, H. (2018). Multisite inhibitors for enteric coronavirus: Antiviral cationic carbon dots based on curcumin. *ACS Applied Nano Materials, 1*(10), 5451–5459. https://doi.org/10.1021/acsanm.8b00779 (accessed on 4th July 2025).

Udugama, B., Kadhiresan, P., Kozlowski, H. N., Malekjahani, A., Osborne, M., Li, V. Y. C., Chen, H., Mubareka, S., Gubbay, J. B., & Chan, W. C. W. (2020). Diagnosing COVID-19: The disease and tools for detection. *ACS Nano, 14*(4), 3822–3835. https://doi.org/10.1021/acsnano.0c02624 (accessed on 4th July 2025).

Verdex Technologies. (2020). Face masks | Verdex Technologies. https://verdextech.com/applications/face-masks/ (accessed on 4th July 2025).

Vu, M. N., Kelly, H. G., Kent, S. J., & Wheatley, A. K. (2021). Current and future nanoparticle vaccines for COVID-19. *EBioMedicine, 74*, 103699. https://doi.org/10.1016/j.ebiom.2021.103699 (accessed on 4th July 2025).

Wang, D., Hu, B., Hu, C., Zhu, F., Liu, X., Zhang, J., Wang, B., et al. (2020). Clinical characteristics of 138 hospitalized patients with 2019 novel coronavirus–infected pneumonia in Wuhan, China. *JAMA, 323*(11), 1061. https://doi.org/10.1001/jama.2020.1585 (accessed on 4th July 2025).

Wang, L., Wang, Y., Ye, D., & Liu, Q. (2020). Review of the 2019 novel coronavirus (SARS-CoV-2) based on current evidence. *International Journal of Antimicrobial Agents, March,* 105948. https://doi.org/10.1016/j.ijantimicag.2020.105948 (accessed on 4th July 2025).

Wang, P., Chen, K., Zhu, S., Wang, P., & Zhang, H. (2020). Severe air pollution events not avoided by reduced anthropogenic activities during COVID-19 outbreak. *Resources, Conservation and Recycling, 158*, 104814. https://doi.org/10.1016/j.resconrec.2020.104814 (accessed on 4th July 2025).

Wang, Z., Chen, X., Lu, Y., Chen, F., & Zhang, W. (2020). Clinical characteristics and therapeutic procedure for four cases with 2019 novel coronavirus pneumonia receiving combined Chinese and Western medicine treatment. *Bioscience Trends, 14*(1), 64–68. https://doi.org/10.5582/bst.2020.01030 (accessed on 4th July 2025).

Wit, E. de, Feldmann, F., Cronin, J., Jordan, R., Okumura, A., Thomas, T., Scott, D., Cihlar, T., & Feldmann, H. (2020). Prophylactic and therapeutic remdesivir (GS-5734) treatment in the rhesus macaque model of MERS-CoV infection. *Proceedings of the National Academy of Sciences, 117*(12), 6771–6776. https://doi.org/10.1073/pnas.1922083117 (accessed on 4th July 2025).

Woo, P. C. Y., Lau, S. K. P., Lam, C. S. F., Lau, C. C. Y., Tsang, A. K. L., Lau, J. H. N., Bai, R., et al. (2012). Discovery of seven novel mammalian and avian coronaviruses in the genus *Deltacoronavirus* supports bat coronaviruses as the gene source of *Alphacoronavirus* and *Betacoronavirus* and avian coronaviruses as the gene source of *Gammacoronavirus* and *Deltacoronavirus*. *Journal of Virology, 86*(7), 3995–4008. https://doi.org/10.1128/JVI.06540-11 (accessed on 4th July 2025).

Mining (2020). Graphene ink may be used to fight coronavirus. *MINING.COM* (blog). https://www.mining.com/graphene-ink-may-be-used-to-fight-novel-coronavirus/ (accessed on 4th July 2025).

NewPages (2020). Shepros nano silver multipurpose sanitizer disinfection products Johor Bahru (JB), Malaysia supply, supplier & wholesaler | Ideallex Sdn Bhd. https://m.ide.my/index.php?ws=showproducts&products_id=2968064 (accessed on 4th July 2025).

Yadavalli, T., & Shukla, D. (2017). Role of metal and metal oxide nanoparticles as diagnostic and therapeutic tools for highly prevalent viral infections. *Nanomedicine: Nanotechnology, Biology and Medicine, 13*(1), 219–230. https://doi.org/10.1016/j.nano.2016.08.016 (accessed on 4th July 2025).

Yamashin-Filter Corp. (2020). *Home | YAMASHIN-FILTER CORP.* http://www.yamashin-filter.co.jp/eng/ (accessed on 4th July 2025).

Yang, G., Chen, S., & Zhang, J. (2019). Bioinspired and biomimetic nano therapies for the treatment of infectious diseases. *Frontiers in Pharmacology, 10* (July). https://doi.org/10.3389/fphar.2019.00751 (accessed on 4th July 2025).

Yang, X. X., Li, C. M., & Huang, C. Z. (2016). Curcumin modified silver nanoparticles for highly efficient inhibition of respiratory syncytial virus infection. *Nanoscale, 8*(5), 3040–3048. https://doi.org/10.1039/C5NR07918G (accessed on 4th July 2025).

Yao, T. T., Qian, J. D., Zhu, W. Y., Wang, Y., & Wang, G. Q. (2020). A systematic review of lopinavir therapy for SARS coronavirus and MERS coronavirus—A possible reference for coronavirus disease-19 treatment option. *Journal of Medical Virology, 92*(6), 556–563. https://doi.org/10.1002/jmv.25729 (accessed on 4th July 2025).

Yetisen, A. K., Qu, H., Manbachi, A., Butt, H., Dokmeci, M. R., Hinestroza, J. P., Skorobogatiy, M., Khademhosseini, A., & Yun, S. H. (2016). Nanotechnology in textiles. *ACS Nano, 10*(3), 3042–3068. https://doi.org/10.1021/acsnano.5b08176 (accessed on 4th July 2025).

Zhai, P., Ding, Y., Wu, X., Long, J., Zhong, Y., & Li, Y. (2020). The epidemiology, diagnosis and treatment of COVID-19. *International Journal of Antimicrobial Agents, March*, 105955. https://doi.org/10.1016/j.ijantimicag.2020.105955 (accessed on 4th July 2025).

Zhang, B., Liu, S., Tan, T., Huang, W., Dong, Y., Chen, L., Chen, Q., et al. (2020). Treatment with convalescent plasma for critically ill patients with SARS-CoV-2 infection. *Chest, March*. https://doi.org/10.1016/j.chest.2020.03.039 (accessed on 4th July 2025).

Zhong, H., Zhu, Z., Lin, J., Cheung, C. F., Lu, V. L., Yan, F., Chan, C. Y., & Li, G. (2020). Reusable and recyclable graphene masks with outstanding superhydrophobic and photothermal performances. *ACS Nano, 14*(5), 6213–6221. https://doi.org/10.1021/acsnano.0c02250 (accessed on 4th July 2025).

Zorzitto, J., Galligan, C. L., Ueng, J. J. M., & Fish, E. N. (2006). Characterization of the antiviral effects of interferon-α against a SARS-like coronavirus infection *in vitro*. *Cell Research, 16*(2), 220–229. https://doi.org/10.1038/sj.cr.7310030 (accessed on 4th July 2025).

CHAPTER 9

Nano-Based Analytics for Early Detection and Diagnosis of Viral Infections

VINITHA RANI[1] and ASHWINI PRABHU[2,*]

[1]*Department of Material Science and Engineering, University of Central Florida, Florida, USA*

[2]*Division of Cell and Molecular Biology, Central Research Laboratory, Srinivas University, Mangalore, India*

*Corresponding author

ABSTRACT

Viral infections pose a serious threat to human life and represent a significant risk factor globally. Diagnosis of such viral infections remains a major concern in many developing and underdeveloped countries, where patients often face significant challenges in accessing appropriate healthcare due to the lack of diagnostic facilities and inadequate treatment options. Currently, researchers are dedicated to developing point-of-care devices for the rapid and cost-effective detection of viral pathogens, bypassing the need for expensive and time-consuming conventional diagnostic procedures. This book chapter focuses on the technological advancements in the detection of these viral pathogens, highlighting the role of nanotechnology in this field.

9.1 INTRODUCTION

One of the major concerns in many developing countries, in terms of medical care, is the struggle in coping with adverse health issues, both communicable and non-communicable diseases (Kumar et al., 2021). The limited availability

Nanotechnological Management of Viral Infections.
Radhakrishnan EK, Shiji Mathew, and Riya Alex (Eds.)

DOI: 10.1201/9781779640895-9

of diagnostic kits or laboratory testing facilities is a major cause of high mortality rates. In the case of any infectious disease, the fundamental basis of the treatment protocol is solely the identification of the disease through reliable and accurate diagnostic tools. Currently, the available conventional diagnostic tools are based on microscopy, polymerase chain reaction, and immunological reactions. These methods have contributed to diagnostics and clinical breakthroughs but still pose many limitations pertaining to the processing speed, cost, and reliability (Granger et al., 2017; Kumar et al., 2021). Even though several advancements have been implemented by the government to foster healthcare systems, numerous factors challenging their proper implementation cause a major hindrance in their smooth functioning. The most common obstacle involves the cost-effectiveness of the healthcare models and the diagnostic kits. Apart from the economic hindrance, technical competencies such as the implementation of technological advancements, commercial availability, and end-user acceptability also aid in hindrance (Mahato et al., 2017). Hence, to uplift healthcare services, several private sectors and pharmaceutical companies have come forward to promote various campaigns and awareness pertaining to the early detection and diagnosis of diseases that can enable them to track and monitor their prevalence rate. Current-day technological advancements have shifted the paradigm of clinical diagnosis to the biomolecular basis, wherein emphasis is laid on the detection of biomarkers in the pre-symptomatic period. However, several conventional detection methods are being challenged by modern rapid kit-based techniques that solely rely on the principle of molecular recognition, in order to enable accurate results in recognizing infections and diseases (Yu et al., 2011).

Infectious diseases tend to cause significant human pathogenesis and mortality throughout the world, surpassing even cardiovascular disease and cancer worldwide. Although developing countries have made significant progress in technological advancements and maintaining sanitation protocols, they still lack enough resources to tackle problems pertaining to the identification of the most infectious diseases related to contaminated food, water, and hospital-acquired infections (Kaittanis et al., 2010). However, in underdeveloped and developing countries, infectious diseases still seem to be a major problem, not only due to a lack of sanitation protocols but also due to poor facilities in identifying and treating these infections in a timely manner. Therefore, improving the standard of living and diagnostic protocols in developing and underdeveloped countries is critical in controlling the spread of diseases before they become a worldwide pandemic (Batt 2007; Kaittanis et al., 2010).

In the current scenario, nanotechnology plays a vital role in providing a great opportunity to develop fast, accurate, and cost-effective diagnostic tools for the detection of pathogens responsible for causing infection. The nanomaterials comprise unique properties that can aid in the fabrication of nanodevices, which, when modified, can detect the biomarkers that are overexpressed in pathological conditions (Rosi et al., 2005). This book chapter focuses on reviewing some of the most promising nanotechnological devices used for the detection of viral infections.

Viruses are infectious agents that can cause infections such as chickenpox, acquired immune deficiency syndrome, severe acute respiratory syndrome, influenza, Ebola, and so forth. Since these diseases spread at an alarming rate, there is a need for a well-timed diagnosis. The detection of viruses is very difficult and requires skilled technicians to carry out the process of viral culturing, antigen or antibody detection, hemagglutination assays, and gene sequencing. The above-mentioned assays are time-consuming and require intensive labor. Therefore, the diagnosis procedure is often expensive, prompting exploration for a rapid and accurate method for the detection of these pathogenic agents (Mokhtarzadeh et al., 2018). The virus usually exists in different morphological forms ranging from 20 nm–900 nm in size. They are composed of different units of proteins and nucleic acids that assemble to form nanoparticulate structures called virions. The viral proteins are usually arranged in the form of a surface layer called the capsid. Sometimes, an outer envelope surrounding an inner core of nucleic acids can also be found. Viruses, due to their minute size, pose several complications in their isolation and visualization compared to other microorganisms such as bacteria, protozoans, and fungi. Viruses can be visualized only under an electron microscope with high magnification power. Hence, electron microscopy remains a crucial requirement for viral research. However, due to its high cost and maintenance, it cannot be routinely used in clinical diagnosis (Draz et al., 2018). Recently, there has been a growing demand for the usage of biosensors in biomedical applications for the detection of viral pathogens.

Biosensors are highly accurate devices that can determine even lower analyte concentrations in biological samples. These devices can produce signals based on their interaction with the corresponding antigen or antibody, after which the signals are then converted into measurable electrical parameters by means of a transducer, which ensures fast diagnosis along with the treatment of illness and detection of pathogens (Cecchini et al., 2016; Mokhtarzadeh et al., 2017; Vidic et al., 2017) (Table 9.1).

TABLE 9.1 Comparison of Common Virus Detection Methods

Technique	Detection Principle	Time	Advantages	Disadvantages
Cell culture	Infectivity assay	Days to weeks	Broad spectrum; inexpensive	Difficulty in maintaining cell cultures; Contamination problems
Electron microscopy	Viral particle	Hours	Broad spectrum; rapid method	Necessity for presence of around 106 viral particles/mL for detection; similarity of morphologies
Hemagglutination assay	Viral protein	Hours	Easy; inexpensive	Poor sensitivity; necessity for fresh reagents
ELISA	Viral protein	Hours	Only one incubation step; no hook effect at high analyte concentrations	Limited concentration range in which the analyte can be quantified without sample dilution; and that the antigen or antibody produce the same response and not distinguishable in one step
PCR	Viral nucleic acid	Hours	Extremely high sensitivity; Easy to set up	Extremely liable to contamination; Not easy to quantitate results; High degree of operator skill required

Source: Reprinted and reused with permission from Mokhtarzadeh et al. (2018). Copyright @ Elsevier (2022).

9.2 NANOMATERIAL-BASED BIOSENSORS

Advancements in the field of nanotechnology have led to the development of diagnostic biosensors called nano-biosensors, which play a pivotal role in the early detection of biomarkers in viral infections (Yockell-Lelièvre et al., 2016). These nano-biosensors can be fabricated on a small-scale to large-scale basis, ranging between 1 and 100 nm, without altering the biosensing properties. Several nanomaterials such as quantum dots, graphene oxide, metal nanoparticles, carbon nanotubes, nanorods, and thin films have been explored for their functional, electrical, and mechanical properties in biomedical applications. Nanosensors can interact with the biological elements present in pathogens, allowing for the detection and diagnosis of infections or diseases (Jianrong et al., 2004). Some of the most commonly used nanomaterials for detecting pathogenic viruses are discussed in the subsections.

9.2.1 GOLD NANOPARTICLE-BASED BIOSENSORS

Colloidal gold nanoparticles are among the most frequently utilized nanomaterials in biomedical applications. Gold nanocarriers are ideal for use in drug delivery applications due to their optical and electrochemical properties. Furthermore, the use of gold nanoparticles in biosensing applications can enhance the detection signal for biomarkers that are present in low concentrations in a given sample (Su et al., 2017). The color change pattern observed in gold nanoparticles is due to interparticle plasmon coupling, a phenomenon widely exploited in the field of biosensors. When the nanoparticles are well dispersed, the gold nanoparticle solution appears red, but it turns deep blue or purple when they aggregate. This property has been used to design a series of biosensors for detecting biological molecules such as DNA, RNA, and proteins in various samples. The recognition of the target molecule is based on the principle of self-assembly recognition of biomolecules on gold nanoparticles, which has been instrumental in biosensor design (Lin et al., 2013).

Liu et al. demonstrated the efficacy of antibody-functionalized gold nanoparticles in the detection of the influenza A virus. The researchers developed a colorimetric immunosensor for the influenza A virus, utilizing a monoclonal anti-hemagglutinin antibody as the tag. The conjugation of influenza-specific antibodies with gold nanoparticles produced an antibody-gold nanoparticle probe. Due to the aggregation between the monoclonal antibody and gold nanoparticles, a red shift in the absorption spectrum was observed, detectable by the naked eye and confirmed by transmission electron and dynamic light scattering. The study suggested that the developed immunosensor exhibited high specificity, accuracy, and good stability against the influenza A virus (Liu et al., 2015).

Muniz et al. conducted a similar study, fabricating a gold nanoparticle-based electrochemical magneto immunosensor for the rapid detection of the hepatitis B virus in human serum. The study utilized magnetic beads as bioreaction platforms and gold nanoparticles as electroactive labels for the detection of human immunoglobulin G antibody and anti-hepatitis B surface antibody (see Figure 9.1). The detection assay was based on the principle of catalytic attraction towards hydrogen evolution in an acidic medium. This quick and accurate detection process offers an alternative to traditional detection methods (De et al., 2010).

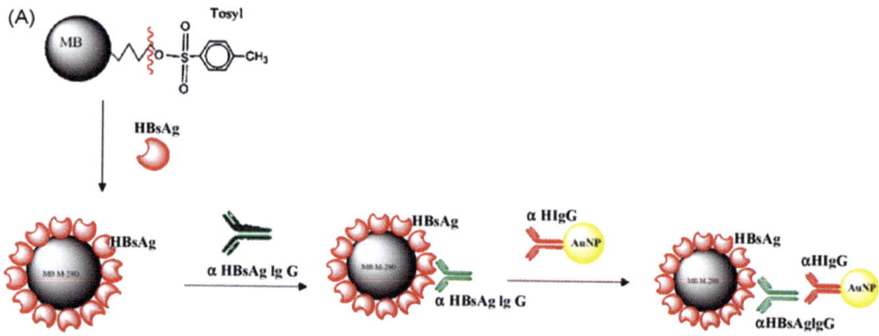

FIGURE 9.1 Scheme of the experimental procedure performed. HBsAg captured on the surface of magnetic beads, incubation with human serum containing HBsAg IgG antibodies and recognition with AuNPs conjugated with goat-human IgG antibodies.

Source: Reprinted and reused with permission from De et al. (2010). Copyright @ Elsevier (2022).

Similarly, dengue is a mosquito-borne disease prevalent in more than a 100 countries. This viral disease is known to infect around 50–100 million people annually, leading to approximately 24,000 deaths. Dengue is caused by the single-stranded positive-sense RNA dengue virus, resulting in fever that may progress to life-threatening dengue hemorrhagic fever. Diagnosing the dengue virus is often challenging, as the initial clinical symptoms resemble those of influenza, measles, yellow fever, and other viral infections. To address this problem, Yrad et al. developed a lateral flow biosensor for the detection of Dengue-1 RNA using gold nanoparticles. Lateral flow biosensors are paper-based testing devices that enable rapid one-step detection of infections. These pre-fabricated strips contain dry reagents that are activated when fluid samples are applied to them. The team created a colorimetric lateral flow biosensor to detect Dengue-1 RNA using dextrin-capped gold nanoparticles. The detection principle was based on the nucleic acid sandwich-type hybridization of a gold nanoparticle-labeled DNA reporter probe, Dengue-1 RNA, and Dengue-1 specific DNA capture probe immobilized on a nitrocellulose membrane. Upon loading the samples onto the strip, a positive test generated a red test line on the strip, visible to the naked eye. This study provided a promising diagnostic platform for the accurate detection of dengue infection (Yrad et al., 2019).

9.2.2 *GRAPHENE OXIDE-BASED BIOSENSORS*

Graphene is the thinnest and lightest sp2 carbon nanomaterial, exhibiting desirable properties such as fast electron mobility, high current density, thermal conductivity, and mechanical strength. These characteristics make graphene an ideal nanomaterial for the fabrication of nanoelectronics, nanodevices, and nanocomposites. Consequently, in recent years, graphene-based biosensors have garnered significant attention for providing a novel sensor platform capable of analyzing and targeting biomolecules with high sensitivity and selectivity. Chemically derived single-layered graphene oxide sheets also provide a large surface area ranging from 20–200 μm, offering an additional benefit in fabricating graphene-based electrochemical biosensors (Liu et al., 2012; Liu et al., 2013; Novoselov et al., 2004; Wang et al., 2010).

Joshi et al. conducted a study to fabricate low-cost reduced graphene oxide using a biopolymer to detect the presence of the influenza virus. The team synthesized a reduced graphene oxide film from shellac through thermal treatment. The thermally decomposed flakes obtained from the thin film were dispersed in indium tin oxide glass electrodes to create electrochemical immunosensors for detecting the influenza virus H1N1 (*see* Figure 9.2). The fabricated biosensor exhibited high sensitivity

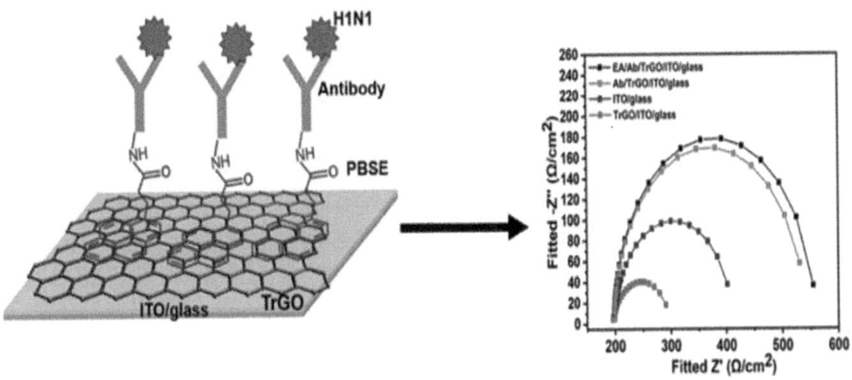

FIGURE 9.2 Schematic representation of the proposed thermally-decomposed reduced graphene oxide (TrGO)-based immunosensor for the detection of the influenza virus H1N1. The electrochemical impedance spectroscopy was used in the study as the final signal for the detection of influenza H1N1 viruses.

Source: Reprinted and reused with permission from Joshi et al. (2020. Copyright @ Elsevier (2022).

and stability. Thermally decomposed graphene oxide, owing to the presence of the phenolic OH moiety, could detect the plaque-forming units of the virus, demonstrating the potential activity of the nanomaterial-based biosensor in clinical applications (Joshi et al., 2020).

Lee et al. also conducted a similar study to fabricate a graphene oxide-based molecular diagnostic biomarker for the detection of Zika and dengue viruses. The team developed a graphene oxide-based tool for the differential diagnosis of Zika and dengue viruses by targeting the potent viral nucleic acid visualized by fluorometric detection, integrated with loop-mediated isothermal amplification to ensure increased sensitivity. When the sample is loaded onto the biosensor, in the presence of the target virus, the fluorescent probes tend to recognize the single-stranded loop of the virus, thereby allowing the detection of viral nucleic acid (Lee et al., 2020).

Omar et al. carried out a study to fabricate cadmium sulfide quantum dots-amine functionalized graphene oxide thin films tagged with a specific monoclonal antibody immunoglobulin M to detect the E-protein of the dengue virus. The biosensor exhibited an excellent detection limit ranging from 0.001 nM–1 pM of the viral protein. The results of the study indicated that the biosensor showed high potential sensitivity and strong binding affinity towards the dengue E protein (Omar et al., 2019). Reddy et al. also conducted a similar study to fabricate MXene-nickel oxide-reduced graphene oxide nanocomposite bioelectrode for the detection of H1N1 and H5N2 viral proteins. The detection strategy is based on the interaction between the H1N1 and H5N1 binding peptides and the electrode. If the test sample contains the viral proteins, when loaded on the biosensor, it reacts to form the protein hemagglutinin, thereby resulting in a fluctuation of the peak in the sensor. The results from this study demonstrated the benefits of peptide biosensors in clinical applications as screening tools for the detection of the virus from clinical samples (Reddy et al., 2022).

9.2.3 CARBON NANOTUBE-BASED BIOSENSORS

Carbon nanotubes are seamless hollow tubes composed of rolling graphite sheets and are subcategorized into single and multiwalled carbon nanotubes. A single-walled carbon nanotube consists of a single sheet of graphite ranging from 0.75–3 nm, while a multiwalled carbon nanotube is made up of two or more curly graphite sheets ranging from 2–30 nm, sometimes extending up to 100 nm. Carbon nanotube-based biosensors are considered to be the next-generation building blocks of ultra-sensitive biosensing systems (Kong et al., 2000; Odom et al., 1998; Yang et al., 2015). Wasik et al. fabricated a heparin-functionalized carbon nanotube biosensor for the detection of the dengue virus. The dengue virus, transmitted by Aedes mosquitoes, can cause severe hemorrhagic disorders in humans and non-human primates. Heparin, an analog of heparan sulfate proteoglycan, which serves as the receptors for the dengue virus, was used in the biosensor as the biorecognition element instead of the traditional antibody (Figure 9.3). The study highlighted the potential use of heparin in clinical diagnosis to improve point-of-care diagnostics for dengue infection (Wasik et al., 2017).

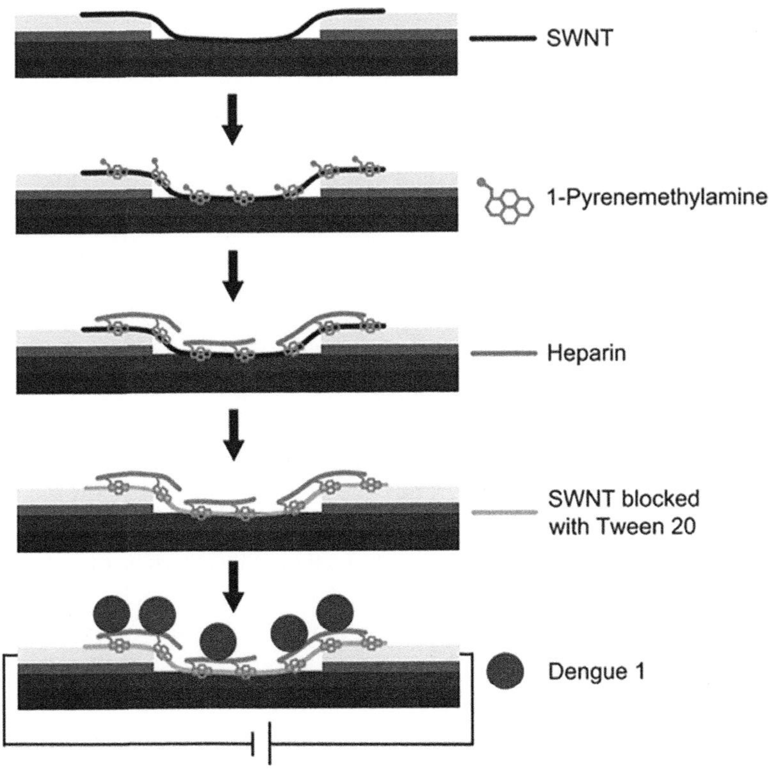

FIGURE 9.3 Schematic representation of the fabrication of chemiresistor used for detection of Dengue virus.

Source: Reprinted and reused with permission from Wasik et al. (2017). Copyright @ Elsevier (2022).

Bhattacharya et al. developed carbon nanotube biosensors using a layer-by-layer technique to investigate the interaction between antibodies specific to avian metapneumovirus. Gold electrodes tagged with silicon and silicon dioxide substrates coated with polyelectrolyte multilayer films functionalized with single-walled carbon nanotubes were employed. The viral antibodies were immobilized between the electrodes and further coated with poly L-lysine to enhance the binding of the antibody to the surface. The conductance of the device was observed to change when the antigen specific to the immobilized antibody reacted with the device (Bhattacharya et al., 2011). Similarly, Fu et al. developed chemiresistive carbon nanotube biosensors for the detection of DNA sequences derived from the avian influenza virus H5N1. The team used two semiconducting single-walled carbon nanotubes and nitrogen-doped multiwalled carbon nanotubes to detect the viral particle. Sensor nanotubes were positioned between interdigitated metal electrodes functionalized with a DNA probe sequence that could rapidly detect DNA target sequences of H5N1, with concentrations ranging from 2 pM–2 nM. The fabricated biosensor exhibited promising results for point-of-care applications in clinical diagnostics (Fu et al., 2017).

9.2.4 QUANTUM DOT-BASED BIOSENSORS

Quantum dots are semiconductor nanocrystals that consist of elements from the periodic groups II-VI, III-V, or IV-VI. Quantum dots have unique optical and electronic properties, such as narrow and symmetric emission spectra, as well as broad absorption spectra that stimulate the excitation of multiple fluorescent colors. They are also resistant to photobleaching when compared to other nanomaterials (Adegoke et al., 2016; Algar et al., 2010; Hong et al., 2018). Norouzi et al. fabricated a quantum dot-based biosensor to detect human T-lymphotropic virus-1. Two probes, namely biotin-labeled acceptor and NH2 reporter probes, with the target DNA, were fused together, after which the resulting sandwich complex was immobilized using streptavidin. The emission spectra of the quantum dot solution after adding it to the sandwich complex were recorded. The biosensor could detect the viral protein concentration ranging from 10 pg/μL–0.24 ng/μL, with a detection limit of 19.5 pg/μL (Norouzi et al., 2017).

Nazrin et al. conducted similar work to detect influenza virus H1N1 using quantum dot-gold nanocomposites. The team fabricated a biosensor using cadmium-zinc-selenium-sulfur quantum dots conjugated with gold nanoparticles for the detection of the H1N1 virus (Figure 9.4). The path distance between gold nanoparticles and quantum dots was linked with a peptide chain consisting of 18 amino acids. When the viral particles bind onto the peptide chain, they induce steric hindrance due to which the fluorescence of the quantum dots gets quenched (Nasrin et al., 2020).

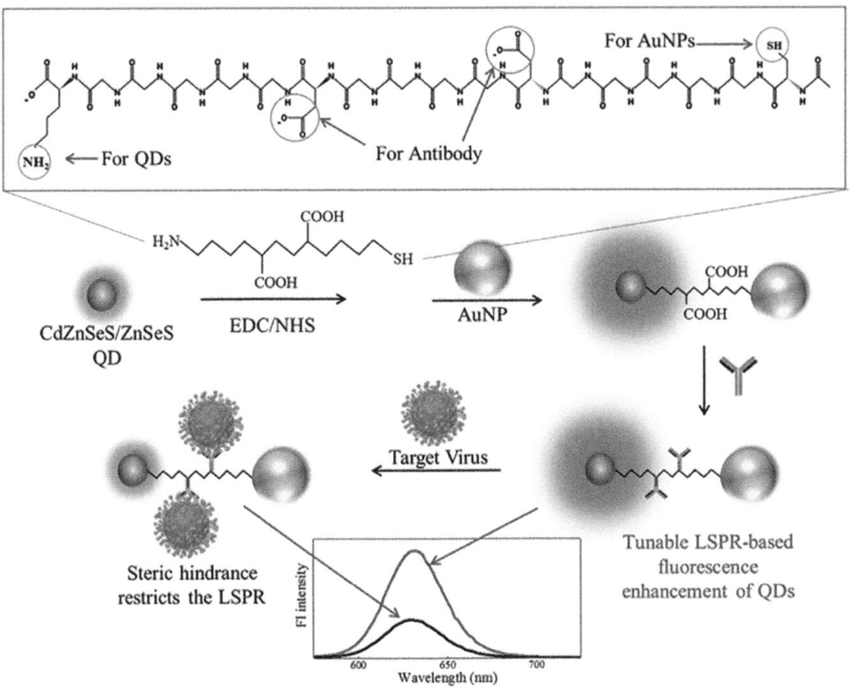

FIGURE 9.4 Schematic diagram for the preparation of CdZnSeS/ZnSeS QD-peptide-AuNP nanocomposite and its detecting mechanism towards influenza virus. AuNPs and QDs are conjugated by peptide linker.

Source: Reprinted and reused with permission from Nasrin et al. (2020).

Similarly, Stringer et al. conducted a study to develop an optical biosensor using gold nanoparticles and quantum dots to detect porcine reproductive and respiratory syndrome virus (PRRSV). The team fabricated the biosensor consisting of two labeled biomolecules: PRRSV-specific antibody tagged with a fluorescent dye bound with quantum dots, along with PRSV-specific antibody labeled with a fluorescent dye tagged with gold nanoparticles. When the viral particle was exposed to PRSV, a coupled reaction occurred between the viral particle and the antibody, resulting in a conformational change in the biosensor, leading to a change in the fluorescence spectrum of the sensor and effectively detecting the viral particle in the sample (Stringer et al., 2008).

Achadu et al. synthesized plasmonic magnetic molybdenum trioxide and graphite carbon nitride quantum dots to detect influenza virus. Specific antibodies targeting the influenza A virus were conjugated onto the surface of the biosensor. When the sample was poured into the biosensor, an immunocomplex was formed between the antibody-conjugated nanomaterials, resulting in a modulation and gradual enhancement in the fluorescence intensity. The fluorescence intensity increased as the concentration of the viral particle increased (Achadu et al., 2020).

9.2.5 SILICA NANOPARTICLE-BASED BIOSENSORS

Recent developments in controlling the surface property and particle morphology in drug delivery and biosensing have led to the exploration of new materials to attain the maximum benefit. One such material is mesoporous silica, which possesses a high surface area and desired pore volume that enhances the biocompatibility of these materials in biological systems. Several techniques have been adapted to functionalize both the internal and exterior pores of these particle surfaces to possess a narrow pore size distribution ranging from 2–30 nm (Bapat et al., 2016; Jafari et al., 2019; Kell et al., 2011; Qhobosheane et al., 2001; Trewyn et al., 2007).

Cha et al. conducted work to detect hepatitis B virus DNA using a silica nanoparticle microcantilever sensor. A 243-mer nucleotide of the hepatitis B virus DNA precursor region was used as the target DNA molecule. The team fabricated a biosensor where the detection probe was conjugated with silica nanoparticles that could specifically target the DNA from the virus (Figure 9.5). To enhance the sensitivity of detection, the size of the silica nanoparticles and the dimension of the microcantilever were optimized by binding the silica nanoparticles through DNA hybridization. When the viral sample was loaded onto the biosensor, the resonant frequency shifts were found to be linearly correlated with the viral concentration present in the sample (Cha et al., 2009).

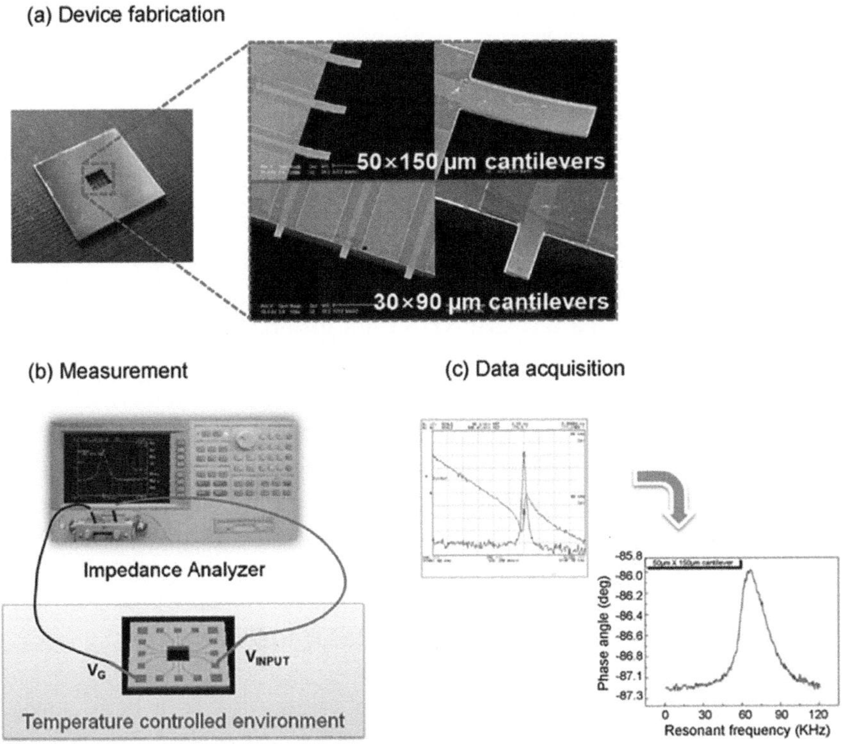

FIGURE 9.5 Dynamic microcantilevers and the data acquisition process for measuring the resonant frequency: (a) photograph of the single device with 12 microcantilevers and SEM images of two types of microcantilevers, (b) schematic diagram of the equipment used to measure the resonant frequency from the dynamic microcantilevers, which utilizes an impedance analyzer, and (c) resonant frequency data obtained from the impedance signal.

Source: Reprinted and reused with permission from Cha et al. (2009).

Singhal et al. fabricated a genosensor for the detection of the hepatitis C virus in human serum. The biosensor was immobilized with DNA complementary to the hepatitis C virus on the surface of methylene blue-doped silica nanoparticles modified with fluorine-doped tin oxide electrodes. The electrodes in the biosensor served as an electrochemical indicator for the detection of the hepatitis C virus in serum samples with a detection limit of 90 copies/mL (Singhal et al., 2017).

Studies carried out by Tuna et al. reveal the potency of probe-gated silica nanoparticles in the direct detection of the SARS-CoV-2 virus from swab samples. The team fabricated fluorescein-loaded mesoporous silica nanoparticles tagged with a specific gene sequence probe on the surface of the nanoparticle, which, upon hybridization with the target viral genome, released fluorescein molecules from the mesoporous nanoparticles. The detection could be carried out within 15 minutes and showed 84% sensitivity (Tuna et al., 2022).

On the other hand, Bamrungsap et al. fabricated a sensitive lateral flow immunoassay for detecting influenza antigens using fluorescently-doped silica nanoparticles. Cy5 fluorophores were covalently bound to organosilane through a reactive NHS ester group, enabling the successful encapsulation of the dyes within the silica matrix. The nanoparticles were then modified with carboxyl silane, providing active carboxyl groups for further conjugation. To achieve specific targeting ability, the monoclonal antibody specific to influenza A nucleoprotein was conjugated with the nanoparticles. When the antibody reacted with the specific antigen, the viral proteins could be easily detected (Bamrungsap et al., 2014).

9.2.6 MAGNETIC NANOPARTICLE-BASED BIOSENSORS

Magnetic nanoparticles have unique properties such as a large surface-to-volume ratio and high saturation magnetization that can be easily manipulated by applying an external magnetic field (Chemla et al., 2000; Khizar et al., 2020; Tang et al., 2020). Magnetic nanoparticles of different sizes can be synthesized in the laboratory and can be coated with desired molecules to achieve targeted drug delivery with biosensing ability. Magnetic nanoparticles can be synthesized using iron oxides or alloys of pure metals. The size and properties of the magnetic nanoparticles can be easily manipulated with respect to biological molecules like DNA, proteins, and nucleic acids (Alavijeh et al., 2019; Fernandes et al., 2014; Fornara et al., 2008; Rabehi et al., 2018; Sepehri et al., 2019).

Islam and Ahsan conducted a study for the rapid detection of SARS-CoV-2 using a magnetic nanoparticle biosensor. The team fabricated a giant magnetoresistive biosensor to detect viral genome +ssRNA and S (spike) protein containing SARS-CoV-2. The principle behind the detection of magnetoresistance-based immunoassay depends on the alteration of magnetization with the changing electrical resistance from high to low, due to the spin collision at the interface between the magnetic and non-magnetic (viral) biomolecules leading to the change in electrical resistance. The fabricated biosensor is more sensitive, cost-effective, and less time-consuming compared to other conventional testing devices (Islam et al., 2020). Similarly, Durmus et al., through their study, explain the importance of magnetic nanoparticle-based electrochemical immunosensing technology for the detection of the SARS-CoV-2 virus and its variants in nasopharyngeal swabs (Figure 9.6) (Durmus et al., 2022).

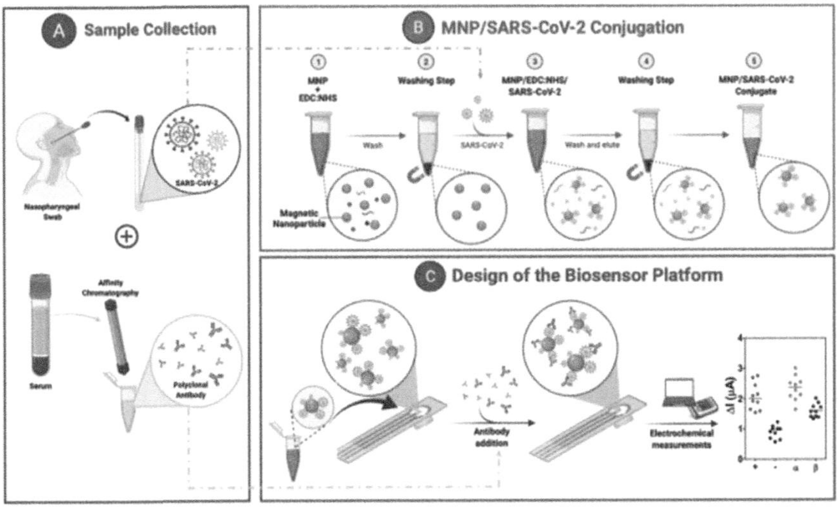

FIGURE 9.6 Illustration of the MNP-based electrochemical immunosensor platform for detecting COVID-19 (and its variants). (A) Nasopharyngeal samples were obtained from patients and identified using RT-PCR for SARS-CoV-2 and its variants. At the same time, antibodies were purified from positive human sera using affinity chromatography and confirmed via specific SARS-CoV-2 ELISA. (B) Conjugation steps of the magnetic nanoparticles (MNPs) for sample preparation. (C) Design and application of the electrochemical sensor in the detection of SARS-CoV-2.

Source: Reprinted and reused with permission from Durmus et al. (2022).

Magnetic nanoparticles, when used for sensing applications, should possess a strong magnetic moment to induce superparamagnetic behavior and avoid any form of magnetic aggregation. It is always preferred that the nanoparticles be passivated either by a hydrophilic or biocompatible coating to prevent the aggregation of the nanocarriers in an aqueous medium or biological system (Haun et al., 2010; Jun et al., 2005; Krishna et al., 2016; Lee et al., 2007; Ravalli et al., 2015). Small magnetic nanocarriers possess an upper hand when compared to larger nanoparticles due to their higher solution stability and ability to pack more closely, achieving maximum surface coverage (Brooks et al., 2002; Miguel et al., 2007; Peng et al., 2006; Perez et al., 2004; Sun et al., 2006).

Hassen et al. conducted a study to fabricate an impedimetric DNA sensor using functionalized magnetic nanoparticles for detecting human immunodeficiency virus and hepatitis B virus. The team synthesized gold electrodes using standard silicon, where the silicon wafers were oxidized using thermal energy to form an 800 nm thick field oxide, followed by the addition of a 30 nm thick titanium layer along with a 300 nm thick gold layer. Finally, the fabricated gold electrode was functionalized using magnetic nanoparticles, after which it was dipped into an acidic etching solution consisting of pure water and hydrochloric acid. The gold surfaces were then rinsed with pure water and incubated in an alkaline etching solution consisting of pure water, hydrogen peroxide, and ammonium hydroxide at high temperatures. The gold surface modification was carried out using magnetic beads along with biotin-modified DNA probes immobilized on streptavidin. The results of the study showed good immobilization of the DNA probes and the hybridization with different concentrations of complementary DNA. It was possible to detect 50 pM of hepatitis B virus DNA and 160 pM of human immunodeficiency virus DNA (Hassen et al., 2008).

9.2.7 SILVER NANOPARTICLE-BASED BIOSENSORS

Similar to gold nanocarriers, silver nanoparticles have also gained importance in the field of drug delivery and biosensing. They possess favorable properties such as high thermal and chemical stability, electrical conductivity, and catalytic activity (Ramanathan et al., 2017; Ravindran et al., 2013; Tan et al., 2021; Velusamy et al., 2016). Several studies indicate that silver nanoparticles can be easily attached to the surface of sensing devices through the simple electrostatic force of attraction. Regarding biosensing and bioimaging applications, silver nanoparticles tend to have a low refractive index, resulting in an increment of the local refractive index that can be detected by the silver extinction shift. Silver nanoparticles, when coated with silica, show excellent improvement in biomolecular detection (Alaqad et al., 2016; Iravani et al., 2014; Koedrith et al., 2015; Sabela et al., 2017; Sharonova et al., 2016).

Lim et al. conducted a study to fabricate a silver nanoparticle-based sensing probe to detect Japanese Encephalitis viral antigens. The team synthesized silver nanoparticles using a silver nitrate solution subjected to heat by the reflux method, followed by the dropwise addition of sodium citrate solution to the boiling silver nitrate solution. The formation of silver nanoparticles was confirmed by the indication of a brownish-yellow color change in the solution. After the formation of silver nanoparticles, these carriers were deposited on a glass slide. The glass slides were then immersed in 3-aminopropyl triethoxysilane for further amine group functionalization. The glass slides were then immersed in a silver nanoparticle suspension overnight for the deposition of the carriers on the glass side. The glass slide was subjected to gentle rinsing to remove excess deposition. Finally, about 55 μg/mL of specific antibodies were dropped onto the silver nanoparticle-coated slides and incubated for 2 hours at 37°C, followed by a gentle wash with phosphate buffer saline to remove the unbound antibodies. The test sample containing the antigen was dropped onto the glass slide and incubated for 1 hour at 37°C. The antigen was detected by measuring the changes in the surface plasmon absorbance at a wavelength of 466 nm (Lim et al., 2017).

Jia et al. also conducted a similar study pertaining to the fabrication of electrochemical biosensors for the detection of influenza A virus (H1N1) and SARS-CoV-2 virus using a silver nanoparticle zirconium-based metal polymer. The biosensor was prepared using a hybrid of polyether polymer ligands using 1,4-benzene dicarboxylic acid and silver nanoparticles as dopants. Specific antibodies for H1N1 and SARS-CoV-2 were separately adsorbed onto the biosensor by means of electrochemical activity. The biosensor was capable of detecting H1N1 and SARS-CoV-2 viruses even at low concentrations and showed good reproducibility in results (Jia et al., 2021).

9.2.8 POLYSTYRENE-BASED BIOSENSORS

Polystyrene is an aromatic polymer that forms due to the polymerization of styrene monomers catalyzed by the dehydrogenation of ethylbenzene. Polystyrene possesses favorable characteristics such as translucency and high durability (Kik et al., 2020). It has found enormous applications in the field of biosensors, photonics, and drug delivery. These carriers also exhibit biocompatible properties and do not show any adverse effects on the biological system (Florence et al., 2004; Loos et al., 2014; Rogach et al., 2000).

Dong et al. conducted a study to fabricate an effective biosensor for detecting the H5N1 virus using polydiacetylene vesicles deposited on polystyrene microspheres. The team immobilized polyacetylene vesicles onto the surface of polystyrene microspheres by applying electric charges to form a composite structure, which was then subjected to a thorough wash and separated by means of centrifugation. The composite was then passed through a 200 μm diameter channel. The purified composite material was then conjugated with anti-H5N1 antibodies using hydroxy succinimide and 1-ethyl 3-(3-dimethylaminopropyl) carbodiimide. When a sample solution containing H5N1 antigen was added onto the composite, it could easily be detected by visualization. The composite was even able to detect 1 ng/mL of the viral particle present in the solution (Dong et al., 2013).

A similar study was carried out by Liu et al. in fabricating a strip test for the optical determination of the H3 subtype in the influenza virus by using gold nanoparticles coated with polystyrene latex microspheres. The team synthesized gold nanoparticles coated with polystyrene latex microspheres conjugated with monoclonal antibodies against the influenza virus. When the strip was loaded with the corresponding H3 viral strain, due to the hemagglutination between the antigen and the antibody, the viral strain could be easily identified. It was also observed that the polystyrene-coated gold nanoparticle strip was specific only to the H3 antigen and showed negative results for other subtype strains (Goud et al., 2021).

9.3 CHALLENGES IN FABRICATING BIOSENSORS TO DETECT VIRAL DISEASES

Electrochemical biosensors are the most reliable and sensitive analytical devices, providing low-level detection of the target analyte and delivering excellent reproducibility and accuracy. These sensors are sometimes even referred to as point-of-care detection devices (Rasouli et al., 2018; Reddy et al., 2020; Sin et al., 2014). Infectious diseases are an ideal application for emerging biosensor technologies. In developing countries, infectious diseases pose a threat in terms of public health, thus there is an urgent need for quick diagnosis at an early stage to improve the quality of life of people (Chin et al., 2012; Lu et al., 2012; Menon et al., 2020; Ritzi-Lehnert, 2012; Singh et al., 2021). Although there have been significant improvements in research studies related to electro-sensing, the commercialization of biosensors is still in its infancy stage. The most commonly followed two techniques in sensing are by using label-free and labeled assays. However, both techniques have their pros and cons. The label-free assay follows some of the easy protocols in sample preparation and quantitative real-time measurements but lacks non-specific bindings, whereas the labeled assays follow multistep protocols, but the incorporation of multiple binding events tends to increase the specificity and sensitivity. Labeled assays always have an upper hand over label-free assays for clinical translation in dealing with real-world samples. Most of the biosensors show excellent performance with pure bacterial or viral cultures from isolated clinical samples. However, the problem arises upon the onset of an active infection in the patient sample. For instance, in the case of healthy urine, only a few cells such as erythrocytes, leukocytes, bacteria, and epithelial cells, in addition to lipid droplets and crystals, can be found. Yet, after an encounter with an infection, the color of the urine can change from a clear solution to a cloudy mixture containing pathogenic viruses and bacteria, white blood cells, and a few epithelial cells. This change in the viscosity of the sample can cause clogging of the microchannels and therefore a reduction in the signal. Hence, there is a need to fabricate the most promising sensors for the detection of viral particles in infected biological samples (D'Orazio et al., 2011; França et al., 2013; Keçili et al., 2019; Park et al., 2011; Qureshi et al., 2020; Sadighbayan et al., 2020; Saylan et al., 2019; Syedmoradi et al., 2017; Xu et al., 2016; Zhuang et al., 2020).

9.4 CONCLUSION AND FUTURE PERSPECTIVES

This book chapter primarily focuses on nano-based analytical devices used in detecting viral infections. It provides insight into various nanocarriers used in fabricating biosensors and their applications in clinical scenarios. The chapter also highlights studies conducted by various research groups and their outcomes related to the detection of viral proteins using biosensors. Despite several challenges, nano-based analytics play a significant role in detecting viral infections at an early stage. The increasing demand for biosensing applications has led to the fabrication of wearable chips, disc chips, paper chips, and paper electrodes. Although several research studies show promising results, only a few biosensor devices pass the trials and are available in the market. To overcome these limitations, innovative detection techniques require collaboration between scientists, funding agencies, and pharmaceutical agencies, enabling them to transform their ideas and thoughts into action.

KEYWORDS

- **biomedical applications**
- **biosensors**
- **early detection**
- **nano-analytics**
- **nanotechnology**
- **viral infections**
- **viral pathogens**

REFERENCES

Achadu, O. J., Takemura, K., Khoris, I. M., & Park, E. Y. (2020). Plasmonic/magnetic molybdenum trioxide and graphitic carbon nitride quantum dots-based fluoroimmunosensing system for influenza virus. *Sensors and Actuators B: Chemical, 321*, 128494.

Adegoke, O., Seo, M. W., Kato, T., Kawahito, S., & Park, E. Y. (2016). An ultrasensitive SiO_2-encapsulated alloyed CdZnSeS quantum dot-molecular beacon nano biosensor for norovirus. *Biosensors and Bioelectronics, 86*, 135–142.

Alaqad, K., & Saleh, T. A. (2016). Gold and silver nanoparticles: Synthesis methods, characterization routes and applications towards drugs. *Journal of Environmental and Analytical Toxicology, 6*(4), 525–2161.

Alavijeh, A. A., Barati, M., Barati, M., & Dehkordi, H. A. (2019). The potential of magnetic nanoparticles for diagnosis and treatment of cancer based on body magnetic field and organ-on-the-chip. *Advanced Pharmaceutical Bulletin, 9*(3), 360.

Algar, W. R., Tavares, A. J., & Krull, U. J. (2010). Beyond labels: A review of the application of quantum dots as integrated components of assays, bio probes, and biosensors utilizing optical transduction. *Analytica Chemical Acta, 673*(1), 1–25.

Bamrungsap, S., Apiwat, C., Chantima, W., Dharakul, T., & Wiriyachaiporn, N. (2014). Rapid and sensitive lateral flow immunoassay for influenza antigen using fluorescently-doped silica nanoparticles. *Microchemical Acta, 181*(1), 223–230.

Bapat, G., Labade, C., Chaudhari, A., & Zinjarde, S. (2016). Silica nanoparticle-based techniques for extraction, detection, and degradation of pesticides. *Advances in Colloid and Interface Science, 237*, 1–4.

Batt, C. A. (2007). Food pathogen detection. *Science, 316*(5831), 1579–1580.

Bhattacharya, M., Hong, S., Lee, D., Cui, T., & Goyal, S. M. (2011). Carbon nanotube-based sensors for the detection of viruses. *Sensors and Actuators B: Chemical, 155*(1), 67–74.

Brooks, R. A. (2002). T2-shortening by strongly magnetized spheres: A chemical exchange model. *Magnetic Resonance in Medicine: An Official Journal of the International Society for Magnetic Resonance in Medicine, 47*(2), 388–391.

Cecchini, F., Fajs, L., Cosnier, S., & Marks, R. S. (2016). *Vibrio cholerae* detection: Traditional assays, novel diagnostic techniques and biosensors. *TrAC Trends in Analytical Chemistry, 79*, 199–209.

Cha, B. H., Lee, S. M., Park, J. C., Hwang, K. S., Kim, S. K., Lee, Y. S., Ju, B. K., & Kim, T. S. (2009). Detection of Hepatitis B virus (HBV) DNA at femtomolar concentrations using a silica nanoparticle-enhanced microcantilever sensor. *Biosensors and Bioelectronics, 25*(1), 130–135.

Chemla, Y. R., Grossman, H. L., Poon, Y., McDermott, R., Stevens, R., Alper, M. D., & Clarke, J. (2000). Ultrasensitive magnetic biosensor for homogeneous immunoassay. *Proceedings of the National Academy of Sciences, 97*(26), 14268–14272.

Chin, C. D., Linder, V., & Sia, S. K. (2012). Commercialization of microfluidic point-of-care diagnostic devices. *Lab on a Chip, 12*(12), 2118–2134.

de la Escosura-Muñiz, A., Maltez-da Costa, M., Sánchez-Espinel, C., Díaz-Freitas, B., Fernández-Suarez, J., González-Fernández, Á., & Merkoçi, A. (2010). Gold nanoparticle-based electrochemical magneto immunosensor for rapid detection of anti-Hepatitis B virus antibodies in human serum. *Biosensors and Bioelectronics, 26*(4), 1710–1714.

Dong, W., Luo, J., He, H., & Jiang, L. (2013). A reinforced composite structure composed of polydiacetylene assemblies deposited on polystyrene microspheres and its application to H5N1 virus detection. *International Journal of Nanomedicine, 8*, 221.

D'Orazio, P. (2011). Biosensors in clinical chemistry—2011 update. *Clinica Chemical Acta, 412*(19–20), 1749–1761.

Draz, M. S., & Shafiee, H. (2018). Applications of gold nanoparticles in virus detection. *Theragnostic, 8*(7), 1985.

Durmus, C., Hanoglu, S. B., Harmanci, D., Moulahoum, H., Tok, K., Ghorbanizamani, F., Sanli, S., Zihnioglu, F., Evran, S., Cicek, C., & Sertoz, R. (2022). Indiscriminate SARS-CoV-2 multivariant detection using magnetic nanoparticle-based electrochemical immunosensing. *Talanta, 243*, 123356.

Fernandes, A. C., Duarte, C. M., Cardoso, F. A., Bexiga, R., Cardoso, S., & Freitas, P. P. (2014). Lab-on-chip cytometry based on magneto resistive sensors for bacteria detection in milk. *Sensors, 14*(8), 15496–15524.

Florence, A. T. (2004). Issues in oral nanoparticle drug carrier uptake and targeting. *Journal of Drug Targeting, 12*(2), 65–70.

Fornara, A., Johansson, P., Petersson, K., Gustafsson, S., Qin, J., Olsson, E., Ilver, D., Krozer, A., Muhammed, M., & Johansson, C. (2008). Tailored magnetic nanoparticles for direct and sensitive detection of biomolecules in biological samples. *Nano Letters, 8*(10), 3423–3428.

França, R. F., Da Silva, C. C., & De Paula, S. O. (2013). Recent advances in molecular medicine techniques for the diagnosis, prevention, and control of infectious diseases. *European Journal of Clinical Microbiology & Infectious Diseases, 32*(6), 723–728.

Fu, Y., Romay, V., Liu, Y., Ibarlucea, B., Baraban, L., Khavrus, V., Oswald, S., Bachmatiuk, A., Ibrahim, I., Rümmeli, M., & Gemming, T. (2017). Chemi resistive biosensors based on carbon nanotubes for label-free detection of DNA sequences derived from avian influenza virus H5N1. *Sensors and Actuators B: Chemical, 249*, 691–699.

Goud, K. Y., Reddy, K. K., Khorshed, A., Kumar, V. S., Mishra, R. K., Oraby, M., Ibrahim, A. H., Kim, H., & Gobi, K. V. (2021). Electrochemical diagnostics of infectious viral diseases: Trends and challenges. *Biosensors and Bioelectronics, 180*, 113112.

Granger, D., Leo, Y. S., Lee, L. K., & Theel, E. S. (2017). Serodiagnosis of dengue virus infection using commercially available antibody and NS1 antigen ELISAs. *Diagnostic Microbiology and Infectious Disease, 88*(2), 120–124.

Hassen, W. M., Chaix, C., Abdelghani, A., Bessueille, F., Leonard, D., & Jaffrezic-Renault, N. (2008). An impedimetric DNA sensor based on functionalized magnetic nanoparticles for HIV and HBV detection. *Sensors and Actuators B: Chemical, 134*(2), 755–760.

Haun, J. B., Yoon, T. J., Lee, H., & Weissleder, R. (2010). Magnetic nanoparticle biosensors. *Wiley Interdisciplinary Reviews: Nanomedicine and Nanobiotechnology, 2*(3), 291–304.

Hong, S., & Lee, C. (2018). The current status and future outlook of quantum dot-based biosensors for plant virus detection. *The Plant Pathology Journal, 34*(2), 85.

Iravani, S., Korbekandi, H., Mirmohammadi, S. V., & Zolfaghari, B. (2014). Synthesis of silver nanoparticles: Chemical, physical and biological methods. *Research in Pharmaceutical Sciences, 9*(6), 385.

Islam, M. A., & Ahsan, M. Z. (2020). Plausible approach for rapid detection of SARS-CoV-2 virus by magnetic nanoparticle-based biosensors. *American Journal of Nanoscience, 6*(6).

Jafari, S., Derakhshankhah, H., Alaei, L., Fattahi, A., Varnamkhasti, B. S., & Saboury, A. A. (2019). Mesoporous silica nanoparticles for therapeutic/diagnostic applications. *Biomedicine & Pharmacotherapy, 109*, 1100–1111.

Jia, Q., Lou, Y., Rong, F., Zhang, S., Wang, M., He, L., Zhang, Z., & Du, M. (2021). Silver nanoparticle embedded polymer–zirconium-based metal–organic framework (polyUiO-66) for electrochemical biosensors of respiratory viruses. *Journal of Materials Chemistry C, 9*(40), 14190–14200.

Jianrong, C., Yuqing, M., Nongyue, H., Xiaohua, W., & Sijiao, L. (2004). Nanotechnology and biosensors. *Biotechnology Advances, 22*(7), 505–518.

Joshi, S. R., Sharma, A., Kim, G. H., & Jang, J. (2020). Low-cost synthesis of reduced graphene oxide using biopolymer for influenza virus sensor. *Materials Science and Engineering: C, 108*, 110465.

Jun, Y. W., Huh, Y. M., Choi, J. S., Lee, J. H., Song, H. T., Kim, S., Yoon, S., Kim, K. S., Shin, J. S., Suh, J. S., & Cheon, J. (2005). Nanoscale size effect of magnetic nanocrystals and their utilization for cancer diagnosis via magnetic resonance imaging. *Journal of the American Chemical Society, 127*(16), 5732–5733.

Kaittanis, C., Santra, S., & Perez, J. M. (2010). Emerging nanotechnology-based strategies for the identification of microbial pathogenesis. *Advanced Drug Delivery Reviews, 62*(4, 5), 408–423.

Keçili, R., Büyüktiryaki, S., & Hussain, C. M. (2019). Advancement in bioanalytical science through nanotechnology: Past, present and future. *TrAC Trends in Analytical Chemistry, 110*, 259–276.

Kell, A. J., Pagé, L., Tan, S., Charlebois, I., Boissinot, M., LeClerc, M., & Simard, B. (2011). The development of a silica nanoparticle-based label-free DNA biosensor. *Nanoscale, 3*(9), 3747–3754.

Khizar, S., Ben Halima, H., Ahmad, N. M., Zine, N., Errachid, A., & Elaissari, A. (2020). Magnetic nanoparticles in microfluidic and sensing: From transport to detection. *Electrophoresis, 41*, 1206–1224.

Kik, K., Bukowska, B., & Sicińska, P. (2020). Polystyrene nanoparticles: Sources, occurrence in the environment, distribution in tissues, accumulation and toxicity to various organisms. *Environmental Pollution, 262*, 114297.

Koedrith, P., Thasiphu, T., Weon, J. I., Boonprasert, R., Tuitemwong, K., & Tuitemwong, P. (2015). Recent trends in rapid environmental monitoring of pathogens and toxicants: Potential of nanoparticle-based biosensor and applications. *The Scientific World Journal.*

Kong, J., Franklin, N. R., Zhou, C., Chapline, M. G., Peng, S., Cho, K., & Dai, H. (2000). Nanotube molecular wires as chemical sensors. *Science, 287*(5453), 622–625.

Krishna, V. D., Wu, K., Perez, A. M., & Wang, J. P. (2016). Giant magnetoresistance-based biosensor for detection of influenza A virus. *Frontiers in Microbiology, 7*, 400.

Kumar, S., Nehra, M., Khurana, S., Dilbaghi, N., Kumar, V., Kaushik, A., & Kim, K. H. (2021). Aspects of point-of-care diagnostics for personalized health wellness. *International Journal of Nanomedicine, 16*, 383.

Lee, J. H., Huh, Y. M., Jun, Y. W., Seo, J. W., Jang, J. T., Song, H. T., Kim, S., Cho, E. J., Yoon, H. G., Suh, J. S., & Cheon, J. (2007). Artificially engineered magnetic nanoparticles for ultra-sensitive molecular imaging. *Nature Medicine, 13*(1), 95–99.

Lee, J. S., Kim, J., Shin, H., & Min, D. H. (2020). Graphene oxide-based molecular diagnostic biosensor for simultaneous detection of Zika and dengue viruses. *2D Materials, 7*(4), 044001.

Lim, L. S., Chin, S. F., Pang, S. C., Sum, M. H., & Perera, D. (2017). A novel silver nanoparticles-based sensing probe for the detection of Japanese encephalitis virus antigen. *Sains Malaysia, 46*(12), 2447–2454.

Lin, M., Pei, H., Yang, F., Fan, C., & Zuo, X. (2013). Applications of gold nanoparticles in the detection and identification of infectious diseases and biothreats. *Advanced Materials, 25*, 3490–3496.

Liu, F., Kim, Y. H., Cheon, D. S., & Seo, T. S. (2013). Micropatterned reduced graphene oxide-based field-effect transistor for real-time virus detection. *Sensors and Actuators B: Chemical, 186*, 252–257.

Liu, Y., Dong, X., & Chen, P. (2012). Biological and chemical sensors based on graphene materials. *Chemical Society Reviews, 41*(6), 2283–2307.

Liu, Y., Zhang, L., Wei, W., Zhao, H., Zhou, Z., Zhang, Y., & Liu, S. (2015). Colorimetric detection of influenza A virus using antibody-functionalized gold nanoparticles. *Analyst, 140*(12), 3989–3995.

Loos, C., Syrovets, T., Musyanovych, A., Mailänder, V., Landfester, K., Nienhaus, G. U., & Simmet, T. (2014). Functionalized polystyrene nanoparticles as a platform for studying bio–nano interactions. *Beilstein Journal of Nanotechnology, 5*(1), 2403–2412.

Lu, C. H., Zhang, Y., Tang, S. F., Fang, Z. B., Yang, H. H., Chen, X., & Chen, G. N. (2012). Sensing HIV related protein using epitope imprinted hydrophilic polymer coated quartz crystal microbalance. *Biosensors and Bioelectronics, 31*(1), 439–444.

Mahato, K., Srivastava, A., & Chandra, P. (2017). Paper based diagnostics for personalized health care: Emerging technologies and commercial aspects. *Biosensors and Bioelectronics, 96*, 246–259.

Menon, S., Mathew, M. R., Sam, S., Keerthi, K., & Kumar, K. G. (2020). Recent advances and challenges in electrochemical biosensors for emerging and re-emerging infectious diseases. *Journal of Electroanalytical Chemistry, 878*, 114596.

Miguel, O. B., Gossuin, Y., Morales, M. P., Gillis, P., Muller, R. N., & Veintemillas-Verdaguer, S. (2007). Comparative analysis of the 1H NMR relaxation enhancement produced by iron oxide and core-shell iron–iron oxide nanoparticles. *Magnetic Resonance Imaging, 25*(10), 1437–1441.

Mokhtarzadeh, A., Eivazzadeh-Keihan, R., Pashazadeh, P., Hejazi, M., Gharaatifar, N., Hasanzadeh, M., Baradaran, B., & de la Guardia, M. (2017). Nanomaterial-based biosensors for detection of pathogenic virus. *TrAC Trends in Analytical Chemistry, 97*, 445–457.

Nasrin, F., Chowdhury, A. D., Takemura, K., Kozaki, I., Honda, H., Adegoke, O., & Park, E. Y. (2020). Fluorometric virus detection platform using quantum dots-gold nanocomposites optimizing the linker length variation. *Analytica Chemical Acta, 1109*, 148–157.

Norouzi, M., Zarei Ghobadi, M., Golmimi, M., Mozhgani, S. H., Ghourchian, H., & Rezaee, S. A. (2017). Quantum dot-based biosensor for the detection of human T-lymphotropic virus-1. *Analytical Letters, 50*(15), 2402–2411.

Novoselov, K. S., Geim, A. K., Morozov, S. V., Jiang, D. E., Zhang, Y., Dubonos, S. V., Grigorieva, I. V., & Firsov, A. A. (2004). Electric field effect in atomically thin carbon films. *Science, 306*(5696), 666–669.

Odom, T. W., Huang, J. L., Kim, P., & Lieber, C. M. (1998). Atomic structure and electronic properties of single-walled carbon nanotubes. *Nature, 391*(6662), 62–64.

Omar, N. A., Fen, Y. W., Abdullah, J., Zaid, M. H., Daniyal, W. M., & Mahdi, M. A. (2019). Sensitive surface plasmon resonance performance of cadmium sulfide quantum dots-amine functionalized graphene oxide based thin film towards dengue virus E-protein. *Optics & Laser Technology, 114*, 204–208.

Park, S., Zhang, Y., Lin, S., Wang, T. H., & Yang, S. (2011). Advances in microfluidic PCR for point-of-care infectious disease diagnostics. *Biotechnology Advances, 29*(6), 830–839.

Peng, S., Wang, C., Xie, J., & Sun, S. (2006). Synthesis and stabilization of monodisperse Fe nanoparticles. *Journal of the American Chemical Society, 128*(33), 10676–10677.

Perez, J. M., Josephson, L., & Weissleder, R. (2004). Use of magnetic nanoparticles as nano sensors to probe for molecular interactions. *ChemBioChem, 5*(3), 261–264.

Qhobosheane, M., Santra, S., Zhang, P., & Tan, W. (2001). Biochemically functionalized silica nanoparticles. *Analyst, 126*(8), 1274–1278.

Qureshi, A., & Niazi, J. H. (2020). Biosensors for detecting viral and bacterial infections using host biomarkers: A review. *Analyst, 145*(24), 7825–7848.

Rabehi, A., Garlan, B., Achtsnicht, S., Krause, H. J., Offenhäusser, A., Ngo, K., Neveu, S., Graff-Dubois, S., & Kokabi, H. (2018). Magnetic detection structure for lab-on-chip applications based on the frequency mixing technique. *Sensors, 18*(6), 1747.

Ramanathan, S., & Gopinath, S. C. (2017). Potentials in synthesizing nanostructured silver particles. *Microsystem Technologies, 23*(10), 4345–4357.

Rasouli, E., Shahnavaz, Z., Basirun, W. J., Rezayi, M., Avan, A., Ghayour-Mobarhan, M., Khandanlou, R., & Johan, M. R. (2018). Advancements in electrochemical DNA sensor for detection of human papilloma virus—A review. *Analytical Biochemistry, 556*, 136–144.

Ravalli, A., & Marrazza, G. (2015). Gold and magnetic nanoparticles-based electrochemical biosensors for cancer biomarker determination. *Journal of Nanoscience and Nanotechnology, 15*(5), 3307–3319.

Ravindran, A., Chandran, P., & Khan, S. S. (2013). Biofunctionalized silver nanoparticles: Advances and prospects. *Colloids and Surfaces B: Bio Interfaces, 105*, 342–352.

Reddy, K. K., Bandal, H., Satyanarayana, M., Goud, K. Y., Gobi, K. V., Jayaramudu, T., Amalraj, J., & Kim, H. (2020). Recent trends in electrochemical sensors for vital biomedical markers using hybrid nanostructured materials. *Advanced Science, 7*(13), 1902980.

Reddy, Y. V., Shin, J. H., Hwang, J., Kweon, D. H., Choi, C. H., Park, K., Kim, S. K., Madhavi, G., Yi, H., & Park, J. P. (2022). Fine-tuning of MXene-nickel oxide-reduced graphene oxide nanocomposite bioelectrode: Sensor for the detection of influenza virus and viral protein. *Biosensors and Bioelectronics, 214*, 114511.

Ritzi-Lehnert, M. (2012). Development of chip-compatible sample preparation for diagnosis of infectious diseases. *Expert Review of Molecular Diagnostics, 12*(2), 189–206.

Rogach, A., Susha, A., Caruso, F., Sukhorukov, G., Kornowski, A., Kershaw, S., Möhwald, H., Eychmüller, A., & Weller, H. (2000). Nano-and microengineering: Three-dimensional colloidal photonic crystals prepared from sub micrometer-sized polystyrene latex spheres pre-coated with luminescent polyelectrolyte/nanocrystal shells. *Advanced Materials, 12*(5), 333–337.

Rosi, N. L., & Mirkin, C. A. (2005). Nanostructures in bio diagnostics. *Chemical Reviews, 105*(4), 1547–1562.

Sabela, M., Balme, S., Bechelany, M., Janot, J. M., & Bisetty, K. (2017). A review of gold and silver nanoparticle-based colorimetric sensing assays. *Advanced Engineering Materials, 19*(12), 1700270.

Sadighbayan, D., Hasanzadeh, M., & Ghafar-Zadeh, E. (2020). Biosensing based on field-effect transistors (FET): Recent progress and challenges. *TrAC Trends in Analytical Chemistry, 133*, 116067.

Saylan, Y., Erdem, Ö., Ünal, S., & Denizli, A. (2019). An alternative medical diagnosis method: Biosensors for virus detection. *Biosensors, 9*(2), 65.

Sepehri, S., Agnarsson, B., Zardán Gómez de la Torre, T., Schneiderman, J. F., Blomgren, J., Jesorka, A., Johansson, C., Nilsson, M., Albert, J., Strømme, M., & Winkler, D. (2019). Characterization of binding of magnetic nanoparticles to rolling circle amplification products by turn-on magnetic assay. *Biosensors, 9*(3), 109.

Sharonova, A., Loza, K., Surmeneva, M., Surmenev, R., Prymak, O., & Epple, M. (2016). Synthesis of positively and negatively charged silver nanoparticles and their deposition on the surface of titanium. In *IOP Conference Series: Materials Science and Engineering, 116*, 012009. IOP Publishing.

Sin, M. L., Mach, K. E., Wong, P. K., & Liao, J. C. (2014). Advances and challenges in biosensor-based diagnosis of infectious diseases. *Expert Review of Molecular Diagnostics, 14*(2), 225–244.

Singh, A., Sharma, A., Ahmed, A., Sundramoorthy, A. K., Furukawa, H., Arya, S., & Khosla, A. (2021). Recent advances in electrochemical biosensors: Applications, challenges, and future scope. *Biosensors, 11*(9), 336.

Singhal, C., Ingle, A., Chakraborty, D., Pn, A. K., Pundir, C. S., & Narang, J. (2017). Impedimetric genosensor for detection of hepatitis C virus (HCV1) DNA using viral probe on methylene blue doped silica nanoparticles. *International Journal of Biological Macromolecules, 98*, 84–93.

Stringer, R. C., Schommer, S., Hoehn, D., & Grant, S. A. (2008). Development of an optical biosensor using gold nanoparticles and quantum dots for the detection of Porcine Reproductive and Respiratory Syndrome Virus. *Sensors and Actuators B: Chemical, 134*(2), 427–431.

Su, H., Li, S., Jin, Y., Xian, Z., Yang, D., Zhou, W., Mangaran, F., Leung, F., Sithamparanathan, G., & Kerman, K. (2017). Nanomaterial-based biosensors for biological detections. *Advanced Health Care Technologies, 3*, 19–29.

Sun, E. Y., Josephson, L., Kelly, K. A., & Weissleder, R. (2006). Development of nanoparticle libraries for biosensing. *Bioconjugate Chemistry, 17*(1), 109–113.

Syedmoradi, L., Daneshpour, M., Alvandipour, M., Gomez, F. A., Hajghassem, H., & Omidfar, K. (2017). Point of care testing: The impact of nanotechnology. *Biosensors and Bioelectronics, 87*, 373–387.

Tan, P., Li, H., Wang, J., & Gopinath, S. C. (2021). Silver nanoparticle in biosensor and bioimaging: Clinical perspectives. *Biotechnology and Applied Biochemistry, 68*(6), 1236–1242.

Tang, C., He, Z., Liu, H., Xu, Y., Huang, H., Yang, G., Xiao, Z., Li, S., Liu, H., Deng, Y., & Chen, Z. (2020). Application of magnetic nanoparticles in nucleic acid detection. *Journal of Nanobiotechnology, 18*(1), 1–9.

Trewyn, B. G., Giri, S., Slowing, I. I., & Lin, V. S. (2007). Mesoporous silica nanoparticle based controlled release, drug delivery, and biosensor systems. *Chemical Communications, 2007*(31), 3236–3245.

Tuna, B. G., Durdabak, D. B., Ercan, M. K., Dogan, S., Kavruk, M., Dursun, A. D., Tekol, S. D., Celik, C., & Ozalp, V. C. (2022). Detection of viruses by probe-gated silica nanoparticles directly from swab samples. *Talanta, 246*, 123429.

Velusamy, P., Su, C. H., Venkat Kumar, G., Adhikary, S., Pandian, K., Gopinath, S. C., Chen, Y., & Anbu, P. (2016). Biopolymers regulate silver nanoparticle under microwave irradiation for effective antibacterial and antibiofilm activities. *PLoS One, 11*(6), e0157612.

Vidic, J., Manzano, M., Chang, C. M., & Jaffrezic-Renault, N. (2017). Advanced biosensors for detection of pathogens related to livestock and poultry. *Veterinary Research, 48*(1), 1–22.

Wang, S., Ang, P. K., Wang, Z., Tang, A. L., Thong, J. T., & Loh, K. P. (2010). High mobility, printable, and solution-processed graphene electronics. *Nano Letters, 10*(1), 92–98.

Wasik, D., Mulchandani, A., & Yates, M. V. (2017). A heparin-functionalized carbon nanotube-based affinity biosensor for dengue virus. *Biosensors and Bioelectronics, 91*, 811–816.

Xu, Y., Liu, M., Kong, N., & Liu, J. (2016). Lab-on-paper micro-and nano-analytical devices: Fabrication, modification, detection and emerging applications. *Microchimica Acta, 183*(5), 1521–1542.

Yang, N., Chen, X., Ren, T., Zhang, P., & Yang, D. (2015). Carbon nanotube-based biosensors. *Sensors and Actuators B: Chemical, 207*, 690–715.

Yockell-Lelièvre, H., Bukar, N., Toulouse, J. L., Pelletier, J. N., & Masson, J. F. (2016). Naked-eye nanobiosensor for therapeutic drug monitoring of methotrexate. *Analyst, 141*(2), 697–703.

Yrad, F. M., Castañares, J. M., & Alocilja, E. C. (2019). Visual detection of dengue-1 RNA using gold nanoparticle-based lateral flow biosensor. *Diagnostics, 9*(3), 74.

Yu, J., Ge, L., Huang, J., Wang, S., & Ge, S. (2011). Microfluidic paper-based chemiluminescence biosensor for simultaneous determination of glucose and uric acid. *Lab on a Chip, 11*(7), 1286–1291.

Zhuang, J., Yin, J., Lv, S., Wang, B., & Mu, Y. (2020). Advanced "lab-on-a-chip" to detect viruses–Current challenges and future perspectives. *Biosensors and Bioelectronics, 163*, 112291.

CHAPTER 10

Nanovaccinology: Current and Future Approaches Against Viruses

SHERIN JOY PARAPPILLY, DONA V. IDICULA, JITHASHA BALAN, and SUMI MARY GEORGE*

Post Graduate and Research Department of Microbiology, Sree Sankara College, Kalady, Ernakulam, Kerala, India

*Corresponding author

ABSTRACT

Infectious diseases have a universal impact on society, mental health, politics, healthcare, and the economy. This impact has been particularly evident since the 2019 COVID-19 pandemic that continues to affect us. Despite the significant advancements in science and technology in the 21st century, we continue to face numerous challenges in managing diseases and infections. To address these challenges, it has become imperative to explore different mechanisms of viral infections and develop innovative strategies for their treatment and prevention. This book chapter focuses on current and future approaches to nanovaccines against life-threatening viral infections.

10.1 INTRODUCTION

Vaccination involves the administration of a biological preparation that triggers active immunity against infectious or malignant diseases. It is also referred to as inoculation or immunization and is prepared using microorganisms such as viruses or bacteria, which are either killed or modified to

Nanotechnological Management of Viral Infections.
Radhakrishnan EK, Shiji Mathew, and Riya Alex (Eds.)

DOI: 10.1201/9781779640895-10

provide resistance against diseases in the human body. Vaccination serves to offer ongoing protection against infectious diseases and activates the host's immune system to develop a robust defense mechanism. Vaccination programs across the globe have successfully eradicated various diseases like poliomyelitis, diphtheria, neonatal tetanus, and smallpox from both developing and developed countries.

Throughout history, humanity has sought diverse methods to protect individuals from life-threatening illnesses. Presently, vaccination plays a critical role in preventing infectious diseases and improving overall health. It is widely recognized as an effective and cost-efficient approach to boosting immunity and well-being. In May 1796, Edward Jenner, an English physician, developed the world's first vaccine against smallpox. Today, numerous vaccines against various infectious agents are available, licensed for production, and distributed worldwide.

The development of lifelong immunity against antigens specific to cancer cells or pathogenic microorganisms is achieved through the generation of cytotoxic T cells and antibodies. The process of vaccination involves the initial uptake of adjuvants or antigens from the surface of Antigen Presenting Cells (APCs) and their maturation, culminating in the binding of antigens with specific T or B cells, leading to the production of cytotoxic T cells and antibodies (D'Amico et al., 2021; Korenkov et al., 2018). Figure 10.1 illustrates the activation of immune cells after vaccination.

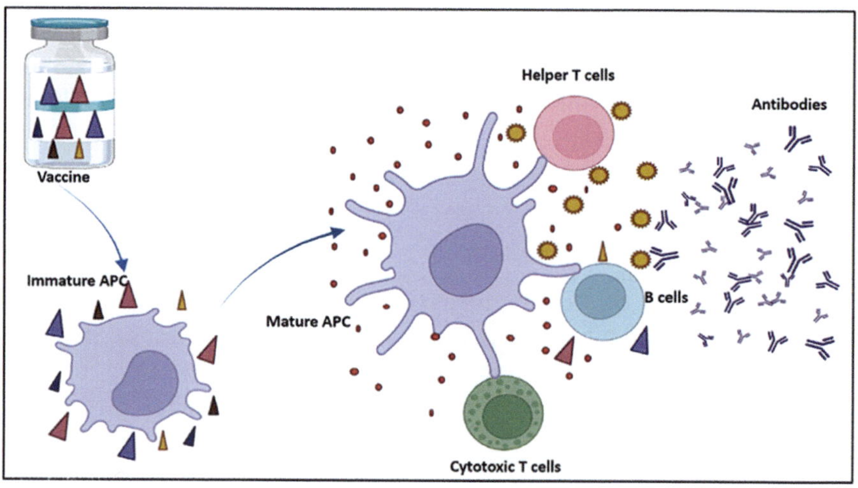

FIGURE 10.1 Activation of the immune cells after the vaccination.

10.2 NANOTECHNOLOGY

Nanotechnology, the scientific study of nanoparticles and their extensive applications in various fields, is truly fascinating. Presently, the use of nanotechnology in the development of targeted vaccines has gained significant traction. Nanovaccines, comprising polymers, biological macromolecules, metal particles, and other substances sized between 1 and 100 nm, find wide-ranging applications in biomedicine, including diagnostics, drug screening, targeted drug delivery, protein or gene delivery, vaccine production, and the study of infectious organism toxicity (Aljabali et al., 2020; Oun et al., 2020; Yaqoob et al., 2020; Youssef et al., 2019). Furthermore, various types of nanomaterials have been devised to reduce contamination and pollution in soil, air, and water (Al Saber et al., 2021; Anjum et al., 2019; Biswas et al., 2021; Masciangioli and Zhang, 2003; Rahman et al., 2020).

The administration of nanoparticles into the human body, following meticulous planning and design, is a matter of significant concern. Owing to their small size and biocompatible nature, nanoparticles can easily penetrate cells and exhibit high sensitivity in medical applications (Zaman et al., 2013). This has led to the manufacture of drug delivery systems, analytical tools, contrast agents, and diagnostic devices utilizing nanomaterials.

Immunization, also known as inoculation or vaccination, involves the deliberate stimulation of the immune system against microorganisms causing infectious diseases. It confers prolonged protection against diseases. Nanovaccines, formulated with nanoparticles and other components requiring an immune response, not only strengthen the immune system to provide protection against infectious diseases but also prevent their spread. However, the development of potent vaccines against certain infectious diseases such as hepatitis C, malaria, HIV, and tuberculosis remains a challenge. The advantages of nanovaccines include fewer side effects, enhanced bioavailability, and site-specific antigen delivery (Zolnik et al., 2010). In comparison with other vaccines, nanovaccines can elicit and target specific immune responses, making them highly effective (Zaman et al., 2013). They also find applications in cancer treatment due to their target-specific responses (Hellström et al., 2001; Kasturi et al., 2011; Moon et al., 2011; Moon et al., 2012).

10.3 NANOVACCINES

Engineered nanoparticles interact with various immune cells such as phagocytic or B cells, making them an excellent target for vaccine development (Zaheer et al., 2021). Nanoparticles display antigens on their surface for direct interaction with immune cells (Irvine and Read, 2020). While traditional vaccines act throughout the body, nanovaccines target specific areas or parts of the body affected by the infection or disease, reducing the vaccine dosage and maintaining the stability of therapeutic agents such as proteins, peptides, nucleic acids, and antigens against degradation (Shahbazi and Santos, 2015; Stammers et al., 2013). Another advantage is the controlled release of antigens and protection of the antigen from gastrointestinal degradation (Galindo-Rodriguez et al., 2005; Shi et al., 2005; Yang et al., 2010). Due to their small size, nanoparticles can easily penetrate cells through the process of cell endocytosis, and targeted delivery is achievable by coating the nanovaccines with antibodies that recognize specific receptors on target cells (Gheibi Hayat and Darroudi, 2019; Luo et al., 2017; Paulis et al., 2013).

Nanovaccines can activate both cellular and humoral immune systems, thereby cross-presenting their antigens through Major Histocompatibility Complex (MHC) class I. This makes them more efficient than conventional vaccines. Nanoparticles can move toward the lymph nodes, the central site for immune cell activation, without the assistance of peripheral dendritic cells (Gheibi Hayat and Darroudi, 2019; Ma et al., 2011). Nanovaccines are less expensive compared to conventional vaccines and are easier to use, as they are available in spray form (Gheibi Hayat and Darroudi, 2019).

10.3.1 CONSTRUCTION OF NANOVACCINE RELEASE SYSTEM

In constructing the nanovaccine release system, several points must be considered: (i) type of antigen; (ii) adjuvants; and (iii) release system (Bhardwaj et al., 2020; Raphael et al., 2015).

1. **Type of Antigen:** The antigenicity depends on the high molecular weight, structural complexity, and foreignness. Proteins and polysaccharides serve as effective antigens. Most vaccines induce the host to produce an antigen in its own cells (DNA and RNA vaccines), whereas others deliver an antigen in protein form (DNA and RNA vaccines). Polysaccharide-based vaccines have been effective in conferring protective immune responses against meningitis and

pneumonia caused by *Streptococcus pneumonia*(Celis-Giraldo et al., 2021).

2. **Adjuvants:** Adjuvants should possess antigen trapping properties and act as immunopotentiators. Nanovaccines formulated with adjuvants developed using alum can induce the secretion of IL-4, while those utilizing manganese nanomaterials can induce IL-18 and IL-1 secretion. Lower doses of nanovaccines with manganese nanoadjuvants containing the SARS-CoV-2 spike protein receptor binding domain have demonstrated strong cellular immune responses (Wang et al., 2021; Zhang et al., 2021).
3. **Release System:** Nanovaccines with reduced degradation and increased antigen stability lead to sustained antigen release, creating an antigen reservoir that remains at the application site for an extended period, allowing efficient immune cell function (Zaheer et al., 2021). Nanovaccines with particle sizes less than 10 μm diameter can easily enter cells using endocytosis (Mohammed et al., 2021). For example, a nanovaccine constructed in 2020, consisting of a rhabdovirus mannosylated antigen, and the antigen-presenting cells' mannose receptor in fish showed an immediate immune response and a 63.5% survival rate (Zhang et al., 2020).

Nanovaccines interact with NK (natural killer) cells, macrophages, neutrophils, and dendritic cells, with their constituents getting degraded and endocytosed based on the route of immunization (Bhardwaj et al., 2020). The adjuvant activity exhibited by nanoparticles activates immune responses through cationic liposomes or the PGLA component, leading to the activation and maturation of dendritic cells, as well as the release of chemokines and cytokines (Li et al., 2021). The use of nanoadjuvants and nanovaccines fosters a lifelong pathogen-specific memory, enabling the host to recognize and eliminate pathogenic microorganisms it encounters (El-Sayed and Kamel, 2020; Mohammed et al., 2021).

10.3.2 MODERN APPROACHES FOR PRODUCING NANOVACCINES

The current pandemic situation has highlighted the urgent need to expedite the development of vaccines against emerging COVID-19 outbreaks. The adverse effects of synthetic agents, such as drug resistance, tolerance, and severe side effects, have become a universal health concern, especially considering the current pandemic, and the emergence of new virus variants through evolution has further complicated the situation (Kaufmann et al., 2018; Metcalf and Lessler, 2017; Mohamed et al., 2022). Although not a panacea, the future of nanovaccine research and development can potentially uncover shared aspects or commonalities to create a unique platform to confront new virus variants in the future.

Recent advances in vaccine development have utilized nanoformulations such as nucleic acid vaccines encapsulated in viral vector vaccines (VVV), virus-like particles (VLP), and lipid or protein-based nanoparticles. Viruses exhibit different affinities towards various organs, cells, tissues, and environments, necessitating a comprehensive understanding of various criteria for achieving targeted and selective delivery. Consequently, the utilization of viral shells as a nanocarrier for the production of nanovaccines has gained significant traction. One of the most recent applications of nanovaccines using nanoparticles is the SARS-CoV-2 vaccine for human use (Mohamed et al., 2022).

Nanovaccines are created using various types of biological macromolecules or nanoformulations such as proteins and lipids (Figure 10.2). There are different types of nanovaccines available.

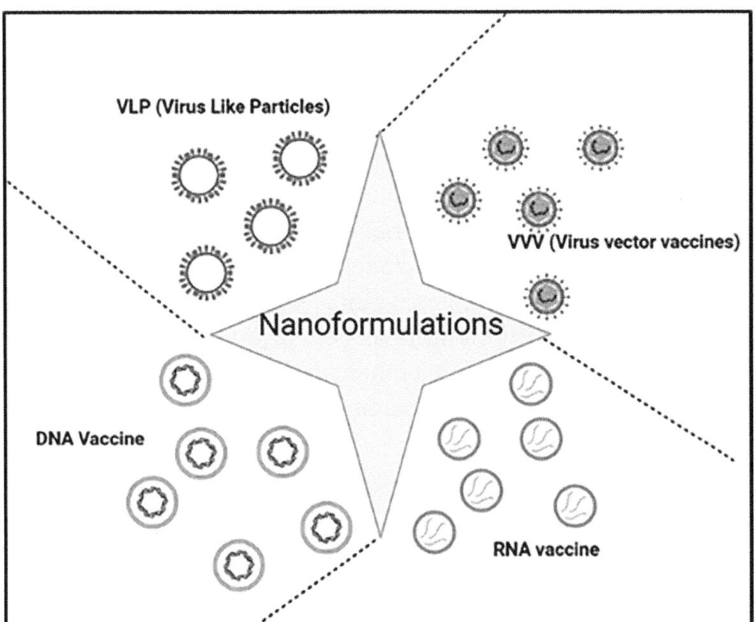

FIGURE 10.2 Different vaccines with nanoformulation.

10.3.2.1 NUCLEIC ACID VACCINES (DNA AND RNA VACCINES)

In lipid-based nanovaccines, the antigens can be presented in the membrane with a fatty acid, glycosylphosphatidylinositol (GPI), or prenyl chains or diacylglycerol, which facilitates easy incorporation into the membrane during the formation of the liposomes. Alternatively, chemically cross-linked or tagged anchors can be used in the bilayer (Karch and Matyas, 2021; Nisini et al., 2018).

Liposomes are a specific type of lipid-based nanomaterials, characterized as unilamellar (phospholipid bilayer) or multilamellar (multiple phospholipid bilayers) surrounded by an aqueous core (Alving et al., 2016). A particular subtype of liposome is the virosome (used as a vaccine carrier), which contains a phospholipid bilayer and viral glycoproteins, enabling the virosomes to target various types of cells (Corthésy and Bioley, 2018). An example of a lipid-based nanovaccine is the influenza-based virosome, which contains antigens as well as neuraminidase and hemagglutinin. Similar to liposomes, virosomes can also carry immunomodulatory particles or drugs (Corthésy and Bioley, 2018).

Lipid nanoparticles (LNP) resemble liposomes but lack a bilayer and appear as a single-layer micelle, providing protection to their nucleic acid from nucleases (Karch and Matyas, 2021) (Figure 10.3).

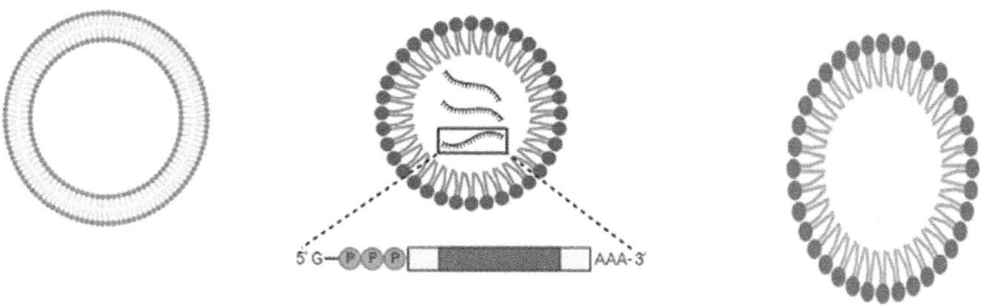

FIGURE 10.3 Lipid-based nanoparticles (LNPs): A. Liposomes; B. Nanoparticles with mRNA; C. Micelle.

Source: Created with BioRender.com.

10.3.2.2 NUCLEIC ACID VACCINES (DNA AND RNA VACCINES)

In this type of vaccine, nucleic acid vaccines (DNA and RNA vaccines) are encapsulated in lipid-based nanoparticles. RNA vaccines are the most potent vaccines and are categorized into two types: self-amplifying mRNA (sa-mRNA) and non-replicating mRNA. They resemble mRNA and are developed from linear DNA molecules with certain chemical modifications made to the nucleotides to enhance stability before the development of the vaccines (Pardi et al., 2018). Genetically engineered nucleic acid molecules were used for the development of sa-mRNA vaccines derived from self-replicating single-stranded RNA viruses that lack the ability to produce virions, making a lower concentration and a single dose of this vaccine sufficient (Bloom et al., 2021; Mohamed et al., 2022).

At the time of immunization, antigen-presenting cells (monocytes and DCs) engulf this mRNA molecule and transport it to the lymph nodes (Lindsay et al., 2019), where type B lymphocytes interact with the antigens, leading to the production of antibodies and differentiation of type B cells (Mesin et al., 2016). The inadequate stability of the mRNA vaccine is one of its major disadvantages, while the lipid-based nanoformulations enhance targeted delivery, nucleic acid durability (Suschak et al., 2017), and protect the mRNA integrity, offering advantages to this vaccine. During recent pandemic situations, mRNA vaccines have demonstrated appreciable efficiency in terms of immunogenicity; however, multiple doses are recommended to maintain immunity.

DNA vaccines are based on the plasmid vector, in which the gene of interest is inserted and transcribed into RNA after immunization, transducing proteins. DNA vaccines function in the nucleus, while RNA vaccines function within the cytoplasm (Lee et al., 2018; Qin et al., 2021). For efficient target delivery of DNA vaccines, physical methods such as microneedle array-based delivery, gene gun delivery, jet injectors, and electroporation, as well as other techniques like virosomes, liposomes, and various natural and synthetic nanomaterials, have been employed (Mohamed et al., 2022; Shafaati et al., 2022). Compared with mRNA vaccines, the immunogenicity of DNA vaccines is lower, requiring multiple doses, and the generation of anti-DNA antibodies is an adverse effect. The advantages of nucleic acid vaccines include their low-cost production, rapid development from design to manufacturing, better adaptations, absence of anti-vector immunity, and non-residual infectivity (Jafari et al., 2022).

Nucleic acids are protected by the lipid nanoparticles from degradation, preserving nucleic acid release and cellular uptake. The lipid components used for COVID-19 vaccine preparation were an ionizable cationic lipid, DSPC (a neutral lipid distearoylphosphatidylcholine), polyethylene glycol

(PEG)–lipid, and cholesterol. In 2022, Mohamed et al. reviewed that the lipid components such as cholesterol and neutral lipid provide fusogenic and bilayer stability to the nanoparticles, while PEG-lipids help protect against particle aggregation and fusion, maintaining the particle size. Ionizable lipids are the major components of mRNA lipid vaccines, as they serve as promising delivery vectors for DNA (forming lipid/DNA complexes), reducing the toxicity of nanoparticles associated with cationic charges, increasing effective encapsulation of mRNA (which is negatively charged), and maintaining neutral charges of the nanoparticles at physiological pH (Papi et al., 2022). Ionizable lipid-DNA complexes can be used to activate various components of the immune system and help target macrophages, as well as protect DNA from being digested by nucleases (Tejeda-Mansir et al., 2019). Additionally, lipid-based nanoparticles can enhance the efficiency of DNA and mRNA delivery.

10.3.2.3 PROTEIN-BASED NANOVACCINE (VLP-VIRUS-LIKE PARTICLE)

Due to the simplicity of manipulation and the variety in secondary designs, most nano-based vaccines have focused on protein-based nanovaccines (Butkovich et al., 2021). VLPs are self-assembled nanostructures that are single, double, or multiple proteins, either non-enveloped or enveloped, with viral proteins such as envelopes, coral viral proteins, and capsids, lacking genetic material (Donaldson et al., 2018; Karch and Matyas, 2021; Nooraei et al., 2021). They are suitable for the targeted delivery of peptides or proteins, genes, and drugs (Chung et al., 2020). Currently, VLPs are made from recombinant viral proteins using different expression systems such as baculovirus/insect cells, avian and mammalian (Vero9, HEK293, CAP-T) cell lines, plants, and yeast (Fuenmayor et al., 2017; Mohamed et al., 2022). VLPs are commonly developed by assembling proteins from viruses; however, chimeric VLPs are prepared by incorporating different proteins from different viruses. For example, different viral proteins from HCV (Hepatitis C virus), HIV (Human immunodeficiency virus), HBV (Hepatitis B virus), bacteriophages, and adeno-associated viruses were used by incorporating nanoparticles (lipids), enhancing the uptake of target cells, encapsulation, and viral binding (Somiya et al., 2017). The first VLPs were synthesized against the hepatitis B virus (Nooraei et al., 2021).

The advantages of VLPs are that they lack a virus genome, have morphological resemblance to the parent virus, come in a variety of sizes and shapes, and are non-pathogenic (Dai et al., 2018; Mohamed et al., 2022). Drawbacks of VLPs are associated with formulations, stability, immunogenicity, purification, and so on (Donaldson et al., 2018).

10.3.2.4 VIRAL VECTOR VACCINES (VVV)

VVV include harmless, non-pathogenic, genetically modified viruses, in which the virulence gene is removed and inserted into the gene of interest (Gebre et al., 2021). The drawback of VVVs is the requirement for booster doses with another serotype. The commonly used viral vectors are adenovirus, poxvirus, Sendai virus, cytomegalovirus, and so forth (Ura et al., 2014). Nanoparticles were prepared with viral and synthetic components that act as standard delivery particles. Plant-based viruses and bacteriophages are commonly used over mammalian viruses, which reduce side effects. VVVs have an effective drug delivery system.

10.3.2.5 POLYMERIC NANOPARTICLES (PNPS)

Natural polymers such as alginate, gelatin, chitosan, and hyaluronic acid, as well as other biodegradable and biocompatible synthetic polymers such as PLGA (poly lactic-co-glycolic acid), PAMAM (polyamidoamine), polyesters, and PLA (polylactic acid), are used as nanocarriers (multifunctional) for the preparation of nanoparticles, interacting with immunocompetent cells to activate life-long immune responses and modulate immunostimulatory functions (Diego-González et al., 2020). These nanoparticles containing nanovaccines act against pathogens, with increased uptake by APCs, thereby enhancing immune responses and preventing antigen clearance and degradation (Chan et al., 2021; Pippa et al., 2021). Polymeric nanoparticles are generally used for delivering nucleic acids and act as carriers and adjuvants with potent practical applications (Dewangan, 2020; Ho et al., 2021; Jin et al., 2019).

10.3.2.6 INORGANIC AND OTHER NANOPARTICLES

Biodegradable nanomaterials such as polyanhydride nanoparticles or micelles with properties such as mucosal adhesion, low toxicity, immune regulation, safety, and biocompatibility; AuNPs (gold nanoparticles) are suitable for mRNA/DNA vaccine delivery. TiO_2 nanoparticles, essential oils, and oil-in-water nanoemulsions appear to have antiviral activity (Celis-Giraldo et al., 2021). Nowadays, nanotechnology aids in vaccine development using nanoparticles with encapsulation properties. Due to their small surface area and size, they act as effective immunostimulatory agents as well as efficient antigen delivery vehicles. Using recombinant technology, the first vaccine was developed in 1985 for human use against the hepatitis B virus and was prepared by inclusion in VLPs (s), which were found to be more immunogenic. Various types of nanomaterials have also been created with structural similarity to DNA, ligands, proteins, and various receptors. Nanoparticle size influences immune system interaction and nanovaccine distribution; smaller particles with sizes less than 100 nm have been found to be more effective. Advantages of nanomaterials include acting as efficient adjuvants for the activation of both cellular and humoral responses, protecting biomaterials from degradation, or increasing bioavailability (Celis-Giraldo et al., 2021; Kheirollahpour et al., 2020).

Animals and humans come into contact with numerous microorganisms in the environment, and this host-pathogen interaction will determine the various perspectives they have with each other. This interaction may lead to infection after a series of events, such as the entry of microorganisms, their colonization, tissue invasion and damage, and finally the evasion of the immune system (Maina et al., 2020; Mukhopadhyay et al., 2020; Shepherd and McLaren, 2020; Tomlin and Piccinini, 2018). The host immune response to pathogenic microorganisms can be summarized in four steps: triggering defense mechanisms through innate and adaptive immune responses, the progression of pathological changes, persistent tissue lesions and infections, evasion of host immune mechanisms, and finally protection or promotion of infections (Gan et al., 2021; Opriessnig et al., 2021; Thakur et al., 2019). Nanoparticle-based vaccine development is a promising approach for medical science, owing to the significant advantages they offer after attachment to immune cells, inducing both cellular and humoral immunity by upregulating genes and providing long-lasting antigen functionality and stability.

10.4 ACTIVATION OF THE IMMUNE SYSTEM

When nanoparticles attach to the antigen-presenting cell system, both cell-mediated and humoral immune responses can be induced (Diaz-Arévalo and Zeng, 2020). Characteristics of nanoparticles such as shape, size, and distribution greatly affect their interaction with cell membranes. Metal nanoparticles like gold, silver, and nickel can activate humoral immunity, thereby inducing cytokine production and APCs. When designing nanovaccines, the antigen loaded inside the nanoparticles and its aggregation in the blood are very important because they affect cellular uptake. Additionally, the glycoproteins outside the surface are considered key factors for cell entry. Surface glycoproteins play a major role in the design of nanovaccines, offering great function and immune responses (Mohamed et al., 2022). In the case of lipid-based nanovaccines, after immunization, APCs such as monocytes and dendritic cells (DCs) engulf the RNA vaccines (Lindsay et al., 2019), while DNA vaccines induce humoral and cellular immune responses in the APC (Mohamed et al., 2022). Virus-like particles directly recognize pathogenic microorganisms through pathogen recognition receptors found on membrane surfaces. Viral vector vaccines have high immune responses, as they resemble viruses. Immediately after target delivery, these VVVs target macrophages and DCs, activating a type 1 response and inducing both $CD8^+$ and $CD4^+$ T cells (Mohamed et al., 2022).

10.5 NANOVACCINES FOR SEVERE ACUTE RESPIRATORY SYNDROME CORONAVIRUS 2 (SARS-COV-2)

The enveloped beta coronavirus SARS-CoV-2 has four structural proteins: E (envelope) protein, M (membrane) protein, nucleocapsid (N), and S (spike) protein (Satarker and Nampoothiri, 2020). The spike glycoprotein is the most potent for viral infection. Currently available nanovaccines for SARS-CoV-2 include Comirnaty by Pfizer, Vaxzevria by AstraZeneca and the University of Oxford, Nuvaxoid by Novavax, Spikevax by Moderna Therapeutics Inc. and the National Institute of Allergy and Infectious Diseases (NIAID), and COVID-19 Vaccine Janssen by Janssen Pharmaceuticals, Companies of Johnson & Johnson (Mohamed et al., 2022).

10.6 SUMMARY AND CONCLUSION

Globally, infectious diseases are the major cause of death, significantly affecting the socioeconomic and public health development of human beings. Overuse of medicines has led to the emergence of side effects and drug resistance by pathogenic microorganisms to available treatments. Hence, there is a need for novel and potent treatment techniques to be developed. The emergence of nanovaccines and nanomedicine as critically controlled target-specific drug delivery mechanisms has transformed the landscape of biomedical research worldwide. The current use of SARS-CoV-2 virus nanovaccine is a good example of successful innovative nanovaccines, developed over years of vaccine technology combined with nanotechnology. The rise of zoonotic infections and endemics transitioning from animals to humans increases the need for new active vaccines capable of preventing or blocking future threats and transmissions.

ACKNOWLEDGMENTS

The authors acknowledged DIST-FIST, KSCSTE –SARD, for the financial assistance in the form of a Project grant. Management – Sree Sankara College, Kalady, for providing research facilities in the department. Dr. Sherin Joy Parappilly is grateful to University Grants Commission (UGC)–Maulana Azad National Fellowship for minority students, for providing fellowship for her research work.

KEYWORDS

- **antibodies**
- **immune system**
- **infectious diseases**
- **nanoparticles**
- **nanotechnology**
- **nanovaccines**
- **pathogenic microorganisms**

REFERENCES

Al Saber, M., Biswas, P., Dey, D., Kaium, M. A., Islam, M. A., Tripty, M. I. A., & Kim, B. (2021). A comprehensive review of recent advancements in cancer immunotherapy and generation of CAR T cell by CRISPR-Cas9. *Processes, 10*(1), 16. https://doi.org/10.3390/pr10010016 (accessed on 4th July 2025).

Aljabali, A. A. A., Bakshi, H. A., Hakkim, F. L., Haggag, Y. A., Al-Batanyeh, K. M., Al Zoubi, S. S., & Tambuwala, M. M. (2020). Albumin nano-encapsulation of piceatannol enhances its anticancer potential in colon cancer via down regulation of nuclear p65 and HIF-1α. *Cancers, 12*(1), 113. https://doi.org/10.3390/cancers12010113 (accessed on 4th July 2025).

Alving, C. R., Beck, Z., Matyas, G. R., & Rao, M. (2016). Liposomal adjuvants for human vaccines. *Expert Opinion on Drug Delivery, 13*(6), 807–816. https://doi.org/10.1517/17425247.2016.1151871 (accessed on 4th July 2025).

Anjum, M., Miandad, R., Waqas, M., Gehany, F., & Barakat, M. A. (2019). Remediation of wastewater using various nano-materials. *Arabian Journal of Chemistry, 12*(8), 4897–4919. https://doi.org/10.1016/j.arabjc.2016.10.004 (accessed on 4th July 2025).

Bhardwaj, P., Bhatia, E., Sharma, S., Ahamad, N., & Banerjee, R. (2020). Advancements in prophylactic and therapeutic nanovaccines. *Acta Biomaterialia, 108*, 1–21. https://doi.org/10.1016/j.actbio.2020.03.020 (accessed on 4th July 2025).

Biswas, P., Hasan, M. M., Dey, D., dos Santos Costa, A. C., Polash, S. A., Bibi, S., & Uddin, M. S. (2021). Candidate antiviral drugs for COVID-19 and their environmental implications: A comprehensive analysis. *Environmental Science and Pollution Research, 28*(42), 59570–59593. https://doi.org/10.1007/s11356-021-16096-3 (accessed on 4th July 2025).

Biswas, P., Polash, S. A., Dey, D., Kaium, M. A., Mahmud, A. R., Yasmin, F., & Hasan, M. N. (2023). Advanced implications of nanotechnology in disease control and environmental perspectives. *Biomedicine & Pharmacotherapy, 158*, 114172. https://doi.org/10.1016/j.biopha.2022.114172 (accessed on 4th July 2025).

Bloom, K., van den Berg, F., & Arbuthnot, P. (2021). Self-amplifying RNA vaccines for infectious diseases. *Gene Therapy, 28*(3, 4), 117–129. https://doi.org/10.1038/s41434-020-00204-y (accessed on 4th July 2025).

Butkovich, N., Li, E., Ramirez, A., Burkhardt, A. M., & Wang, S. W. (2021). Advancements in protein nanoparticle vaccine platforms to combat infectious disease. *Wiley Interdisciplinary Reviews: Nanomedicine and Nanobiotechnology, 13*(3), e1681. https://doi.org/10.1002/wnan.1681 (accessed on 4th July 2025).

Celis-Giraldo, C. T., López-Abán, J., Muro, A., Patarroyo, M. A., & Manzano-Román, R. (2021). Nanovaccines against animal pathogens: The latest findings. *Vaccines, 9*(9), 988. https://doi.org/10.3390/vaccines9090988 (accessed on 4th July 2025).

Chan, Y., Ng, S. W., Singh, S. K., Gulati, M., Gupta, G., Chaudhary, S. K., & Dua, K. (2021). Revolutionizing polymer-based nanoparticle-linked vaccines for targeting respiratory viruses: A perspective. *Life Sciences, 280*, 119744. https://doi.org/10.1016/j.lfs.2021.119744 (accessed on 4th July 2025).

Chung, Y. H., Cai, H., & Steinmetz, N. F. (2020). Viral nanoparticles for drug delivery, imaging, immunotherapy, and theranostic applications. *Advanced Drug Delivery*

Reviews, 156, 214–235. https://doi.org/10.1016/j.addr.2020.06.024 (accessed on 4th July 2025).

Corthésy, B., & Bioley, G. (2018). Lipid-based particles: Versatile delivery systems for mucosal vaccination against infection. *Frontiers in Immunology, 9*, 431. https://doi.org/10.3389/fimmu.2018.00431 (accessed on 4th July 2025).

D'Amico, C., Fontana, F., Cheng, R., & Santos, H. A. (2021). Development of vaccine formulations: Past, present, and future. *Drug Delivery and Translational Research, 11*, 353–372. https://doi.org/10.1007/s13346-021-00924-7 (accessed on 4th July 2025).

Dai, S., Wang, H., & Deng, F. (2018). Advances and challenges in enveloped virus-like particle (VLP)-based vaccines. *Journal of Immunological Sciences, 2*(2).

Dewangan, H. K. (2020). Rational application of nanoadjuvant for mucosal vaccine delivery system. *Journal of Immunological Methods, 481*, 112791. https://doi.org/10.1016/j.jim.2020.112791 (accessed on 4th July 2025).

Diaz-Arévalo, D., & Zeng, M. (2020). Nanoparticle-based vaccines: Opportunities and limitations. In *Nano Pharmaceuticals* (pp. 135–150). https://doi.org/10.1016/B978-0-12-817778-5.00007-5 (accessed on 4th July 2025).

Diego-González, L., Crecente-Campo, J., Paul, M. J., Singh, M., Reljic, R., Alonso, M. J., & Simón-Vázquez, R. (2020). Design of polymeric nano capsules for intranasal vaccination against *Mycobacterium tuberculosis*: Influence of the polymeric shell and antigen positioning. *Pharmaceutics, 12*(6), 489. https://doi.org/10.3390/pharmaceutics12060489 (accessed on 4th July 2025).

Donaldson, B., Lateef, Z., Walker, G. F., Young, S. L., & Ward, V. K. (2018). Virus-like particle vaccines: Immunology and formulation for clinical translation. *Expert Review of Vaccines, 17*(9), 833–849. https://doi.org/10.1080/14760584.2018.1516552 (accessed on 4th July 2025).

El-Sayed, A., & Kamel, M. (2020). Advanced applications of nanotechnology in veterinary medicine. *Environmental Science and Pollution Research, 27*, 19073–19086. https://doi.org/10.1007/s11356-018-3913-y (accessed on 4th July 2025).

Fuenmayor, J., Gòdia, F., & Cervera, L. (2017). Production of virus-like particles for vaccines. *New Biotechnology, 39*, 174–180. https://doi.org/10.1016/j.nbt.2017.07.010 (accessed on 4th July 2025).

Galindo-Rodriguez, S. A., Allemann, E., Fessi, H., & Doelker, E. (2005). Polymeric nanoparticles for oral delivery of drugs and vaccines: A critical evaluation of *in vivo* studies. *Critical Reviews™ in Therapeutic Drug Carrier Systems, 22*(5).

Gan, Y., Li, C., Peng, X., Wu, S., Li, Y., Tan, J. P., & Ding, X. (2021). Fight bacteria with bacteria: Bacterial membrane vesicles as vaccines and delivery nanocarriers against bacterial infections. *Nanomedicine: Nanotechnology, Biology and Medicine, 35*, 102398. https://doi.org/10.1016/j.nano.2021.102398 (accessed on 4th July 2025).

Gebre, M. S., Brito, L. A., Tostanoski, L. H., Edwards, D. K., Carfi, A., & Barouch, D. H. (2021). Novel approaches for vaccine development. *Cell, 184*(6), 1589–1603. https://doi.org/10.1016/j.cell.2021.02.030 (accessed on 4th July 2025).

Gheibi Hayat, S. M., & Darroudi, M. (2019). Nanovaccine: A novel approach in immunization. *Journal of Cellular Physiology, 234*(8), 12530–12536. https://doi.org/10.1002/jcp.28120 (accessed on 4th July 2025).

Hellström, I., Ledbetter, J. A., Scholler, N., Yang, Y., Ye, Z., Goodman, G., & Hellström, K. E. (2001). CD3-mediated activation of tumor-reactive lymphocytes from patients with advanced cancer. *Proceedings of the National Academy of Sciences, 98*(12), 6783–6788. https://doi.org/10.1073/pnas.021557498 (accessed on 4th July 2025).

Ho, W., Gao, M., Li, F., Li, Z., Zhang, X. Q., & Xu, X. (2021). Next-generation vaccines: Nanoparticle-mediated DNA and mRNA delivery. *Advanced Healthcare Materials, 10*(8), 2001812. https://doi.org/10.1002/adhm.202001812 (accessed on 4th July 2025).

Irvine, D. J., & Read, B. J. (2020). Shaping humoral immunity to vaccines through antigen-displaying nanoparticles. *Current Opinion in Immunology, 65*, 1–6. https://doi.org/10.1016/j.coi.2020.01.007 (accessed on 4th July 2025).

Jafari, A., DaneshPouya, F., Niknam, Z., Abdollahpour Alitappeh, M., Rezaei-Tavirani, M., & Rasmi, Y. (2022). Current advances and challenges in COVID-19 vaccine development: From conventional vaccines to next-generation vaccine platforms. *Molecular Biology Reports, 49*(6), 4943–4957. https://doi.org/10.1007/s11033-022-07132-7 (accessed on 4th July 2025).

Jin, Z., Gao, S., Cui, X., Sun, D., & Zhao, K. (2019). Adjuvants and delivery systems based on polymeric nanoparticles for mucosal vaccines. *International Journal of Pharmaceutics, 572*, 118731. https://doi.org/10.1016/j.ijpharm.2019.118731 (accessed on 4th July 2025).

Karch, C. P., & Matyas, G. R. (2021). The current and future role of nano vaccines in HIV-1 vaccine development. *Expert Review of Vaccines, 20*(8), 935–944. https://doi.org/10.1080/14760584.2021.1945448 (accessed on 4th July 2025).

Kasturi, S. P., Skountzou, I., Albrecht, R. A., Koutsonanos, D., Hua, T., Nakaya, H. I., & Pulendran, B. (2011). Programming the magnitude and persistence of antibody responses with innate immunity. *Nature, 470*(7335), 543–547. https://doi.org/10.1038/nature09737 (accessed on 4th July 2025).

Kaufmann, S. H., Dorhoi, A., Hotchkiss, R. S., & Bartenschlager, R. (2018). Host-directed therapies for bacterial and viral infections. *Nature Reviews Drug Discovery, 17*(1), 35–56. https://doi.org/10.1038/nrd.2017.162 (accessed on 4th July 2025).

Kheirollahpour, M., Mehrabi, M., Dounighi, N. M., Mohammadi, M., & Masoudi, A. (2020). Nanoparticles and vaccine development. *Pharmaceutical Nanotechnology, 8*(1), 6–21. https://doi.org/10.2174/2211738507666191024162042 (accessed on 4th July 2025).

Korenkov, D., Isakova-Sivak, I., & Rudenko, L. (2018). Basics of CD8 T-cell immune responses after influenza infection and vaccination with inactivated or live attenuated influenza vaccine. *Expert Review of Vaccines, 17*(11), 977–987. https://doi.org/10.1080/14760584.2018.1541407 (accessed on 4th July 2025).

Lee, J., Kumar, S. A., Jhan, Y. Y., & Bishop, C. J. (2018). Engineering DNA vaccines against infectious diseases. *Acta Biomaterialia, 80*, 31–47. https://doi.org/10.1016/j.actbio.2018.08.033 (accessed on 4th July 2025).

Lee, W., Kingstad-Bakke, B., Paulson, B., Larsen, A., Overmyer, K., Marinaik, C. B., & Suresh, M. (2021). Carbomer-based adjuvant elicits CD8 T-cell immunity by inducing a distinct metabolic state in cross-presenting dendritic cells. *PLoS Pathogens, 17*(1), e1009168. https://doi.org/10.1371/journal.ppat.1009168 (accessed on 4th July 2025).

Li, Y., Xiao, Y., Chen, Y., & Huang, K. (2021). Nano-based approaches in the development of antiviral agents and vaccines. *Life Sciences, 265*, 118761. https://doi.org/10.1016/j.lfs.2020.118761 (accessed on 4th July 2025).

Lindsay, K. E., Bhosle, S. M., Zurla, C., Beyersdorf, J., Rogers, K. A., Vanover, D., & Santangelo, P. J. (2019). Visualization of early events in mRNA vaccine delivery in non-human primates via PET–CT and near-infrared imaging. *Nature Biomedical Engineering, 3*(5), 371–380. https://doi.org/10.1038/s41551-019-0378-3 (accessed on 4th July 2025).

Luo, M., Samandi, L. Z., Wang, Z., Chen, Z. J., & Gao, J. (2017). Synthetic nano vaccines for immunotherapy. *Journal of Controlled Release, 263*, 200–210. https://doi.org/10.1016/j.jconrel.2017.03.033 (accessed on 4th July 2025).

Ma, W., Smith, T., Bogin, V., Zhang, Y., Ozkan, C., Ozkan, M., & Minev, B. (2011). Enhanced presentation of MHC class Ia, Ib and class II-restricted peptides encapsulated in biodegradable nanoparticles: A promising strategy for tumor immunotherapy. *Journal of Translational Medicine, 9*(1), 1–10. https://doi.org/10.1186/1479-5876-9-34 (accessed on 4th July 2025).

Maina, T. W., Grego, E. A., Boggiatto, P. M., Sacco, R. E., Narasimhan, B., & McGill, J. L. (2020). Applications of nanovaccines for disease prevention in cattle. *Frontiers in Bioengineering and Biotechnology, 8*, 608050. https://doi.org/10.3389/fbioe.2020.608050 (accessed on 4th July 2025).

Masciangioli, T., & Zhang, W. X. (2003). Peer reviewed: Environmental technologies at the nanoscale.

Mesin, L., Ersching, J., & Victora, G. D. (2016). Germinal center B cell dynamics. *Immunity, 45*(3), 471–482. https://doi.org/10.1016/j.immuni.2016.09.001 (accessed on 4th July 2025).

Metcalf, C. J. E., & Lessler, J. (2017). Opportunities and challenges in modeling emerging infectious diseases. *Science, 357*(6347), 149–152. https://doi.org/10.1126/science.aam8335 (accessed on 4th July 2025).

Mohamed, N. A., Abou-Saleh, H., Mohamed, H. A., Al-Ghouti, M. A., Crovella, S., & Zupin, L. (2022). Think like a virus: Toward improving nano vaccine development against SARS-CoV-2. *Viruses, 14*(7), 1553. https://doi.org/10.3390/v14071553 (accessed on 4th July 2025).

Mohammed, G. M., ElZorkany, H. E., Farroh, K. Y., Abd El-Aziz, W. R., & Elshoky, H. A. (2021). Potential improvement of the immune response of chickens against *E. coli* vaccine by using two forms of chitosan nanoparticles. *International Journal of Biological Macromolecules, 167*, 395–404. https://doi.org/10.1016/j.ijbiomac.2020.11.200 (accessed on 4th July 2025).

Moon, J. J., Huang, B., & Irvine, D. J. (2012). Engineering nano- and microparticles to tune immunity. *Advanced Materials, 24*(28), 3724–3746. https://doi.org/10.1002/adma.201200446 (accessed on 4th July 2025).

Moon, J. J., Suh, H., Bershteyn, A., Stephan, M. T., Liu, H., Huang, B., & Irvine, D. J. (2011). Interbilayer-crosslinked multilamellar vesicles as synthetic vaccines for potent humoral and cellular immune responses. *Nature Materials, 10*(3), 243–251. https://doi.org/10.1038/nmat2960 (accessed on 4th July 2025).

Mukhopadhyay, D., Arranz-Solís, D., & Saeij, J. P. (2020). Influence of the host and parasite strain on the immune response during *Toxoplasma* infection. *Frontiers in Cellular and Infection Microbiology, 10*, 580425. https://doi.org/10.3389/fcimb.2020.580425 (accessed on 4th July 2025).

Nisini, R., Poerio, N., Mariotti, S., De Santis, F., & Fraziano, M. (2018). The multirole of liposomes in therapy and prevention of infectious diseases. *Frontiers in Immunology, 9*, 155. https://doi.org/10.3389/fimmu.2018.00155 (accessed on 4th July 2025).

Nooraei, S., Bahrulolum, H., Hoseini, Z. S., Katalani, C., Hajizade, A., Easton, A. J., & Ahmadian, G. (2021). Virus-like particles: Preparation, immunogenicity and their roles as nano vaccines and drug nanocarriers. *Journal of Nanobiotechnology, 19*(1), 1–27. https://doi.org/10.1186/s12951-021-00806-7 (accessed on 4th July 2025).

Opriessnig, T., Mattei, A. A., Karuppannan, A. K., & Halbur, P. G. (2021). Future perspectives on swine viral vaccines: Where are we headed. *Porcine Health Management, 7*(1), 1–16. https://doi.org/10.1186/s40813-020-00179-7 (accessed on 4th July 2025).

Oun, A. A., Shankar, S., & Rhim, J. W. (2020). Multifunctional nanocellulose/metal and metal oxide nanoparticle hybrid nanomaterials. *Critical Reviews in Food Science and Nutrition, 60*(3), 435–460. https://doi.org/10.1080/10408398.2018.1536966 (accessed on 4th July 2025).

Papi, M., Pozzi, D., Palmieri, V., & Caracciolo, G. (2022). Principles for optimization and validation of mRNA lipid nanoparticle vaccines against COVID-19 using 3D bioprinting. *Nano Today, 43*, 101403. https://doi.org/10.1016/j.nantod.2022.101403 (accessed on 4th July 2025).

Pardi, N., Hogan, M. J., Porter, F. W., & Weissman, D. (2018). mRNA vaccines—A new era in vaccinology. *Nature Reviews Drug Discovery, 17*(4), 261–279. https://doi.org/10.1038/nrd.2017.243 (accessed on 4th July 2025).

Paulis, L. E., Mandal, S., Kreutz, M., & Figdor, C. G. (2013). Dendritic cell-based nano vaccines for cancer immunotherapy. *Current Opinion in Immunology, 25*(3), 389–395. https://doi.org/10.1016/j.coi.2013.03.001 (accessed on 4th July 2025).

Pippa, N., Gazouli, M., & Pispas, S. (2021). Recent advances and future perspectives in polymer-based nano vaccines. *Vaccines, 9*(6), 558. https://doi.org/10.3390/vaccines9060558 (accessed on 4th July 2025).

Pollard, A. J., & Bijker, E. M. (2021). A guide to vaccinology: From basic principles to new developments. *Nature Reviews Immunology, 21*(2), 83–100. https://doi.org/10.1038/s41577-020-00479-7 (accessed on 4th July 2025).

Qin, F., Xia, F., Chen, H., Cui, B., Feng, Y., Zhang, P., & Luo, M. (2021). A guide to nucleic acid vaccines in the prevention and treatment of infectious diseases and cancers: From basic principles to current applications. *Frontiers in Cell and Developmental Biology*, 830. https://doi.org/10.3389/fcell.2021.633776 (accessed on 4th July 2025).

Rahman, M. A., Rahman, M. H., Hossain, M. S., Biswas, P., Islam, R., Uddin, M. J., & Rhim, H. (2020). Molecular insights into the multifunctional role of natural compounds: Autophagy modulation and cancer prevention. *Biomedicines, 8*(11), 517. https://doi.org/10.3390/biomedicines8110517 (accessed on 4th July 2025).

Rambe, D. S., Del Giudice, G., Rossi, S., & Sanicas, M. (2015). Safety and mechanism of action of licensed vaccine adjuvants. *International Current Pharmaceutical Journal, 4*(8), 420–431. https://doi.org/10.3329/icpj.v4i8.24024 (accessed on 4th July 2025).

Raphael, I., Nalawade, S., Eagar, T. N., & Forsthuber, T. G. (2015). T cell subsets and their signature cytokines in autoimmune and inflammatory diseases. *Cytokine, 74*(1), 5–17. https://doi.org/10.1016/j.cyto.2014.09.011 (accessed on 4th July 2025).

Satarker, S., & Nampoothiri, M. (2020). Structural proteins in severe acute respiratory syndrome coronavirus-2. *Archives of Medical Research, 51*(6), 482–491. https://doi.org/10.1016/j.arcmed.2020.05.012 (accessed on 4th July 2025).

Shafaati, M., Saidijam, M., Soleimani, M., Hazrati, F., Mirzaei, R., Amirheidari, B., & Ahmadyousefi, Y. (2022). A brief review on DNA vaccines in the era of COVID-19. *Future Virology, 17*(1), 49–66. https://doi.org/10.2217/fvl-2021-0170 (accessed on 4th July 2025).

Shahbazi, M. A., & Santos, H. A. (2015). Revolutionary impact of nano vaccines on immunotherapy. *New Horizons in Translational Medicine, 2*(2), 44–50. https://doi.org/10.1016/j.nhtm.2014.11.058 (accessed on 4th July 2025).

Shepherd, F. R., & McLaren, J. E. (2020). T cell immunity to bacterial pathogens: Mechanisms of immune control and bacterial evasion. *International Journal of Molecular Sciences, 21*(17), 6144. https://doi.org/10.3390/ijms21176144 (accessed on 4th July 2025).

Shi, R., Hong, L., Wu, D., Ning, X., Chen, Y., Lin, T., & Wu, K. (2005). Enhanced immune response to gastric cancer specific antigen peptide by coencapsulation with CpG oligodeoxynucleotides in nano emulsion. *Cancer Biology & Therapy, 4*(2), 226–232. https://doi.org/10.4161/cbt.4.2.1472 (accessed on 4th July 2025).

Somiya, M., Liu, Q., & Kuroda, S. I. (2017). Current progress of virus-mimicking nanocarriers for drug delivery. *Nanotheranostics, 1*(4), 415. https://doi.org/10.7150%2Fntno.21723 (accessed on 4th July 2025).

Stammers, T. S., Erden, Y. J., & Hunt, G. (2013). The promise and challenge of nanovaccines and the question of global equity.

Suschak, J. J., Williams, J. A., & Schmaljohn, C. S. (2017). Advancements in DNA vaccine vectors, non-mechanical delivery methods, and molecular adjuvants to increase immunogenicity. *Human Vaccines & Immunotherapeutics, 13*(12), 2837–2848. https://doi.org/10.1080/21645515.2017.1330236 (accessed on 4th July 2025).

Tejeda-Mansir, A., García-Rendón, A., & Guerrero-Germán, P. (2019). Plasmid-DNA lipid and polymeric nano vaccines: A new strategic in vaccines development. *Biotechnology and Genetic Engineering Reviews, 35*(1), 46–68. https://doi.org/10.1080/02648725.2018.1560552 (accessed on 4th July 2025).

Thakur, A., Mikkelsen, H., & Jungersen, G. (2019). Intracellular pathogens: Host immunity and microbial persistence strategies. *Journal of Immunology Research, 2019*. https://doi.org/10.1155/2019/1356540 (accessed on 4th July 2025).

Tomlin, H., & Piccinini, A. M. (2018). A complex interplay between the extracellular matrix and the innate immune response to microbial pathogens. *Immunology, 155*(2), 186–201. https://doi.org/10.1111/imm.12972 (accessed on 4th July 2025).

Ura, T., Okuda, K., & Shimada, M. (2014). Developments in viral vector-based vaccines. *Vaccines, 2*(3), 624–641. https://doi.org/10.3390/vaccines2030624 (accessed on 4th July 2025).

Wang, Y., Xie, Y., Luo, J., Guo, M., Hu, X., Chen, X., & Chen, C. (2021). Engineering a self-navigated MnARK nanovaccine for inducing potent protective immunity against novel coronavirus. *Nano Today, 38*, 101139. https://doi.org/10.1016/j.nantod.2021.101139 (accessed on 4th July 2025).

Yang, J., Li, Z., Zhou, J., Chen, R., Cheng, L., Zhou, Q., & Yang, L. (2010). Preparation and antitumor effects of nano vaccines with MAGE-3 peptides in transplanted gastric cancer in mice. *Chinese Journal of Cancer, 29*(4), 359–364.

Yaqoob, A. A., Ahmad, H., Parveen, T., Ahmad, A., Oves, M., Ismail, I. M., & Mohamad Ibrahim, M. N. (2020). Recent advances in metal decorated nanomaterials and their various biological applications: A review. *Frontiers in Chemistry, 8*, 341. https://doi.org/10.3389/fchem.2020.00341 (accessed on 4th July 2025).

Youssef, F. S., El-Banna, H. A., Elzorba, H. Y., & Galal, A. M. (2019). Application of some nanoparticles in the field of veterinary medicine. *International Journal of Veterinary Science and Medicine, 7*(1), 78–93. https://doi.org/10.1080/23144599.2019.1691379 (accessed on 4th July 2025).

Zaheer, T., Pal, K., & Zaheer, I. (2021). Topical review on nano-vaccinology: Biochemical promises and key challenges. *Process Biochemistry, 100*, 237–244. https://doi.org/10.1016/j.procbio.2020.09.028 (accessed on 4th July 2025).

Zaman, M., Good, M. F., & Toth, I. (2013). Nanovaccines and their mode of action. *Methods, 60*(3), 226–231. http://dx.doi.org/10.1016/j.ymeth.2013.04.014 (accessed on 4th July 2025).

Zhang, C., Wang, G. X., & Zhu, B. (2020). Application of antigen presenting cell-targeted nanovaccine delivery system in rhabdovirus disease prophylactics using fish as a model organism. *Journal of Nanobiotechnology, 18*(1), 1–13. https://doi.org/10.1186/s12951-020-0584-x (accessed on 4th July 2025).

Zhang, R., Wang, C., Guan, Y., Wei, X., Sha, M., Yi, M., & Jiang, Z. (2021). Manganese salts function as potent adjuvants. *Cellular & Molecular Immunology, 18*(5), 1222–1234. https://doi.org/10.1038/s41423-021-00669-w (accessed on 4th July 2025).

Zolnik, B. S., González-Fernández, Á., Sadrieh, N., & Dobrovolskaia, M. A. (2010). Minireview: Nanoparticles and the immune system. *Endocrinology, 151*(2), 458–465. https://doi.org/10.1210/en.2009-1082 (accessed on 4th July 2025).

Index

D

E

F

G

I

J

K

L

O

P

Q

R

S

T

W

X

Y

Z

For Product Safety Concerns and Information please contact our
EU representative GPSR@taylorandfrancis.com Taylor & Francis
Verlag GmbH, Kaufingerstraße 24, 80331 München, Germany